Your
Magical Child

Your Magical Child

FIRST EDITION
First Printing 1994

Programming of Tables: Rique Pottenger
Cover Painting: Molly A. Sullivan
Book Design: Daryl Fuller
Illustrations: Maria Kay Simms

Library of Congress Catalog Card Number 94-072198

ISBN 0-935127-30-5

ACS Publications
An Imprint of Astro Communications Services, Inc.
P.O. Box 34487
San Diego, CA 92163-4487

Your

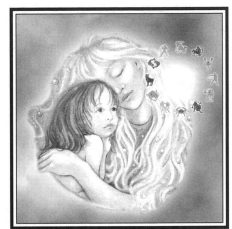

*M*agical Child

by

*M*aria Kay Simms

ACS Publications
San Diego, CA

Other books by Maria Kay Simms:

Twelve Wings of the Eagle
Dial Detective
Search for the Christmas Star (with Neil F. Michelsen)
The Witch's Circle
Future Signs

Dedicated

To
Shannon
Molly
Elizabeth
Tessa
and
Hayley

with lots of love!

Author's Note on the Second Edition

Since the first publication of *Your Magical Child* in 1994, many things have, of course, changed—change being the one fact of life that is inevitable! This book looks considerably smaller than its first incarnation, but in regard to its text, it is actually slightly bigger. I've added short house interpretations for all of the planets, as well as a few other additions, particularly in Chapter 10. There, a greater emphasis has been placed on how you, as a parent, can use this book with your own chart, and in comparing your special magical style to your child's. The major deletion is in the complexity of the look-up tables, and in the type size, in order to make the book more easily accessible to young parents who may have no previous knowledge of astrology. There's still a free chart coupon for a fully calculated birth chart that will enable you to take advantage of every portion of the book.

Acknowledgments

Again, my primary thanks go to my immediate family, for without all of you, this book simply could not exist.

Thanks to Mom (Anne Simms) for all the very good advice I asked for and got—and also for understanding when not to advise! And thanks to Dad, whom I know still watches over us, from the invisible realms, for all your understanding supportiveness.

Thanks to Shannon, Molly and Elizabeth for reading my manuscript and giving me your permission to tell all those stories about you—even the slightly embarrassing ones—but most of all, thanks for just being you! Special thanks to Molly for her lovely painting on the cover, and to Shannon and her husband for allowing me to use Tessa's chart as an example to help readers see how to use the look-up tables.

And Tessa, I thank you, too! You knew right away when Momma showed you the cover painting, that it was you two. I hope that when you are older, you'll still be happy about being in this book. But, just in case you aren't, Grandma used only your first name, to protect your privacy.

There are many others, too, who are part of the experiences that form the basis for a book such as this. Thank you for all we've shared together, be it pleasure or sometimes pain, for through it all, I've learned, and because of that, I wouldn't want to go back and change a thing, even if I could.

For particular assistance in pre-publication review of the original manuscript, many thanks to Marion D. March and Zipporah Dobyns, Ph. D. and Jeanne Hall. And last, but most certainly not least, many thanks to the ACS staff, especially Rique Pottenger, Maritha Pottenger, Daryl Fuller and Camille Swiggett-See.

Table of Contents

Chapter One

Understanding Magic

Your magical child? Yes, definitely! That's the first thing any "star parent" needs to know and appreciate. Each baby comes into this world with his or her own special magic, and grows through early childhood instinctively accomplishing marvelous, miraculous feats. Think of what children create before they are even two years old. They learn to know their world, to crawl and then to walk. They even learn to understand and speak a language—more than one language, if others around them are multilingual. They do these things with an ease that would far outstrip any adult learning a comparable task.

The very young regard their world with wonder—studying with transfixed attention your face, their fingers and toes, then perhaps a flower, a butterfly, as they learn at an amazing rate. Of course the child also encounters many mysterious things that puzzle, surprise or startle, things that defy intent or are scary. But with a little understanding support from a friendly adult, these mysteries will be solved, and the little sorcerer or sorceress will again be happily creating a magical world.

I believe in magic—in the miracle of life, and in the power of mind and soul for creative change and growth. Through the mind and soul, you can be whatever and wherever you truly want to be. You can accomplish things that others—and perhaps even previously, yourself—might call improbable …impossible …coincidence …luck. And yet, there you are. What was once only a thought has become reality.

The problem with growing up is that all too often you come to disbelieve in magic. The process is slow, but seems to be, at least to some degree, inevitable. Is it the price we must pay for being "civilized?" Perhaps.

Childhood is also very full of "shoulds" and "shouldn'ts" and "can'ts" and "musts" from bigger people who seem very powerful to the child. These powerful beings may have the best of intents, and of course, many of the things they insist be done or not done are quite necessary. The child needs to be protected from dangers he or she does not understand, and also needs to learn to function harmoniously with others. Unfortunately, it's a fine line between "civilizing" and "stifling" that all too often can result in a grown-up who has lost the joy and creativity of childhood, and has either forgotten the magical powers that once came so easily, or believes they never existed at all.

My first year of teaching art was in an elementary school, and it was there that I remember first really noticing the creeping effects of "reality" vs. magic. In kindergarten, first and (for the most part) second grade, the children's art was truly magical—uninhibited, creative and wonderful. No need to speak of composition here. Absolutely everyone filled however large a page was available with lively, colorful and bold designs. They were marvelous artists!

By the fourth grade, "reality" had set in for nearly every one of them. Their art was inhibited and painfully conventional—every picture with a narrow band of green across the bottom for grass, with tiny people, trees that looked like lollipops with brown stems and green tops, little box houses with a peaked roof. At the top of the page was a blue band for sky, with perhaps a white, puffy cloud or two, and maybe a little curved v-shaped object for a bird. Lots of empty space glared out from between ground and sky.

How hard I worked that year to "loosen" those kids up, in trying to restore some of the natural creativity that had been lost to conformity and inhibitions acquired through too many adult opinions (and peer opinions, influenced by adults) of how things "should" look in order to be "real."

Grownups can recreate the art of magic in their lives, with faith in themselves and through training the mind and soul to clearly focus intent and purpose. I know—I've seen it happen. It's easier if the magic of their inner child can be released. It's easier if the magic of their inner child was never stifled in the first place!

I hope to give you some added insight into how to keep magic alive in your child's life—and in your own, too. This aging "sorceress" has a little extra formula for that magical mix, too, that you might not find in the other child rearing books you've read. First, though, you deserve to know just a little bit more about "where I'm coming from." The personal world view of anyone who claims to offer you advice on anything is important for you to know. What people say about what "works" or "doesn't work" is always influenced by what that person believes, and don't let anyone ever try to tell you differently. Even when someone offers you all kinds of empirical evidence or even scientific proof that something is true, if you scratch deeply enough you will find a belief, an assumption, a hunch, that the person then set out to confirm with logic. Many of our core beliefs, out of which we form our assumptions, are not even conscious. They may be "programmed" by early experiences that we do not even consciously remember. This is one big reason why early childhood environment is so significant in what a person becomes, and why parental influence is so important.

But... before anyone leaps to the conclusion that I am going to tell you that the kind of person your child becomes ALL depends on your influence (guilt, worry, guilt), let me say, quite emphatically, that nothing is that simple!

A Little Laughter Helps—Guilt Doesn't

One of my favorite newspaper cartoon strips is "Cathy," by Cathy Guisewite, because Cathy is so very good at helping us laugh at our common foibles. (Sometimes laughter is the only thing that DOES help!) Cathy's married friend Andrea has two little kids, a toddler daughter named Zenith, and her baby brother, Gus. Recently I read two consecutive days of the strip that aptly illustrate two major realities that I've experienced—and you probably will, too—of life with children.

In the first strip Andrea and her husband are carrying huge stacks of books on child rearing, and stacking them in a wall around their two kids, who are on the floor, and not too happy about having their freedom curtailed. In the last frame the parents collapse on the sofa behind their wall of books and exclaim to each other, "Do you remember when we actually had the energy to READ?"

On the next day's strip, Andrea and her husband have put Zenith in her crib crying and are walking away, holding Gus, who is also crying. Andrea tells Zenith that she has to have a "time-out" so she'll understand she can't bite her little brother. In the next frame she worries about whether Zenith bit him to express her anger that Andrea leaves her to work all day. Daddy wonders whether Zenith might be sensing his special father-son bond and is bidding for equal attention. They rush back to Zenith. In the final frame both parents and children sit inside the crib with Zenith, Andrea smiling that they "are really coming together as a family" while Dad bemoans "all we need is for someone besides us to be in charge."

I had a good chuckle over both of these strips. Exaggerated? Yes, a bit. But why are they funny? Because they are so TRUE—in basic underlying principle. They illustrate the reality of being a caring Mom or Dad, or any child care-giver, with high expectations of yourselves that you can't match—and it's generally more productive to laugh about it than to cry!

#1 Reality: You never have enough time. All the wonderful theories and intentions you have about how to do everything right by your kids will frequently dissolve into confining the little "rug rats" (your generation slang, so I'm told), or installing them in front of the "boob tube" you swore you wouldn't overuse, just to give yourself a few minutes of peace.

#2 Reality: No matter what well-intentioned thing you do, there will probably be some "expert" theory as to why it wasn't "right" that could someday be offered as a reason why your adult kid has a personality quirk, low self-esteem, self-destructive habit or psychological hang-up.

What you do—and don't do—matters. You know it. That's why you're reading books to help you learn to be a better parent. But never forget that no matter who you are or what you think, your child is not you, nor does the child "belong" to you. That child is uniquely his or her own person, and may ultimately make choices in life that are the last thing you ever expected. (You'd better believe that this daughter gave her small-town midwestern parents a few surprises—fortunately for me they were both loving and resilient!)

As people seek to become more aware of what they believe and why, and increase their education and experience of their world, they often alter some of their beliefs. Other times they think (intellectually) that they have altered them, but then something stressful occurs, old emotional buttons get pushed, and the old beliefs crop out.

For all these reasons, when you evaluate what a book has to offer you, or what any "expert" says, in deciding whether you should adopt their views as workable truths for you, be aware that those views are based both on expertise and on the expert's world view.

This Grandma's World View

Although I've lived past the half-century mark, my world view is very much part of the so-called "new age" in that I believe that each individual has the power within self to create his or her own destiny. Yes, external events may happen over which one has no control, but no force outside the self dictates individual response—whether one laughs or cries, copes or falls apart, learns and grows, etc. Ultimately, the responsibility for creating destiny as it applies to our happiness or unhappiness in life, or our fulfillment or lack of it, lies within each individual.

I believe that everything in the universe partakes of the Life Force, and that God/Goddess is immanent within the Universe and within each individual. Every baby comes into this world not in "original sin" but **good**, and the Earth is good. That baby can learn to be "bad"—or I prefer to say, in disharmony with his or her world. But given a fair chance, the baby will learn to live in harmony, to cope with and learn from challenges, and to make the choices that will lead to a fulfilling life.

It is the job and privilege of parents to provide the love and the resources that will encourage their children's best individual potential— that will allow the child's magic to happen, and continue unsquelched as the child grows. In doing so, the parents must remain open to learning, too (as surely they will!), and they should respect and honor the child's own unique style, temperament, talents and choices, rather than attempt to impose their own preconceived image of what the child should be and do.

In another sense, I must tell you that my world view is not that "new" at all, for in a less clearly articulated form, it's not so different from what, years ago before anyone ever thought of the term "new age," my Mom and

Dad called "common sense." In that, I was a very lucky child—which is not to say that I haven't managed to create my share of problems and make my share of mistakes along the way!

In any case, the most important single ingredient that you can contribute to your child's ability to create magical feats of learning, coping, growing and being happy is love—the kind of love that does not possess, but rather encourages and accepts individual uniqueness. I want to support your efforts to love and honor your child's special uniqueness, and by doing so, influence that child's ability to develop the inner strength that everyone needs to grow, physically, intellectually, emotionally and spiritually.

The child's potential can be described by three different methods, all of which will be dealt with in the next chapter. Your influence is important, but limited, for most of the choices for your child's future will be the child's. In fact, I believe it is quite possible that the child-soul chose you, and that the chart of his or her birth reveals a myriad of choices and alternative possibilities that will lead to more choices that this individual soul "set up" as growth opportunities for this lifetime. Knowledge of the chart does not mean that all obstacles can be cleared from the path, but it can make the way a little smoother.

So be forewarned, underlying everything you read throughout this book, is this Grandma's philosophical blend of "new age" world view and "old age" common sense.

Grandma's Magical "Cookbook"

In the trade jargon of my publishing field, this book will be called a "cookbook." Its "secret ingredient" that you won't find in many other books on child rearing is astrology, and "cookbook" means that it is designed so that even if you have no previous knowledge of astrology, you can still easily look up an interpretive paragraph for every aspect in a horoscope. If you've read this far (for the fact that I am an astrologer was clear from the back cover), you are at least intrigued with the idea. Still, some of you may be thinking, "What on earth can the stars tell me about parenting?" Well, don't run off until you give me a few minutes to tell you. Trust me, you won't be sorry. You might even have some fun!

On the practical side, I'll tell you how to get your child's birth chart, so you can use the ancient and modern art of astrology, even if you have no previous experience with it at all. Easy look-up tables in the appendix will allow you to read interpretations of your child's planetary positions even before you receive the full chart. I'll also tell you a few tales from my own experience (may my children forgive me!), that sometimes agreed and sometimes disagreed with the currently fashionable expert recommendations for child rearing. (Believe me, fashions do change—which can be encouraging or confusing, depending on one's point of view.)

Most importantly, though, I'll do my best to reinforce what you already know—that you have a very special child. I want you to know to the very core of your being what a unique and magical child you have, and how you can encourage that child to reach for his or her highest potential.

Astrological knowledge can help you understand how to get just the right magical blend of guidance and letting well-enough alone that will enable you to increase the happiness and success of your life with your children. It can offer you the insight to understand, guide and accept your child—and yourself. It can be a very affirmative key to awareness and understanding of self and others that will encourage you to take positive steps in allowing your child to reach for his or her full potential. On the other hand, astrology can also help you relax a bit because it demonstrates that there's a mysterious ingredient in addition to heredity and environment that factors into "what happens." In other words, while your influence is very important, what YOU are, or do, or fail to do, will not be the ONLY factor in how your child turns out.

My philosophy, then, is about doing the best you can—and also about a no blame, no guilt and always-forgiving acceptance of that which is beyond your personal control. It's about creative change, because in choosing to devote a large slice of your life to child rearing, you have set your feet on a path that will change you. At the same time you are changing, your baby also changes into tot, then child, then teen-ager, to an adult who, hopefully, will be your mutually supportive friend, as well as your son or daughter—or former student, patient or charge. (The tools in this book are useful for teachers or anyone else who cares for small children.)

You'll hear much more about change—opinions about what you can, what you can't and what you probably shouldn't try, or which would be a waste of your time to try. Much of it can be encapsulated in an often-quoted and much-loved prayer. It's become a time-worn adage, known to millions, which I'll cite below. Read it slowly, and think about it, even if it's already familiar to you. Keep it in mind throughout the years to come. It will help you keep your perspective—and maybe your sanity. Then read on, while I try to conjure a bit of magical "wisdom to know the difference," with the help of a modern application of the ancient wisdom of astrology.

The Serenity Prayer
God grant me the serenity
To accept the things I cannot change,
The courage to change the things I can,
And the wisdom to know the difference.

Chapter Two

Individuality — Fate or Free Will?

Fate vs. Free Will is an age-old dilemma that still rages on today within many schools of thought, the popular versions of which probably aren't thought through very clearly, if at all. By the term "popular," I mean the superficiality with which the masses tend to understand complex subjects. Whether you're speaking in terms of psychology, religion, astrology or whatever topic we could name that attempts to deal with human behavior, that age-old dilemma of fate or free will is a central issue. As an example, I'll pose two general questions, related to the three complex studies I've just named:

1. If there's something about your life that's causing you a large problem, is it your fault or someone/something else's? Superficially understood psychology might allow you to excuse your inability to cope with the problem by blaming a childhood trauma. Superficially understood religion might sigh in resignation that "it is God's will" or perhaps the fault of Satan. Superficially understood astrology allows you to excuse your destructive trait or "bad luck" by saying it's in your horoscope.

2. Conversely, if you are very fortunate, is that due to your own effort or choices, or is it caused by something else — is it because your childhood environment was so supportive an environment, or is it the grace of God, or is it your lucky stars?

An automatic follow-up to that primary issue is this one: whose responsibility is it to improve an undesirable situation? Yours or someone/something else's?

The dilemma of fate vs. free will has been discussed and argued in countless conversations and volumes of writing, and will probably never be resolved. If you think I'm going to resolve it for you, in favor of one or the other, you're wrong. It's not that easy. Like so many things, this polarity of opposites is just not "black" or "white," but gray.

Some people find it more convenient to assign responsibility elsewhere. They find life easier when they absolve themselves and just follow the rules. Other people strongly resist and rebel against any outside influence that they perceive is interfering with their personal control over their destiny. Most of us probably lean toward each of these attitudes at one time or another, or we might prefer to assign "fate" to one area of our lives, but demand "free will" in another. It is important that I tell you upfront what I think, though, because my opinions on this topic are central to the rest of this book, and very relevant to your understanding of what I can tell you about enhancing your life with children — or with yourself, for that matter.

You will find that I don't allow anyone, of any age, very much room for blaming anyone or any situation for very much of anything, certainly not for attitude and response. In my mind, there's a big, big difference between a "reason" for a particular circumstance, and an "excuse" for being a certain way because of it.

There are three basic areas we need to discuss, as a background for understanding fate and free will in terms of just "who" our kids are — or "who" we are, for that matter. I'll take them one by one.

Heredity

There are definitely some aspects of heredity that can be said to be "fated." By this I mean that genealogical makeup determines some limitations with which the individual must cope. This is easier to illustrate with a few examples:

My daughter Molly loved to dance, and from the time she was a kindergartener, she took lessons. As she progressed into the middle grades, she had become an accomplished ballerina, graceful, lithe and expressive, and she dreamed of dancing professionally some day. Then, puberty and her genetic makeup struck. She grew a foot or more taller, seemingly overnight. Although still strikingly beautiful, slender, graceful and sexy to any male who might spot her walking by, as a ballerina she became more like an Amazon — too tall and heavy for a potential male partner to handle. And so the dream took a nose dive and eventually was replaced by another. Today she is an accomplished artist, with her BFA from art school, who sometimes does modern dance primarily for her own enjoyment.

"Fate" was the part of her individual self that said being a professional ballerina was an unrealistic notion. "Free will" was her resilience in coping with her disappointment and finding another dream.

You see or read about many more dramatic examples of that contrast between fate and free will just about any day of the week. Think of the kids who've been covered in the news, or have even had movies made of their lives, who were born with a physical handicap, but nevertheless became shining inspirations of pluck and determination.

I had an acquaintance once who had been struck by a hereditary blindness as he approached young adulthood. He learned Braille, went through college, law school and became a lawyer. I went to college with a blind-from-birth girl who was quite self-sufficiently getting around the campus, pursuing her degree. A lovely young woman who is my second cousin has been deaf and mute from birth. A graduate of Galludet College for the deaf, she now has a successful career as a grade school teacher. She drives, travels around the country by herself and is quite independent.

I'm sure readers also know of other equally handicapped persons who are very dependent, perhaps on some form of government welfare or disability, or even sitting along the street with a collection cup. You probably also know of people whose lives are miserable as they constantly bemoan the fact that it is because they are too fat, too thin, too short, too tall, not pretty enough, too pretty to be taken seriously, not of the majority race, or the preferred sex — and so on and on and on.

Am I being fair, in the case of people such as I've mentioned in that last paragraph? Some of you will say, "No!" Not fair." You might say that heredity might predispose a condition, but the ability to cope with it comes from the environment. You might go on to say that the people who succeeded were raised in the "right" environment; the people who are miserable were raised in an environment that predisposed ("fated") them to fail. Perhaps you may be right — but then again, perhaps the behavioral psychologists don't have all the answers, either. Let's think about the power of the environment.

Environment

I remember my first exposure to the formal study of psychology in college. The particular instructor I had was very sold on the idea that environment determines behavior, and for most of the time, we studied experiments with rats, and occasionally other animals, that were chosen to prove his point. I was less than impressed by the behavior of rats being illustrative of the potential behavior of people, but being environmentally predisposed (at that tender age) to conform to what the powers-that-be (parents, teachers) expected of me, I didn't argue. I gave him the test answers he wanted, in order to assure a good grade in the course.

Now, environment is everything and everyone that is part of an individual's world. "It" is often given credit for things that go right: "My, doesn't he just take after his Daddy! Such a gentleman, and so studious at his work." "What a kind young lady she is. She has learned that from your example." And then, in either case, perhaps, "Such a well-behaved child — comes from **such** a nice home." On the other hand, environment even more often gets blamed for what goes wrong: "What a slob! Well, look at his Dad." "She's such a sassy little brat. But it's no wonder. Her Mom yells at the kids all the time." And: "With the home *that* child comes from, it's no wonder."

Environment makes a terrific excuse for legions of people to explain a myriad of different problems that all boil down to one very basic issue. They are not happy with their lives, and it "helps" — is so-o-o-o "healing," in more of a self-help or "New Age" jargon — to identify the roots of their unhappiness as being **outside** themselves. This can be OK, **but only if** the identifying process is followed through by an acceptance of the personal responsibility to do something to improve the situation. In this case, the environmental problem may be identified as a "reason" but is NOT used as an "excuse."

All too often, however, the follow-through of identifying the roots of unhappiness gets bogged down in blaming whatever person(s), prejudices, childhood deprivation or abuse, accidental circumstance, "act of God" or whatever else is perceived as having "caused" the problem. This can become a victim mentality that engages in self-destructive behavior, or expends more energy in demanding "rights" that are perceived as "due" in compensation, than in making personal changes in attitude that will make self-improvement possible.

Why is it that one child raised in a deprived, even abusive environment, will grow up and succeed in life, and perhaps even say that it was that very deprivation that motivated the will to work harder? Why is it that another raised in a similar environment , even in the same family, will grow up and repeat the abusive behavior, or perhaps be self-destructive, and blame such behavior on that early environment?

Why is it that one small child might sit and pout all afternoon while the other kids are having fun, because of some small perceived unfair treatment? Why is it that a sibling, from the same family environment, will act with aggression toward whoever has been "unfair," while yet a third child, same environment, will laugh it off and join the game? Can this difference in personality ALL be due to the small environmental differences between them, perhaps to birth position? Or is it due to a slightly different genetic make-up? Or could there perhaps be a third, less tangible element that reveals information that may not be so easily evident from a study of either heredity or environment?

I believe there is a third element that is well-worth your consideration, which brings me to that third area of discussion I promised...

Astrology

Nearly everyone would agree that heredity and environment both factor into why people are the way they are, and behave the way they do, even though they might disagree on the relative effect or importance of each. A considerably more controversial supposition is that astrology might be a method of understanding the intangibles that cannot be so easily explained by citing hereditary or environmental influences. Such a supposition all too often tends to be greeted, by people who have never really explored the subject, with attitudes such as, "You don't really believe in that stuff, do you — get serious," or "Tell me something about myself — but don't tell me anything bad!"

At the roots of both these typical attitudes is the same old dilemma of fate vs. free will, fed by a vague fear that if astrology is taken seriously, it means that somehow "fate" has the upper hand — that if the "stars foretell," free will and control of whatever one perceives as reality goes right out the window.

Not true! There is nothing in anyone's horoscope that consigns that person to a particular "fate." Let's face it — life is just not that simple! No, the choices involved in working with one's astrological birth chart (also called horoscope, or in this context, just "chart") are up to the individual, just as the individual must choose how to work with a hereditary trait or an environmental condition. The chart can yield information about personality characteristics, about strengths and weaknesses, about the probable timing of critical life passages, and even minor "ups" and "downs." It is also possible to derive information from the chart about heredity and environment! Contrary to the tabloid "pop" astrologers penchant for wild predictions, however, the horoscope does not dictate if or how something will happen, or just how an individual will cope with what happens.

As has been already illustrated in the examples given previously, free will is not unlimited, but a wide range of responses to limitations are possible.

A few rather silly analogies to a birth chart are commonly used because they make illustrations of the relative importance of fate and free will as to what astrology can "predict" and what it can't.

The birth chart is like a road map. It tells you which roads are available for where you might go, but it does not choose for you which roads you will take to get there.

Or, the chart is like a blueprint of a building, in that it gives a basic plan, but does not dictate the final result, for many choices will be made along the way in regard to quality of workmanship or building materials.

Or, a chart is like a seed that is planted. An apple seed may be destined to grow into an apple tree. It may grow into a healthy tree, not grow at all, or grow poorly. It may someday produce wonderful apples, or wormy ones. It all depends on many things — quality of soil in which it is planted, how much rain it gets, and so on. One thing you can count on is that it won't grow up to be a tomato!

So, none of the three — heredity, environment, astrology — gives you all the answers. Why add astrology to the things you have to consider in guiding your child? Here are four good reasons I can give you:

1. Astrological knowledge can help you fill in some of the gaps that cannot easily be seen through a consideration of heredity or environment.

Why is your little pride and joy not a "chip off the old block"? Why is he so fascinated with things you never cared a bit about, that are not a part of your homelife? Where did he find out about such things, and what motivated him? Why is Susie so outgoing and risk-taking when you are so conservative and quiet?

Many examples could be given, and some might say that if you delve deeply enough, the puzzle could be linked to an environmental or hereditary factor. Perhaps that is true, if you have time to closely analyze each little puzzle — and believe me, you won't. In any case, increased awareness of a reason is only that — awareness — and you can often achieve that easier and more quickly with a little astrological knowledge. It's where you go from there that counts.

2. Astrology can help you relax!

Let's face it. Fair or not fair, right or wrong, parents — and teachers — tend to worry about whether they are doing right by their children. Guilt, guilt, guilt! If you're the biological parents, you even gave the kid his or her genes! It's the environment that you parents provide that will influence the earliest, most formative years. This is true in regard to the environmental influences of your homelife and family interactions, and to a large extent it is also true of the environmental influences that your child encounters away from home, at least in the earlier years when you are making most of the choices of where to go and of who the child's friends, day-care providers, schools, etc., will be. You can do all the "right" things that the experts tell you to do, make all of the best intentioned choices, and still the kid is, in many ways, a puzzle to you. How do you really know what is best for this very unique little individual? How much can you really draw on your own childhood experience, or your experience of other children?

"This is supposed to help me relax!?" you may be saying. Yes, it is! What I am saying, and what astrology can help you see, is that your child has a very unique personality and set of potentials that belongs to him or her alone. You didn't give the child his or her birth chart. Even if you planned the pregnancy, and the delivery was induced or surgical, the very complex combination of factors involved in **your** choice of that one moment of time, at one particular place, are seldom honored by the tiny soul who is making entrance into this world. I believe that babies come when **they** intend to come, despite any pitiful thoughts we might have that we are in control, and it's all part of a mysterious, miraculous, magical process that is beyond the full knowledge of this mortal world.

You didn't choose that horoscope for your child and therefore there are just some things that are truly out of your control. But you can use the child's chart to help you to do your best in providing encouraging environmental influences. This is so very important, and is, to a large extent, within your control. Astrology will help you appreciate and learn to encourage, rather than suppress, your child's special gifts (even if they turn out to be not quite the "blueprint" you would have chosen). Astrology will help you understand how to more easily communicate with

your child, and to guide the more challenging aspects of his or her personality into productive pursuits. Through this tool of awareness you have the key to understanding:
  • What can be changed,
  • What you'd be better off to serenely accept,
  • And the wisdom to know the difference!

3. Astrology puts you ahead of the game, giving you a chance to anticipate opportunities and potential problems.

Detailed studies of the potentials of hereditary influence are beyond the scope of most people — and besides, how many pregnancies are carefully planned, or planned at all. If you have adopted, or if the child or children that motivated you to read this book are your students, you may know little or nothing about their heredity. Some environmental influences have been studied and projected, but the details of environmental effects on a personality are most often discovered in hindsight. Sometimes such things are remembered (blamed) as a parent or teacher's misunderstanding of a child's needs or potentials. The understanding you can achieve through astrology can give you advance knowledge through which you can improve your ability to live happily with your child, while at the same time providing the activities, the encouragement and the acceptance that this very individual, unique and special child needs to grow to full potential.

4. Astrology can help you understand and improve your interactions with the child — your own responses to his or her behavior, and the ways in which you may provoke undesirable behavior.

For this, you need to understand yourself, as well. If you have your chart, you can read the astrological interpretations in this book for yourself, too. (If you don't have your chart, see page 287 for instructions on how to get it.) See how my interpretations relate to your memories of what you were like as a child, and think how some of the same characteristics, interests, strengths and challenges have translated into your adult behavior. By comparing your chart with your child's, you can gain much insight into ways you can improve your interactions and communications with each other. The recommended resource list in the back will direct you to additional sources of astrological self-awareness designed for adults.

Always remember: YOU are the adult. You have the capacity to read a book like this, or use any number of other resources to understand yourself, your own motivations and responses, and make the changes in yourself that will improve your relationships with others and your own personal happiness. Your baby or toddler behaves on instinct, revealed by his or her birth chart and influenced by his genes. As the child grows, another type of "programming" develops through the influence of the environment. In the early years that environment, to a very large extent, is YOU. The child will not be able to delve into astrology or any other complex self-analysis study for many, many years. It's up to you to exercise the mature control over your behavior that the child may lack over his or her own, and to help that child channel instincts into the gifts that will encourage success and happiness, rather than into behavioral habits that cause discouragement and problems.

It's also up to you to develop enough wisdom through awareness of yourself and your needs, and of the uniqueness and special needs of your child, so that you can guide when guidance is warranted and, just as importantly, **let go** when the child's independent choice is the better route. I hope to help you do that by sharing some of my own experiences with children — including some that I feel good about and also a few that I don't — along with my basic astrological knowledge, as it might apply to a small child.

Chapter Three
Those Phases All Kids Go Through

Regardless of heredity, environment or astrology, all kids go through similar phases of development. Yes, it is possible to correlate various phases with astrological cycles, and I'll mention a few of the more broadly understood outer planet cycles that correlate with the development of all children at approximately the same age. For the most part, though, this chapter won't have much to say about astrology. Astrological timing requires a level of study that is beyond the intent of this book, and I think it is more useful to just summarize some of the developmental stages as they have been commonly observed. These are the generally accepted "normal" phases that all babies and children (and their parents) go through (no matter what their individual horoscopes might tell us). It's important that you know something about those phases. Your child's astrological chart will tell you something of the particular **style** in which he or she might handle the phases, but I wouldn't want the astrology to mislead you in any way that the phases won't happen. They will. Individual style will show more as the child gets older than it will with a little baby.

At the same time as I've just said that though, I've also seen, through the years, that fashionably "correct" views change in regard to analyzing what those phases mean and what parents should do or not do about them. With each of my three pregnancies, I was told different things by the obstetricians and pediatricians about what I should do prenatally, and how to handle the care and feeding of the baby. The books and articles by the experts gave different opinions, too. And then there's the advice from friends and relatives. Can this be confusing? You bet.

It will also be obvious, as you read, that this summary of phases is filtered through the perspective of my own experience, and those who have influenced that experience. I'm not even going to try to tell you all about each age, for there are hundreds of books that cover developmental stages and what to do about them in more detail than you'd ever have time to digest. I've listed several of the new ones that I like in the bibliography, but if you find yourself in the position of the parents in the Cathy cartoon, with no time to read, I think you'd do well to keep good, old Dr. Spock handy. He was the easiest and quickest reference for a myriad of major and minor questions when I first needed such a reference 25 years ago. I reviewed his updated "Baby and Child Care" against several recent books, and I think he still makes a lot of sense, and in an easy reference format, too.

One of the things I like best about Dr. Spock is that he starts his book right out with "Trust yourself. You know more than you think you do." Most difficulties I've both experienced as a parent, and observed in others, comes from parental uncertainty and waffling about whether you are doing the "right thing" and trying too hard to measure yourself against some "expert" opinion about what you should do. It's important to trust your own instincts, and personally, I also think that instinct, more often than not, equates with common sense.

In this chapter you will hear about some of my personalized experiences of the various childhood phases, within the framework of the world view I've already expressed, but was still in the process of formulating during much of my children's childhoods. I won't pretend to be addressing an entire spectrum of possible experiences with children. I have had some experience with boys, through my daughters' friends, and also through past teaching experiences in a coop nursery school, a kindergarten, and as the art teacher in all the grades, junior high and high school. For a number of years I had frequently visiting step-sons, aged 11-17, but the only really intimate experience I've had raising children from babyhood on is with girls. Although we lived in quite a few different areas, and at one time or another my daughters have had friends of just about every race, religion, ethnic background and income level, including a few from disadvantaged families, most of our contacts were with families similar to our own, who could be fairly described as middle-class, mostly college-educated parents who were interested in and involved with their children's progress. Of all the dozens of anecdotes I could relate to you, I've tried to choose those that have some bearing on similar experiences I've also known others to have with children going through common stages. Nevertheless, they are definitely personal experiences, not clinical observations.

My experience is mainly that of a Mom, so this chapter is addressed primarily to the Moms, though I'll direct a few points to the rest of you here and there. In the interests of non-sexist language, but avoidance of the constant awkward use of "he and she, his and her," etc., I'm going to freely switch back and forth in referring to a generalized statements about children as "he" in some paragraphs and "she" in others.

When my kids were babies I listened to the pediatricians, and read books by some of them and by child psychologists, of course, but the stronger influence was the advice of my own mother. That was because what the doctors told me sometimes just wasn't nearly as helpful as what Mom said. Not that she said all that much, please understand. For one reason, she lived in a different state than I, and for another, she is not one who is inclined to push her opinions on her adult children unless she is asked for them. Still, her actual experience as a mother was always valuable information when I asked her. I realize that I am very fortunate, on that score, because I know that mother-daughter communication is not always as easy as I've experienced.

I do recommend that you do ask questions and learn from the experiences of your Mom, if you can, and from other older relatives or older friends who have raised children. Remember, they have "been there" — some of those doctors or psychologists are speaking more from an academic perspective, and it's not always the same thing, believe me. Scientific observations of what large numbers of children experience in common can be very useful knowledge, just as astrological observations of common characteristics of certain planetary configurations can be useful. However, both of these approaches must be considered within the framework of the particular dynamics and environment of the individual family, and no kind of book can truly do that for you.

If you are open to the memories of those who have lived through experiences that you now approach, and you ask questions of them and are genuinely interested in what they have to say, you will find that they will tell you a lot that is worthwhile. They'll tell you of their successes, and they are also likely to tell you of their mistakes, and you can learn from both.

There's another reason, too, for talking to your parents (or whoever had strong influence in raising you) even if you're inclined to think they're "old-fashioned" and even if you don't like some of the things they did in regard to you. It's important to be aware of and open to learning more about **how you were raised**, because, I guarantee you, the most significant influence on how you parent your children will be that of how you, as a child, were parented. This will be true even if you hate how you were parented, because then you will be making a concerted effort to do things the opposite way. This may be fine, but it also may not be in the best interests of you and your child, if you are primarily just reacting in opposition rather than being truly aware of what you are doing.

Most people, even if they don't realize they are doing it, fall into patterns with their children that echo the patterns that existed between them and their own parents. The words and the nuances and even the style may be different, but the basic patterns tend to be repeated. If your parent manipulated you with guilt, you will tend to coerce your children with guilt, even if you do it much more subtly, or with different words or techniques. If your parent hit you when angry, you are more likely to "lose it" and hit your kids when you get mad. If your parent trusted you, you will be much more inclined to trust your children... and so on it goes.

If you truly wish to change and do things in a different way, you have to be very aware of how you are really behaving. Those parenting dynamics are buried in your subconscious, part of deeply ingrained patterns that became a part of your life even before the age of conscious memory. If you can "get outside yourself" and watch, you will see what I mean. You will go along for a time quite consciously doing things according to a method you may have adopted from a modern child care expert, for example, and then in a particularly stressful moment you will suddenly hear yourself sounding just like your mother! I know I'm not the only one who's noticed this — even Cathy's cartoons have poked fun at the truth of it all.

The Needs of the Infant

Like the *Cathy* cartoon suggested, once the baby is old enough to move around, you don't have a lot of time to read the child care books anymore. The best time, as I remember, for reading the books was during my pregnancy. Since it's possible that some readers of this book, too, are expectant Moms, I'll start out by talking to you about babies, fashion trends in taking care of them, and about what worked for me, which was not always "in" fashion.

I'll freely admit that for me, babies were by far the easiest part of living with children. The older they got, the more complex were the challenges.

If you're reading this while awaiting a new baby, and are a little afraid of the prospect, I can relate to that. I was scared, too, even though I was 27 years old when pregnant with my first one. I'd never had any experience with babies before. I was never one to "kootchy-koo" other people's kids, and I remember once when I was pregnant and a visitor thrust a new baby into my arms, that my Mom even laughed that I looked "so unnatural." Somehow, though, when my own was put in my arms, it did seem very "natural." Here was this little being, whom I'd been feeling kicking me from inside for months, who was completely dependent on me, and was so very soft and sweet. Bonding began right away.

My observation (unscientific, but still my opinion) is that very small baby behavior depends a lot more on Mom (or other caretakers) than on baby. If you handle a baby calmly and with warm assurance, the baby will be calm and content. If you are unsure and nervous, the baby will pick that up and behave accordingly. Please don't take this wrong, but it's a little like dealing with an animal. Calm, confident friendliness will win over most any small pet, while your fear and uncertainty can be interpreted by the pet as threatening. A horse senses immediately whether the mounting rider is afraid of it or not.

It helps overcome new-mother nervousness to consider the baby's perspective. Life must be pretty confusing. He's just been through the traumatic experience of being thrust out into the world, and he's not sure exactly what is him and what is Mom, except that she, who might be only an extension of himself, is the part that has the food and makes things more comfortable—but is not always right there when he wants her. Quite possibly there are all sorts of past life or pre-birth experiences muddling around in his mind, along with all sorts of new sounds, smells, feelings and sights that he doesn't understand. Why is he in this little body that can't do much of anything and can't make other people understand what he needs? What **does** he need? All that matters is that sometimes he feels safe and comfortable and other times he doesn't. When he cries, perhaps he's only trying to tell us, "Won't someone please make some sense out of all this, and make me feel secure?"

At this point in life, no matter what personality type she may be becoming, the baby is acting on instinct, and an important part of the instinctive need is to feel secure. If you think about how the baby must be feeling, it's a lot easier to get outside yourself, and put any fears you might have secondary to reassuring her that this world is safe and warm.

When my first child was born, 25 years ago, the style was wavering between an out-going fashion for bottle feeding (obviously still favored by some of the hospital nurses, probably for convenience) and an in-coming fashion for breast feeding (generally advised by the pediatricians). My mother firmly advocated breast-feeding, and her taken-for-granted attitude was an enormous reinforcement to my own judgment that the "new" advice made sense. Mom had successfully nursed her children according to the traditions of her family, against an almost universal advocacy of bottle feeding and active discouragement from others around her, along with considerable pain in the early days of breast engorgement, so it was no accident that she had the attitude "of course you can do it."

The first few days can be tough, but if you stick to it, it's really only a few days until it becomes easy, and the rewards are great. It's a close, warm, sensual contact with the baby that increases bonding. Breast milk, being designed by nature for the baby, is much less likely to cause stomach distress than formula. Night feedings are a lot easier, and when bottle feeding friends took baby visiting, they had to haul along a very large and awkward bag. I stuck a spare diaper in my purse.

One thing I didn't agree with the pediatricians about though, was "demand" feeding, which in observing a few recent mothers, still seems to be frequently advocated today. In my observations, both years ago and now, demand feeding most often results in little sleep, a baby that is fat but fussy, and a frazzled mother. With my first new baby Shannon, I followed the more common sense advice received on a phone call to Mom, who suggested that I gradually space the baby's feedings out with calm, a little patience, stroking and reassurance, and a little bottled water, if necessary. I had a contented and calm baby on five feedings a day, who could be counted upon to sleep from midnight until 6 A.M. within just a few weeks after birth. Well before she was two months old, the late feeding just before midnight was eliminated, and she slept peacefully through the entire night.

For those of you who might be leaping ahead to the potential astrological questions inherent in that last statement — mind you, this baby had a Sagittarius Sun, Gemini Moon and Cancer Rising. It was not that **she** was so characteristically calm; it was that **I** was calm, with the firm conviction that "demand" wasn't in her or my best interest, no matter what the doctor had advised. Her Grandma (my Mom), my own instinct and common sense prevailed.

By the time I had my second daughter Molly, two years later, the fashions from pregnancy advice to feeding advice had changed again. Deciding that the way I'd handled my first baby worked fine, I listened to what the experts told me, rejected what was inconsistent with my experience, and did things exactly the way I had done them the first time. Molly was just as calm and contented a baby as Shannon had been, and she slept through the night within a very few weeks of birth. (If it hadn't worked, of course, I'd have gone "back to the books." I'm not **that** stubborn!)

By nine years later, when my youngest daughter Elizabeth was born, the fashions had changed even more, but again, with the same methods as had been successful for me in the past, I had a third "good" and very "easy" baby. When Shannon had my granddaughter Tessa in 1991, she followed the examples of Tessa's Grandma and Great-Grandma and had just as easy a time as we had. In each case, and in each time period, we saw other young mothers around us who, advocating some sort of demand feeding advice, were being kept up through the night, were feeding every two or three hours, and still had very fussy babies.

Were we lucky? Maybe. My limited experience is not enough to dispute the idea that colic or general fussiness is an unexplained thing that can happen to anyone, anytime, for no apparent reason. I do suspect that lack of sleep and increased tension in the caretakers aggravates the colic and fussiness. My motivation in rejecting "demand feeding" is most certainly not to be cold and structured, or to suggest that your time clock is more important than the baby's. It is just that I think what the baby probably wants, in seeming to fuss for breast or bottle every time you turn around, day or night, even if the tummy is full from a very recent feeding, is **security**, much more than food. Security suggests warmth and nurturing, but it also means routine, and dependable expectations. If every time the baby whimpers, you push breast or bottle in mouth, baby will learn that food equals attention. If you give other kinds of positive attention instead, the baby will learn to respond positively to that, and not be "demanding" about food. It does not foster security to have a ragged, worn-out Mom who is nervous from lack of sleep and from being regarded as nothing more than a milk machine. In order to have lots of love energy to give to your baby, you really have to give a little to yourself, too.

There's little that helps you in those early months quite so much as six hours of uninterrupted sleep. The baby needs the sleep, too — lots of it. It won't hurt a bit to gently steer the baby toward a more sustained sleep at a time that's good for you, as well. Of course you won't want to let a baby cry hard without checking to see what's wrong and doing something to reassure him. Just don't assume that food will fix it, if he was just fed less than three hours ago. Try something else first. Also, it won't hurt to wake him for a feeding if he sleeps more than four hours during the day, in order to encourage the longer period of sleep at night.

Whether you feed by breast or bottle, I think it cannot be emphasized enough the importance of cuddling the baby while you feed her. If the baby goes to sleep before she's had enough (20 minutes to 1/2 hour nursing), tickle her cheek and sucking will usually start again. The cuddling is every bit as important as the food. When my baby was fussy I often found that putting her in an infant seat, propped up near where I was working, so I could talk to her as I worked, often made her quite content. It's also very effective to carry baby around in a papoose-type infant carrier. I'll bet the Native American mothers' infants in their papooses didn't cry all that much. If all else fails, try a little water in a bottle or a pacifier before resorting to a too-soon feeding.

If after a month or so your breast-fed baby still insists on waking up at 3 AM or some other such inconvenient hour, offer a few ounces (three or four) of formula at the last feeding as a breast supplement — and don't feel guilty about it! Sometimes breast milk is sparse at the end of a long day. When I decided that it was high time baby gave me a decent night's sleep, I found that the little bit of formula did the trick very nicely, and she was out for the night. This may work for you, too, or maybe not. The point is, don't make such a fetish of doing things only one way to the point that you feel "wrong," or worried about failing, if it seems it might be a good idea to try something else.

While it is of utmost importance to start a baby out in these first very instinctive need-gratification months with the security that his needs will be met, it is also important for the health and well-being of all concerned to strike a balance between the baby's needs and yours. If you can feel sure about that — no guilt — you can relax, and if you relax, I guarantee you that your baby will feel more relaxed, too. To a considerable extent, this same philosophy works, no matter how old the kid gets, but it gets tougher as they get older. All the more important that you both relax now!

I'm a feminist, and a career woman, so I understand those of you who are juggling career goals with motherhood. Still, I strongly recommend that if you can possibly arrange to be home with your baby for **at least** the first few months, you should. Get off the fast track, accept that most of your time belongs to baby, and try to relax into that. The world won't stop if you don't get much of anything else done for a few months. Your body has gone through a lot of changes, and needs some time to recover. Take naps when the baby does, if you're tired. If you just absolutely can't avoid going back to your outside job, let's hope that Dad or a reliable and warm caretaker is available to give **consistent**, nurturing attention to the baby — and you must accept without conflict that a stronger bond may be forged between baby and the person who is there the most. Baby doesn't recognize the blood-bond at this point. It's being made to feel safe, secure and loved by someone that counts.

The security that is established during the early months and the very early years, before the time of conscious memory, is of enormous importance to your child's ability to cope successfully with life, no matter what his or her personality. You won't be able to protect the baby or tot from all potential traumas. Some things happen that are beyond personal control. But a very early relaxed and reassuring environment, you can and must, somehow, provide.

Parents must lobby for more understanding and flex time from employers. No matter what else anyone accomplishes in life, there is nothing more important to the future of our entire society than a good early foundation for our children. This is in everyone's best interests — make sure they know it.

OK, I'll get off the soapbox, now. Except for a word to the Dads. Baby needs you, too, and so does Mom. She needs you to help with the chores that she's too tired to do. And she and the baby need you to hold and pay attention to baby as often as possible. One of the times I was most deeply grateful to my babies' fathers for taking over, was at bedtime. Mom-as-food is not always the best person to settle baby quietly for the night. Baby may have had enough food, but not enough cuddling, Mom is exhausted, and baby wants to keep sucking, primarily because that's a way to continue cuddling. There's nothing like a strong, calm Daddy shoulder with a light patting on the back, to soothe a tired baby into dozing into easy willingness to be tucked in for the night.

The Emerging Individual

Once the first few months are over, and the baby sleeps less during the day, becomes more alert, studies everything intently — your face, his hands and feet, anything else that catches his eyes — the magic of birth truly begins to become the magic of individuality. Baby fully realizes that he is himself, separate from Mom. The books put this at around six months; I found it to be somewhat earlier. Games of hide and seek, peek-a-boo, are part of learning that when Mom and Dad (or objects) disappear, they also reappear. They continue to exist, even when not in sight. Baby learns to sit up, move around by rolling, creeping, crawling. He learns to do and to understand so many things, he is truly a genius, learning and growing more rapidly than he ever will again. His is a magical world of constant new discovery, but also many things that seem inexplicably scary.

One of the more interesting books on the psychology of young children is *The Magic Years* by Selma H. Fraiberg. Her "hook" in discussing the powers, the beliefs and the fears of children is a theme of primitive, superstitious magic, which is gradually defeated by logic and objective reality. The child, she says, lives in a magical world where he believes his actions and thoughts bring about events. Later he believes in "human or super-human causes for natural events or for ordinary occurrences in his life." Because the child so lives in his imagination, Fraiberg goes on, his world is unstable and spooky until subdued and "put into its place by rational thought processes."

Well, perhaps I have a tough little inner child that refuses to grow up, but I have a different slant on magic than Fraiberg. I **still** believe that my actions and thoughts can bring about events. However, I do think her book makes many valuable points, and is well worth reading.

I was amused by Fraiberg's analogy of parents as the missionaries who civilize the primitive savage, but the track I'd like to take on these first "magic years" is a product of my own views on magic. I'd prefer to think of parenting not as the missionary determined to convert the savage, but rather as the more mature magical person who encounters the talented young novice. Let's, for the purpose of this analogy, call the parent the adept — who guides the naturally talented, but untrained, little magician in the understanding, the ethics and the focused use of his powers. The child needs guidance and example in the ways of becoming aware of his world and how things work within it. He needs to learn how to find his own unique style of acting, thinking and **believing in himself** that will allow him to create events in which he can flow in harmony with his world and the other people who inhabit it. You could call this more "civilized," but let's instead call it a more mature kind of magic. No longer merely superstitious, the child becomes more aware and more focused — a fledgling adept.

In assisting the child in finding who she is, and what she can and cannot do, **without** destroying her personal magical style, the parent will learn a great deal, too. One of the most profound things you are likely to learn, very early on in your parenting, is how much patience you have! You will think you have an issue all taken care of, and suddenly the child seems to backtrack. What have you done wrong now? Probably nothing. The child has just arrived at a new stage of development. Individual cases may be a little earlier or later than the books say, but all kids seem to go through somewhat similar experiences. With many of them, the more you try to control, the harder it gets. One of the toughest things to learn is when to leave the kid to her own devices.

Sometimes you'd best stand by and allow a little rage to be expressed, so long as no mayhem is involved. I'm remembering my first small daughter, Shannon, at about eight or nine months, sitting on the floor vehemently determined to force various shaped wooden blocks through corresponding holes in a box, furiously banging them down on the box and crying bitterly. I'd tried once or twice to gently show her how to move the blocks around until the shapes matched and would slide right in, but she was determined to do it her way. So I tuned her out as best I could and went on with my work. She finally cooled off, tried again, got the blocks through, smiled with pride and then went on to something else, having accomplished a tremendously potent little piece of focused magic!

Babies this age are very determined little investigators, full of discovery and learning at the most rapid rate they will ever achieve. Of course you have to protect them from obvious danger, and your house from total destruction, but overprotection of either can stifle learning and create unnecessary fears. I'm for rearranging the house so that only a very few "no-nos" are within reach, lots of interesting OK things are available, potential fall areas like the bottom of stairs are padded, and playpens are only rarely used.

A few safe "no-nos" are good, because it is necessary to learn respect for other's things, and that there are things that he must not do — but baby will test you! I'm visualizing my small granddaughter Tessa at ten months, with gleeful grin at her mother as she reached out time and time again for that framed picture on the end table — testing, testing. Tessa was gently but firmly told "no" and when necessary, either distracted away or removed, and the picture stayed — Shannon's determination with the blocks was still with her, too! The lesson for you, here, is a minor aspect of a major issue that will test you time and again for many years to come. It's **consistency**. You waffle, and the kid has scored. But he hasn't really won, because he has learned that "no" really means "maybe," and what you say isn't dependable. This does not contribute to the child's security.

The older baby is in the business of trying out the whole idea of Self, as separate from parents. He is discovering his individuality, and testing his independence. It's heady, and it's scary. One of the scary things is, "now that I know Mom isn't me, how do I know **for sure** if she'll come back when she goes away?" This is likely why a baby who has been contentedly sleeping through the night for months will suddenly become wakeful, and try to engage parents in a game of staying up until you're all ready to collapse, or coming back at his cries over and over again through the night — if you are willing to play. If you play, the problem will not go away, and you'll have your much needed evenings gone. I don't think it's possible to "spoil" a tiny infant, but you can turn an older baby into a tyrant if you don't keep a balanced perspective.

All of my kids went through the bedtime challenge as tots. The most stubborn was my youngest, Elizabeth. I remember when we decided that enough was enough, and she would just have to cry it out. We reassured her that we were right out in the living room, it was time for her to go to sleep and we would see her in the morning. She screamed for what seemed like an eternity. It was horrible not to go check. Finally silence. We crept in and found her sound asleep, standing up, her hands tightly clenched on the crib rail. We gently laid her down and she slept through the night, and greeted us with happy smiles in the morning. This scenario was repeated for several nights, but after that, all was well again.

One of the things a good child care book is good for (see bibliography for suggestions) is the analysis of **why** (such as fear of separation as a natural stage of development) children behave as they do at fairly standard ages. Toddlers have many little fears that we might think of as irrational, but they are very real to the child, and are quite understandable within a framework of mental development at various stages. Understanding **why** can help you be empathic toward the child and what you do in guiding him, rather than dissolving into frustrated fears or anger yourself.

The So-Called "Terrible Twos"

It's a bad rap, but kids at two, and nearing two, are frequently labeled with this title. The psychologically conscious may cringe, but I'll admit that I've even been known to remark, on a few occasions, that the primary reason Nature generally makes two year olds the cutest they'll ever be in their lives is so that their parents don't strangle them. (It can be therapeutic to admit you are totally exasperated, sometimes, even if you'd never follow through.)

Your guidance of your little magician must be a balance of your own example and kindly but firm guidance in assisting him to develop self-control, and knowing when to hold back and watch for the child's readiness. Pushing doesn't make a whole lot of difference — the baby will do things when he is ready. Your job is to be alert to readiness and provide the environment and atmosphere necessary for him to discover that he can and wants to do the things he eventually must do in order to get along. When my first two were toddlers I was a typically young and enthusiastic parent who was determined to do everything "right." There were a flock of books then on creating super babies — *Teach Your Baby to Read* was one of them, I think. You get the idea. Parents were encouraged to be overly concerned about each stage of development, and goal-oriented me was right in there with my flash cards, sandpaper letters and what have you. OK, so they did just about everything early, could read before kindergarten, and we still had a lot of fun, with the possible exception of potty training. That was not successfully accomplished until well into the "twos" despite my mother's older fashion for beginning it earlier.

The hindsight lesson for me began with Elizabeth, born at a time when I was more career-involved and older (38). I just was no longer enthusiastic about such constant involvement with what she was doing, and was much more relaxed about my ability to survive small children. I wise-cracked, for example, that I didn't remember anyone ever going through a high school graduation in diapers. So I relaxed, waited until she noticed what older people do and showed definite signs of wanting to be dry and clean, and then provided a potty. She trained herself, with practically no effort on my part, at just barely age two, earlier than either of her older sisters with whom I'd been over-involved in the process. Also, with no particular effort on my part, other than reading to her every night, she did everything else just as early as the two older girls had, and also taught herself to read before kindergarten. She did have the advantage of an early home frequently full of adults and near-adults to pay attention to her, and to imitate. She, the child of a second marriage, had several sisters and brothers from her Dad, all ten years or more older, as well as her two older sisters from me.

Two is the prime year that the tot, having discovered his independence, now declares it with a vehement "NO!" Such discovery begins in the second half of the year between the first and second birthdays, but at age two it becomes very emphatic. "No" was among all of my daughters' first words, and my granddaughter's, as I believe it to be of nearly all children. My mother still occasionally comments (yes, even at my age), that my first two complete sentences were "I do it myself" and "Leave the baby alone." I see in her baby book that I have written a note about one of the earliest sentences of my middle daughter Molly — "MO! I do!" — as she stubbornly struggled with trying to dress herself. (Molly mixed up a few consonants at first, as many children do. My favorite was her loud — and in perfect tune! — singing of "Winkle, winkle, little car, Oh my wonder what you are.")

I doubt if anyone who's taken language classes as teen or adult will argue with me of the magic involved in the ease in which a two-year old learns a complex language. You can best assist this particular brand of magic by talking with your child a lot, and reading to him very early, right during the first year. By two, you should be both reading and talking about the books. Name things in the pictures, and ask little questions in order to encourage the child to talk and name things, too.

At two (or almost two) the tot is learning language very rapidly, but not enough to avoid considerable frustration in communication, for you and for him. One fine day soon, he'll all of a sudden string words into sentences and the few cute things he says that you write in baby books will "explode" into a huge vocabulary. After this, some of the frustrations ease up. Communication is a most helpful art.

My first two children were born almost exactly two years apart. They became very different in taste and personality the older they got, which demonstrates how very limiting a Sun-sign approach to astrology can be (they are both Sagittarians), but that's another chapter. As very young children, however, they were sometimes initially mistaken for twins, and they looked so much alike as toddlers that today I have a couple of photos of one of them alone, of which I am not sure which one it is. (Granny, maybe creeping age is showing!) In many ways it was nice having two cute little girls so close in age, but if asked now, I would say spacing babies three years apart is probably better. One good reason for that is the language barrier, and another is the very contradictory nature of the two-year old.

A two year old needs stability because his own inner world is still pretty unstable. He's learning about himself, trying many things, and trying to learn to make decisions. In expressing his independence he contradicts you — "NO" — but often even contradicts himself. Consistency and dependability in his environment are important, and upsets over drastic changes will stay with him for a long time, as part of his subconscious programming. Getting a new sibling is a pretty drastic change.

Shannon handled this and many other big changes in her life very well, considering that there were many moves, divorce, step-father, and other big changes as she grew up. I wonder, though, as I look at her pensive and sad little face as she poses for the photo with me and her little baby sister. In spite of careful preparation as best we could, she became physically ill with a cold and fever when I went to the hospital, separated from her for the first time in her life. Perhaps that experience was the beginning impetus for her becoming the most conservative and traditional of my three children.

Let me insert a small astrological note, here, to encourage you to go to the extra effort it takes to find out about aspects when you get to the astrological look-up section. From a sign interpretation only, Shannon's chart suggests that she would be the most free-spirited of her sisters. Her more conservative, responsible approach is reflected by her Saturn very closely conjunct her Midheaven. Aspects "weigh" much more significantly than signs in a horoscope interpretation. (See page 184.)

Shannon's personality modification also probably has to do with family position. First children get the full intensity of new parent focus on doing everything "right," and then are generally expected to be the "big" boy or girl when siblings come along to demand most of parents' attention. No wonder they tend to be more serious, regardless of what other inherent personality factors might be.

It's nearly impossible to adequately prepare a child for the birth of a sibling before you even have the shared language to talk about it. A three year old is much more ready to deal happily with a new baby, for this is a prime stage of imitation, and little age three may even be a good little Mommy or Daddy in wanting to help you.

Security blankets and similar comforters are often very important to children of around two. (In some cases, this starts in the last half of the first year.) Go along with it. It will pass. If the thing gets incredibly filthy and you're alert, you can probably get it through the wash when the kid is happily occupied with something else. Think about it. You probably have a few possessions that you'd be lost without, too. Shannon had three soft toys — Panda, Doggie and Pooh Bear — that she elaborately arranged next to her each night as her bedtime routine. Woe onto all of us if one of them should be temporarily missing. Molly had a "blanky" and also sucked a knot on her finger and twisted a lock of hair until I sometimes had to trim a bit to get it untangled. Elizabeth attached herself to any piece of nylon nightgown that she could get her hands on. She particularly favored a leopard print one, which I eventually gave up and let her keep, until it was worn to shreds. I think she was still using it for dress up play years later.

Give your "terrible twos" as much stability and consistency in their lives as you can, without unduly hampering their growing independence. Take your time and let them do things their way whenever possible, and maintain a sense of humor. They'll be three sooner than you think, and you'll forever after have those stories of how cute and exasperating and magical they were as tiny tots.

Three to Six

If there's an exception to my previous comment that infants are easy, but it gets more complex the older kids get, it's the blessed age of three. After the "terrible twos," little three-year-old is a special delight. Still at their cutest, they can now converse with you, which makes lots of things easier to handle. At this age they love to imitate Mommy and Daddy and have you both on a pedestal. Which of course means that you had better set a good example! This is true at **any** age, but very intensely so at this one, when the child is so involved in learning by imitation.

This is when most kids identify themselves with the parent of the same sex, so that parent becomes a particularly important role model. The parent of the opposite sex tends to become a romantic ideal, becoming in that sense, the subconscious *anima* or *animus* (in Jungian psychology terms, referring to the inner female and male) that often strongly influences future choices of romantic partners when the child grows up. I don't personally remember any undue jealous conflicts caused because of this, but I know that it does happen in many cases. The child will deal better with either parent alone than with both together. Children tend to compete with the parent of the same sex for the attention of the parent of the opposite sex.

In any case, you-as-role-model becomes very, very important at this age, and it will stay that way for many years to come, so keep this paragraph in mind in regard to any other age group I mention. It's been said that example is not just the **best** way to influence people, it is the **only** way. My experience tells me, as I'm sure yours will, too, when you think about it, that there is nothing any parent or any teacher can possibly **say** that will make as strong an impression as what they **do**.

At this age your child is also very conscious of your approval or lack of it. He doesn't do things especially for their own sake. It's not a matter of conscience yet. He does things in order to please you. Obviously, then, it is going to help the child grow and learn if you look for plenty of opportunities to catch him doing something right — and say so! If criticism is required, phrase it positively, for negative criticism can be very damaging to self-esteem. Very few kids ever bring much of anything to "show you" after they've been put down. More often they're likely to see themselves as demeaned and less worthy. Praise, when deserved, is infinitely more encouraging, and constructive suggestions can lead to an occasion for praise. If you'd like help on language and examples in this area, it's not a bit too early to read books on Parent Effectiveness Training. *The One Minute Mother* would be a good starter.

As your child watches, imitates and tries, he gains in skill and in increased self-control. One of the primary requirements for producing mature magic is self-mastery. This is not the self-control of mere conformity. I am talking about the inner control and increased ability to focus an intent and follow through on it that comes from self-confidence in one's competency. In short, to create magic in your life, you need to believe in yourself.

Three is an expansive age. Expansion is a keyword for the planet Jupiter (see page 129), and it is between the ages of three and four that Jupiter, as it is moving along the zodiac of signs, first comes to a 90° angle, the aspect called a square, from the position it held in your child's birth chart. The child continues to learn very rapidly, and opens up from his own small world primarily at home to a larger world, that should involve play with other children. It's time for them to have the opportunity to learn from a wider range of activities than might be available to them at home, and it is also time to develop the social skills of interacting with other children. Here the "MINE!" of two learns to cooperate and share. Children teach these social skills to each other, for the most part, better than we can teach them. If you stand back and give them the chance, they will often work out their little differences and spats quite nicely.

My daughters all went to pre-school. Since they were all born in fall or winter, they started, in fact, a little before their third birthdays, and continued for half-days every day until they entered elementary school. I was (and still am) a strong advocate of Montessori pre-schools, so much so that I managed to get all three of them into a Montessori school for at least part of their pre-school experience, even though I had little money at the time and really couldn't afford it. I traded paintings and art work in two places, and in another, went in and cleaned the place in trade for tuition. I'm not going to go into a detailed treatise on the method here, for there are plenty of books on the topic. Enough to say that such schools are extremely well organized in methods of allowing each child to develop skills independently at his or her own pace. Toys and tools are marvelously designed to facilitate this with little instruction from the teacher, who is seldom up front directing the class, but rather is quietly moving around observing and guiding only when necessary. Observing a good Montessori class in session is fascinating. The kids have fun, and they learn a lot, without any pressure. All three of mine taught themselves to read and do simple math.

During two of the years we lived in San Francisco in the 70s, we were also in a very good cooperative pre-school. All of the parents worked one-day a week, so the ratio of adults to kids was excellent. It was noisier and not as well organized and richly equipped as a Montessori school, but many of the parents were very creative, artistic people who enthusiastically brought a wide variety of activities to the children. During the second year, the assistant teacher had to leave, and since I had kindergarten teaching experience, I was asked to take over, and was then there for a ½ day session every day. It was a good experience, but also the time when I realized that I was probably better cut out to be the mother of girls!

I could not **believe** how many ways the little boys found to get in trouble. They were creative beyond imagination in that area. The little girls, in groups, were capable of being much noisier, but no six of them could ever think up the mischief that any one boy seemed to be able to devise. Fortunately, the little guys were also cute and sometimes even funny — most of the time — but I'll admit I was relieved to not have to try and keep up with them from morning 'till night.

One of the things I did have trouble with, in regard to the boys, was their propensity for gutter language. They took utter delight in using whatever shock-value words they could come up with. I handled it pretty well at school, using the prescribed tactic of calmly asking them to define the word used, and when they often couldn't, at least not very satisfactorily, we discussed why they should want to use a word for which they didn't know the meaning. Substitutes were suggested. It worked some of the time. What I wasn't prepared for was dealing with my pretty, usually well-behaved, little blond daughter trying out the same words at home. Shannon has always been by far the most outspoken of my daughters, and this was no exception. There were times when I wondered if by the slip of giving her the initials S.A.S. (as in sass), we'd marked her for life! I'm ashamed to admit that one day when she persisted in flinging out one of the worst of the boys' obscenities, I absolutely lost it and washed her mouth out with soap.

She still tells that story once in a while, and we both laugh at it now. But I do consider it one of my mistakes, even if she did modify her language (at least in my presence) after that! And don't get me wrong, she was an exceptional young lady much of the time, and always so in the more public places where she knew it was not appropriate to be otherwise. I tell you this story to demonstrate that shock language is a common bounce-off of pre-school, even in the "nicest" of environments, with parents who do not use such language themselves. Understand it for what it is — another trying out of something new. (In this case, shown by Sun-Uranus, page 162.)

I **don't** recommend handling it like I did with Shannon. The discussion of meaning is better, with perhaps a time-out alone in the child's room if inappropriate behavior persists.

Somewhat related to the above, is an intense interest in sex and where babies come from during the pre-school years. This is a time to be prepared to answer lots of questions. We had one bed time story book that explained in collage type pictures all about how plants were pollinated, how animal babies were born, and how human babies were born. I no longer have the book, so I can't give you the specifics on it. It was more than well-worn with repeat requests. I think it is best to answer questions simply and honestly, but not to volunteer more than is being asked for at that moment. Usually the child is well-satisfied with a very simple answer, and really doesn't want to be overloaded with an entire treatise. Don't worry, you'll get another question soon!

During these years it's also possible you may find that your child has an imaginary friend to whom he talks. Play along with it, and don't worry about it or in any way demean the child or scoff. This happens with a lot of kids, especially imaginative ones. It may be an important comfort, or a way of expressing needed feelings, or a way the child is beginning to deal with new things, fears, conflicts or ambiguities in his life. The stage will probably pass soon, or maybe it won't. But it's very unlikely any harm will come of it. Anyway, don't you ever talk to yourself sometimes? I do!

It's also possible that a child will report that he actually sees people whom others don't. Again, I urge you not to scoff, or to express alarm. Science and objectivity in no way explain everything in this world, no matter what some very logical types might think. A very psychically sensitive child may actually be seeing things that you can't. How do you know, really, all things that are possible or not possible? In any case, it won't help the child for you to insist that something isn't real, when it is most decidedly real to him. If your child, who has slept quite peacefully in the dark for years, now suddenly expresses a fear and wants a night light, give him one. It won't hurt anything, and may help a lot to make him more secure.

Molly first told me at about the age of six that she saw spirits. She had gone into a dark part of the big, old house into which we had just moved. We lived upstairs, and downstairs I had my business, an arts and crafts gallery and metaphysical bookshop. She came running out into the lighted room where I was teaching an art class, and quite alarmed, told me that there were a man and a lady in there. She described them. I went back in with her, looked around, turned on the lights. Nothing. All was locked and secure. I told her, "Maybe you imagined it, or maybe they were spirits, but nothing feels wrong here. Did you feel they were going to hurt you in any way?" "No," she said. "Well, don't worry about it then," I said, "Go on and play." Later, she told me that she had seen them again, and that they came in and sat on her bed at night. She wanted a light on, which I permitted, and she was then able to sleep just fine. One evening when a psychic foundation that held its meetings in my building was assembled, I asked a woman who had been with the group for sometime if anyone had ever seen spirits here. She said, "Oh yes, a man and a woman. They live here. I've seen them often." She went on to give me the same description Molly had.

I never saw the spirits then, nor did Shannon, but who would I be to say that Molly did not? Finally, just once, many years later and in a different house, I was alone in a darkened room with a sleeping Elizabeth who was ill with the flu, and I did see a shimmering lady who came in and briefly bent over Liz, as if to check to see how she was, and then vanished. I was wide awake, with no reason to be hallucinating. This is the only time in my life anything like this has happened to me, but Molly, who was then a teenager, had said several times that there was a lady in that house who appeared in her room sometimes.

As I've said, there are many things we do not know. It would serve no purpose to ridicule a sensitive child. As she grew up, and on into adulthood, Molly has occasionally continued to see beings that most others do not, and is psychically sensitive in other ways, as well. She doesn't make a big thing of it, and perhaps it was a beginning factor in her very creative imagination and of the very strong talent in art that has become her career field. In any case, whatever you believe about these things, I urge you to handle them with sensitivity and understanding — and never ridicule — if your child experiences them. What is "real" is always a matter of individual perception.

Elementary School

Between the ages of six and seven, thereabouts, the planet Saturn will have moved to its first square to the degree of Saturn in your child's birth chart. Among Saturn's primary keywords are responsibility, discipline and limitation (see page 130). This is the time in which the more play-oriented days of pre-school and kindergarten are over and the child settles into the much greater discipline required of elementary school. This may or may not coincide with the opposition of Jupiter to its birth chart position, and your child is expanding at the same time as more limits are being set.

For many of you, it will be possible, if you are interested, to find out exactly when your child experiences each of these aspects by looking ahead in the planetary look-up tables for the positions of Jupiter and Saturn during the years your child will be six or seven, and comparing them with the birth chart positions. These are what astrologers call generational aspects — they happen to most people at about the same age — but the timing varies from year to year, and the more dramatic adjustments in your child's life are likely to be made when the aspects are closest.

Saturn gets a bad rap in some astrological texts, but trust me, it can as easily reflect the "good" experiences as it can the "bad" ones. It does require an increased sense of responsibility and a greater development of self-control. All of my kids handled it very well at this age, and so will most of yours. Each of my three had the aspects time out a different way, so in order to demonstrate how this might vary, I'll tell you a bit about their experiences, as they fit in with normal (what is "normal," anyway?) childhood phases at this age.

Outer planets have cycles that include apparent retrograde motion (backwards) as seen from Earth. They don't really go backward. It's sort of like the optical illusion that happens when you're on one train and you pass another train which is moving in the same direction on the track beside you, but a bit more slowly. For a weird moment it seems that other train is moving backwards. If this retrograde motion period happens when the outer planet is close to the degree of a planet in your chart, the passage (astrologers call it "transit") may take many months.

Shannon had the Saturn square beginning four months before she turned six. This was the September that she started first grade. She'd already learned to read in Montessori, we couldn't afford the first grade program that they wanted her in, and she was a month too young for the public school first grade deadline. The big city kindergarten to which she'd be required to be bussed was a big, urban jungle, in which the kindergartners at the end of the school year were just laboriously learning the ABCs. We decided to send her to the Catholic school that was just two blocks from our home, which we judged, on observation, to have an acceptably creative program, certainly much better than the available public school offered. Still, there was Saturnine limitation and responsibility inherent in switching this bright and independent little girl from the very open Montessori style to a conventional classroom, with uniforms, even. She did very well, though, even shining with her role on stage in a school program, just as she entered the time of her Jupiter opposition shortly after the turn of the year. Saturn, having retrograded several degrees away from her birth chart Saturn, returned to the square in June, as we packed up to leave the San Francisco neighborhood where she'd grown up from the age of three, and moved East.

About every seven years Saturn makes a major aspect to the position it held in the birth chart, and it usually reflects a significant change or "shift of gears" in the person's life. Sometimes this is only an internal change, but other times it is also associated with a life-changing event. This was the case for Shannon.

It's interesting that all three of my daughters experienced a very significant change of residence and circumstances during that first Saturn square, which is certainly not to say that it will be the same in other families, but in some way, expect a "shift of gears" either internally, externally or both, to coincide. For most children, entering first grade is in itself, a very major life change.

Molly, too, had the Jupiter opposition in the spring of her first grade year, while her Saturn square encompassed the entire school year. She, too, started first grade in the fall before she turned six. Her first grade year was marvelous — she loved her teacher and did well in everything, despite the fact that her father and I divorced in the middle of that year. Right at the end of the school year, during the last month of her Saturn transit, we moved to a different town in Connecticut, where I was to start my business, mentioned previously.

For Liz, the Jupiter and Saturn cycles did not coincide. The Jupiter opposition came in the spring of her first grade year. She was doing very well in school, had lots of friends, and seemed happy, but was expanding a bit too much in the weight department. This may have reflected an inner, unexpressed tension over the fact that my second marriage (to her father,) which had been (in hindsight) perhaps too hastily entered, was not working out. That summer, Molly, Liz and I left Connecticut and moved back to my home town in Illinois, where I needed to both get some space from my marriage and see my mother through a serious health crisis. (Shannon went off to a university that year.) Liz's Saturn square began late, the spring of her second grade year in Illinois (she was then seven) and lasted until a bit after her eighth birthday. She was then in third grade in Florida, where I'd taken a job after Mom recovered and my divorce was final. Despite all this change, she flourished, happy in school, very active in Brownies, and was being tested into gifted programs in Florida. In spite of the fact I can see plenty of both flexibility and strength in her chart, I've always been amazed at Liz's ability to adapt. She was in a different school every year until sixth grade, and every summer flew off alone to spend two months with her father, waving 'bye to each of us on either end with not a trace of anxiety, eager for the activities ahead in either place.

During the grade school years, conformity to what the other kids are thinking and doing gradually supersedes the parents-on-the-pedestal of three. The child's world broadens, and ideas are picked up from many sources. Pressures increase, and life can become pretty complex for the kids, and for you. These are years when you may well find that understanding your child astrologically, as well as in other ways, becomes very useful. Just see that you do not seek to use it to control, but rather to understand, and to offer guidance.

I will not even attempt to cover all of the possible issues you could encounter. Best here, to leave my input to the astrological look-ups, which hopefully will prepare you with some insight into what your child's unique style might be. The best kind of guidance will be that which is alert to the child's particular bent, in order to facilitate his or her ability to make the most of it. When unacceptable behavior happens, which it is bound to, to one degree or another, remember the "rule" of consistency, and try not to lose your own self-control.

Besides *One Minute Mother*, there's another new book out that I wish I'd had years ago. It's a light-hearted humor book in cartoons with a very profoundly serious foundation called *Purrfect Parenting*. It has very sound advice, but handled in a way that helps us laugh at ourselves a bit, too. Trust me, if you ever get where you can't laugh at yourself in this game, you're in trouble.

In the conclusion of this book, I'll be telling you a little about how you can use astrology to not only understand your child, but to understand yourself and how you and your child interact. This can be invaluable. Knowing why you and your child sometimes "push each other's buttons" in a way that can send you far off of your own best intentions for parental serenity (sanity?) won't always work, but if it helps even some of the time, it's worthwhile.

Personality mixes between people can also be a factor in your kid's friendships and in how they do with particular teachers. You won't always be able to know the astrology of it, or be able to do anything about it if you do, but greater understanding may help. Molly nearly lost one whole grade, academically, because of an unfortunate mix with her teacher. Sensitive Molly so very much wanted approval, and to be sure of what she was doing, but whenever she asked a question, the much more assertive young teacher would criticize her for not listening carefully enough in the first place. Molly became so intimidated that she quit asking questions at all, consequently made mistakes, felt bad, but didn't complain because she didn't want to make trouble. When I'd ask about her teacher, all she'd ever say is "she's so-o-o pretty." By the time I really understood what was going on (I'm afraid I was too preoccupied with my business that year to tune in as much as I should have), Molly, who started out so academically bright, had decided she wasn't smart at all. It was not until she successfully handled some fairly tough academic courses for her college degree that she really regained her confidence in herself in that area. I could view it, I suppose, that this experience in some way led her to so greatly excel in the arts, but I still consider it one of my major mistakes as a parent that I did not "tune in" earlier in that school year and demand that she be switched to another class.

At around the age of nine children go through their second Jupiter square, and this may also be a significant time of expansion. I can't remember a specific story of Shannon at this age. Molly was nine when Liz was born. She was flourishing in her first real act of independence from her older sister. Molly was always the "little sister," led and often dominated by Shannon. They had both started out in dancing lessons a couple of years before. Shannon wanted to quit, but I could see that Molly didn't really want to follow Shannon this time, so I encouraged her to continue. She loved it and was very good at it, and dance was her favorite activity for several years.

Liz, during the year of her Jupiter square, showed her first clear indications of being an independent thinker who was concerned with causes, expressing the more philosophical side of Jupiter, perhaps. Before she was 11, she had become a vegetarian and animal rights activist. She is still a vegetarian as a teenager — has never budged from her decision, quite independently of peers or family.

Adolescence

The scope of this book's astrological interpretations is intended primarily for small children, up into the early grades, but I'd feel incomplete if I didn't say just a few things about the adolescent crisis.

I'm sure I don't have to remind any of you of the time you went through puberty. I think all of us have some indelible memories of our adolescence. It's not the easiest time for most people, if any. Your body is changing fast; hormones are racing. For many kids the face breaks out in zits, and for others, it must be tiring just growing. I remember when I was teaching junior high school how amazing was the change in the boys from seventh grade to eighth grade. In the seventh grade year they were shrimps, dwarfed by most of the girls, who had already begun puberty with the onset of menstruation at age 11 or 12 and had reached near adult height. We'd break for summer vacation, and on the return to school the next fall, I'd have trouble even recognizing some of the boys, so greatly had they changed in one short summer. Kids who came up to my nose in the spring now towered over me.

At this age, kids are both expanding and testing limits, in ways that are much more mature than before, but in a way that is often not very mature, either, from the perspective of their parents or other adults. The problem is, that to the adolescent, the adults are just old and out of touch with the way things are. I've heard it said (and admittedly, maybe even said it once in a while since I became one of those who is "over the hill" — and that includes all of you who are over 30, too, in kid-view — maybe even over 25) that one never again knows as much about life as one knows at 15.

Well, that's probably not fair. I think we all know, at adolescence, that we know a lot, but certainly don't know everything. We're just reluctant to admit it, at least to our elders. We can see-saw back and forth from bravado to self-consciousness, from confidence to a painful shyness, from being alert and quick to fading off into a dreamy quiet that has our parents asking if we feel well or if anything is wrong. You remember — admit it.

At about age 12, seventh grade for all of my children, Jupiter returns to the same degree as in the natal chart, a full cycle complete and a new one beginning. In astrological books this is often touted as a time of opportunity. It's the beginning of a new cycle of growth, and for many kids that is quite literal. They begin sprouting up at a faster rate. How easily it all goes for both your child and you may depend on whether the Jupiter return coincides with the first opposition of Saturn to its natal position. It's the Saturn opposition that is the classic astrological transit associated with the so-called "adolescent crisis." You can read about this life crisis or passage in books that have nothing to do with astrology. Knowing when the Saturn opposition actually takes place would give you a closer idea of timing.

It seems to me that if the Jupiter return comes early, and the Saturn opposition at a later time, the Jupiter return is an easy, productively expansive time. If they come closely together, the Jupiter expansion and the Saturn opposition become an expansion of the Saturn issues. For me, and all those years later, for Liz, the Jupiter return came in seventh grade, and the Saturn opposition not until high school. For all three of my daughters and for myself, the second Jupiter square of the new Jupiter cycle came at age 15, sophomore year.

For Shannon and Molly the Jupiter Return was very closely followed by the Saturn opposition in eighth grade, which extended into the first part of high school. Shannon had a severe problem with acne as puberty set in, and a lot of problems in her relationship with her step-father, aggravated because she was the most outspoken of my daughters and he was very authoritarian with her. Molly grew herself out of her favorite dance activity, as was related in the last chapter, and then went through an overtly sexy-acting stage that attracted boys who were too old for her. Both girls used far too much make-up for my taste.

Somehow, we got through it all, not without frustration. By the time each became 15, Shannon and Molly had modified their make-up to a tasteful level, and even on occasion, advised me on how to wear mine. Shannon's skin cleared, but her problems with her step-father never really did, expanding right through the Jupiter square at age 15. On the more encouraging side of the age 15 expansive period, she developed a beautiful singing voice, and partially through that, really blossomed. She finished high school a semester early and went off to college. This was just a few months before I left that marriage, for a number of reasons, one of which was our complete inability to reconcile our differences on how to deal with teenagers. Molly, by her sophomore year, coinciding with her Jupiter square, had settled down a great deal and had found her niche in the art department, excelling in what was to become her future career.

I had my own Jupiter return in seventh grade, and that expansive period, encouraged by a favorite teacher who was especially interested in my art work, hallmarked what was to become my first career. I won a prize in a state-wide art contest. At the time of my Saturn opposition, as a Freshman, I decided to go steady with a senior, which I am sure did not thrill my parents, but they did not interfere. Much later, my father related that it was all he could do not to throw him out by the nape of his neck when he saw him with his arms around me. By the end of the year, at the time of my Jupiter square, I broke off what had become a stifling relationship, determined that no boy waiting for me was going to interfere with my decision to get out of that small town and go to college. I never "went steady" again until I became pinned to my future husband as a senior in college. As another phase of my adolescent crisis, I rebelled against the religion I'd been raised in, and very active in, and began a long period of seeking and searching, trial and change, for a spiritual path that made sense to me.

Liz had her Jupiter return in seventh grade, as she became increasingly "at home" in the first school to which she'd gone for two consecutive years since she started. She made friends, did well, and on the day of the last transit of Jupiter exactly on the degree of her natal Jupiter, was honored as one of the seventh graders to have scored superior ratings in the state for taking SAT exams. As of this writing, she has just entered her Saturn opposition. Saturn has been moving more slowly than usual this cycle, and it opposes the natal position in Liz's chart near the end of her sophomore year in high school. Her Jupiter square began in December '93, and due to retrogrades and directs, both aspects carry through the summer, with Saturn continuing into her Junior year. What will happen? So far, so good. Dad is being very understanding of this, his youngest child to become a teen. He is even supporting her growing sense of independence with a ticket for a solo trip to Europe this summer to visit a former classmate. What next? Who knows. By this stage of the game, I trust that she, — and I — will be O.K.

But... at this point, and especially after also having taught in both junior high and high school, nothing any teenager does, thinks or says would surprise me. My words of advice for parents:

1. Don't resist too much. Adolescents will rebel against something — of that you can be sure. Let it be something other than you! This is a natural stage of development in which they must begin to define who they are as differentiated from what all adult authorities say they should be. Whether they merely "test the waters" for a while, or engage in an all-out rebellion may depend upon how much you fight them, and in how many ways. Of course, there are some things you cannot allow, and on these you must be consistent. But let lesser issues go for the time being. Things like dress, hair, make-up, expressions of ideology different from yours — are these things really that critical?

If their music bugs you, which the favored music of any teen-age generation is often inclined to do to the older generation, get them some earphones, or try to soundproof their room. It's not worth fighting about, and it won't change. My older girls were brought up constantly surrounded by opera and classical music (their father is an opera singer). They still went through the loud music stage — Liz, too, and me, a long time ago, though we loved the classics, too. The preferences of youth and most adults seldom agree. Best to agree to disagree. Find a compromise solution.

2. Respect their privacy. I don't think it's fair play to snoop in a kid's diary or room unless it's truly a matter of life and death. Strong suspicion of drugs is life and death, but if you are reasonably alert, you shouldn't have to snoop to know if you have this to worry about. Most anything else is just plain snooping. You wouldn't like it if they did it to you, either.

3. Keep the lines of communication open. Don't lecture, listen. If you're aware, alert and genuinely interested in what they think, and are not pushy, they'll probably talk to you, at least some of the time. If you let them know that you are there for them, no matter what, they probably will talk to you if they have a problem.

4. Trust them. You should have been guiding them in the idea of being responsible for the consequences of their own actions all along. Now, I think it is important to trust them. My parents let me know, without lecturing, what their opinions were on various ethical and moral issues. They trusted me to be mature enough to know how a young lady behaved, and did **not** make rules. I would have done anything not to let them down — even though I didn't always tell them everything. So far, that same element of trust has worked very nicely for me in parenting my kids. I know they haven't told me everything either, but we haven't had a problem that we couldn't work out together, since they have trusted me to be there if needed.

5. Set a good example. No matter how much they disagree with you now, ultimately the main things they will learn from you, for better or for worse, is what you are.

Actually, I think teenagers are very interesting and a lot of fun — even though they worry you to distraction sometimes. Theirs, too, is a truly magical age. They are merging from child to adult before your very eyes, and the experience of sharing that with them is fascinating. If you remain open, they'll teach you more things than you could imagine.

A Few Words about Single Parenting, Divorce and Step-Parenting

In recent years the "traditional family" has become untraditional, and in many school classes, a child living with both parents who are married to each other is an exception rather than the rule. A great many children live with single parents; others live with one parent part of the year and the other parent another part. More often than not, the mother works outside the home, perhaps due to career drive, but more likely due to economic necessity. Since my kids and I have experienced all of these scenarios, of course I have some opinions here, too.

I think it is important for a single parent not to dwell on guilt. Kids can be better off with a single parent than with two parents who are together but tense much of the time because they don't get along. These days too many politicians and pundits seem to feel that all the ills of society could be fixed if we just return to the two parent family. I won't deny that children need role models of both sexes, but if the two parents living together are tense and fighting with each other, or keeping the peace only because one is totally dominant over the other, these can be pretty distorted role models. If you are parenting a child alone, I do think you owe it to that child to see that suitable role models of the opposite sex from yours are available. This could be a teacher, scout leader, relative or friend, but bring some appropriate person or persons into your child's life who will take a real interest in the child. And, no matter how busy you are, it is very important that you make time to do things with and just be with your children, when you are really **there**, communicating with each other, not just occupying the same room.

If you are very unhappy, it's hard to have energy to give to your children. All too often kids will get the brunt of stressed emotions unhappy parents are suppressing toward each other. I know. I'll admit I've been guilty of it on occasion. I didn't like myself very much after yelling at my kids and then realizing later that what they'd done really wasn't significant, but had only just provoked me when I was already feeling stressed and irritable. I am ordinarily a very calm and self-contained temperament. The only people I've ever really screamed at in my life are my kids — fortunately, not too often, but it has happened. It was never so much what they had done, as that I was not in a state of mind to handle it properly at that moment.

I think it's the very best thing, of course, if parents can stay together as partners, lovers and friends. I was very fortunate to be raised by two who did, and thus had good role models in both. But I lived in a different age, and was not so fortunate in my own first two marriages. It was very devastating for me to come to terms the first time with the fact that things just weren't working out, and it was even more difficult when I had to deal with the failed outcome of a too-hastily entered second marriage. I could say that it was apparently necessary for me to work out some major polarity problems that are reflected in my own chart through relationships, but it doesn't really matter here. I did what I did, and left the marriages when it became apparent that I could no longer grow as I wished or live serenely within them.

Having made my decision to leave each time, I also decided that nothing could be gained and much could be lost, for my children, if tension remained. I have maintained friendships with both ex-husbands, standing my ground when necessary, but keeping any disagreements away from the kids if at all possible. I think it is very important to keep the children out of the middle. Don't criticize the other parent to them, and never, never ask your children to take sides. Strive, if at all possible, to present a united front in any disciplinary matter relating to your children, just as you would — should — if you were still married.

I think it is safe to say that my daughters have learned that their Dad(s) and I are human and therefore less than perfect, but still OK. In having an old-memories talk with Shannon a year ago, she commented that one valuable outcome of the unsettled times we'd had through my divorces, was that I had set for them an example of a woman who could stand on her own two feet independently, and was not willing to settle for unhappiness in trade-off for the security of a relationship. She thought that model had already helped to see her through one difficult period prior to her marriage, and had led her to expect and successfully achieve, with less conflict than many of her friends, a more egalitarian type of marriage.

As for step-parenting, this can be touchy. I, personally, had little trouble as a step-parent, possibly because I had once been a teacher of teenagers, and understood them pretty well. The same basic rules as given above under adolescence apply. I never tried to be an authority over my step-children. I talked with them, gave opinions when asked either directly or indirectly, and respected theirs. We got along fine. I can't speak from the experience of step-parenting younger kids because I haven't. My second husband had problems with my two older daughters primarily because he was too authoritarian, and refused to understand adolescents for what they are, which gave him problems with some of his own teenagers as well.

My late husband Neil, with whom I had a very fulfilling relationship, got along fine with Liz, the only child to live with us on an on-going basis, and with Shannon and Molly, too, when they visited. He was a friend to them, did things with them, helped when asked, and did not try to be their father. If he thought something ought to be handled differently in my dynamics with them, he talked with me quietly about it alone, but did not overtly interfere. If he felt they were wrong on anything that directly concerned him, he spoke to them directly about it, quietly but firmly. I think this is the style of step-parenting that works best.

If you are a step-parent, I think it's best for you to leave discipline to the parent in matters that do not directly concern you. In regard to your own rights, however, you should kindly but firmly, stand your ground. When your step-kids of any age are on your turf, you have a right to expect their respect for your property, for the way you wish to run your household, for your private times with your spouse. If your spouse won't back you on these things, you have a problem with the spouse, not the kids. It's toward improving your relationship with your spouse that you need to direct your energy. If, after trying and counseling, if necessary, you just can't resolve your differences, you may be back to where this section began. But don't take it out on the kids. Combined families are complex, and you should consider this carefully before you get into it. No matter what the make-up of your family, though, consistency and a united front from adults who really can agree with each other, will provide the most security for kids.

Chapter Four
Your Child's Birth Chart

In order to learn what astrology has to tell you about your child's personality traits, talents and potential challenges, you will need to have a chart calculated for his or her date of birth, time of birth, and the longitude and latitude of the city in which the birth took place. Your child's birth chart will give you a wealth of insight into his or her own special style of creating magic.

In the appendix of this book you will find easy "do it yourself" tables, so that you can look up some of the things in your child's birth chart, and then look up my interpretations that correspond. Please understand, though, that while this will be accurate information, it will be only partial. It is no substitute for a complete birth chart. I strongly urge you to get a full, accurate birth chart for your child, and the best way to do that these days is to get a computer calculation.

Why is a full birth chart so important? The most unique information about your child—that which individualizes him or her from all other children born on the same day—can only be determined with exact time plus place of birth. It is with the addition of time and place that we can know the houses of the horoscope and the very important positions of Midheaven and Ascendant. As you continue to read, you'll find a whole chapter interpreting planets in relation to the Midheaven and Ascendant, and examples of why I think that the symbolic meaning of a planet close to one of these important points provides information about characteristics that can dominate a personality far more significantly than the zodiac sign of the Sun or any other planet.

Because I want so much for you to have a full, complete chart for your child, I've arranged for you to get a free one! In the back of the book you will find a coupon. All you have to do is tear it out, fill out your child's birth date, time of birth and place of birth, and send it in. (If you want to order additional charts at a low cost, you will find order instructions in the back of this book, or alternatively, you'll find an ad for accurate, low-cost software for your home computer.)

The chart you will receive for your free chart coupon is my special "Magical Child" design, which is illustrated in this chapter. It shows your child's traditional horoscope wheel with symbols of the planets and signs, but right below it will be a list that tells you in "plain English" just which interpretive paragraphs in this book you should read for that child.

Ordering your Chart

Your Child's Birth Data

Fill in the blanks on the coupon with a child's name, birth date, birth time and location. If you don't have the birthtime for the child firmly in your memory, look on his or her birth certificate. Any child born within the United States in the years included in this book's tables (1985-2005) should surely have accurate birthtime recorded on the birth certificate — unless the child was born in some remote place like in an airliner over the Pacific, in which case let's hope the event was dramatic enough that someone had the presence of mind to look at a watch and find out at least approximately where you were (coordinates, time zone). Other countries recording standards vary.

If you were born in the USA, want to get a chart for yourself and don't know your time, it should be recorded in the bureau of vital statistics in the city or county of your birth. For quite a number of years now, since the time of easy photocopying, most requests for birth certificates come as a photocopy of the official record that was filled out by the attending physician. If, instead, you have a short certificate form that was transcribed from the official record book, it may not have the time. In that case, call the office where it came from. Most officials will tell you the time, but occasionally you may get someone who is a stickler for making their extra certificate fee, or is hostile to astrology, and they will refuse to give you any information on the phone. In that case, you'll have to go there personally and ask to see the records, or order a new birth certificate by mail. For mail orders, be sure to specify that you want the time — a copy of the full record. For births in any reasonably sized city in the USA since the mid 1920s, the official record should have the birth time.

Looking at the Chart

Once I've got it — what do I do with it?

On page 45 you will find an illustration of a "Magical Child" chart for my granddaughter Tessa. (Now, just who else do you think a Grandma would choose for an example chart!) I'll go over it with you, just to make sure you understand how to use your child's chart with this book. But first, there are a few general things that you should understand about the "cookbook" interpretations.

Understanding the Interpretations

It is important for you to realize that a "cookbook" such as this one interprets each planet in your child's chart one at a time. The personality theme indicated by one planet may seem to be in contradiction to that of another. In one sense, this is quite understandable, since most people do have contradictions within their personality. On the other hand, it's easy to see why a beginner would find such contradictions confusing. Just what **are** you supposed to think?

The real trick to good astrological interpretation is the **art of synthesis** — being able to pull all the separate pieces of the puzzle into one whole, and make sense of it. If you become sufficiently intrigued by astrology to want to learn a technique of synthesis, I suggest *Astrology: The Next Step* by Maritha Pottenger. Meanwhile, in order to anticipate which characteristics will be most prominent for your child, you should **look for repeated or similar themes**.

A "rule of thumb" many astrologers will cite is "**if you find it three different places in the chart, it's important**." Traits suggested the most frequently will be strongest. Traits only mentioned once may be very minor personality factors.

Below the Chart — Words!

If the graphic on the top of the page strikes you as "that's a bunch of symbols I don't understand and I really don't care. Just tell me what it **means**," that's OK. I'm not particularly inclined toward technical things either. I had to care very, very much to learn to do this — but that's another story. Just look at the bottom half of the page, below the chart graphic. There you will find a list in words that you can follow to know which paragraphs in this book you should read to learn about the individual child whose chart it is. You can then skip, if you like, right past the rest of this chapter and begin reading the specific interpretations that apply to your child!

The Chart Wheel

The chart wheel is provided on your chart form, rather than just the word list alone, so that you will have the "real thing." You (or your child) might someday decide to study more about astrology on your own, or wish to take the chart to an astrologer for further interpretation.

If you haven't looked at a chart wheel before, you probably have some very typical questions. Let's look at Tessa's chart, and I'll tell you why it is drawn as it is, and what the various glyphs and numbers are.

First you see a large circle divided into 12 sections. This graphic represents a map of the solar system as seen from a particular place on Earth at a specific moment in time. On this map are numbers and symbol

☉	Sun	♈	Aries
☽	Moon	♉	Taurus
☿	Mercury	♊	Gemini
♀	Venus	♋	Cancer
♂	Mars	♌	Leo
♃	Jupiter	♍	Virgo
♄	Saturn	♎	Libra
♅	Uranus	♏	Scorpio
♆	Neptune	♐	Sagittarius
♀ or ♇ Pluto		♑	Capricorn
		♒	Aquarius
		♓	Pisces

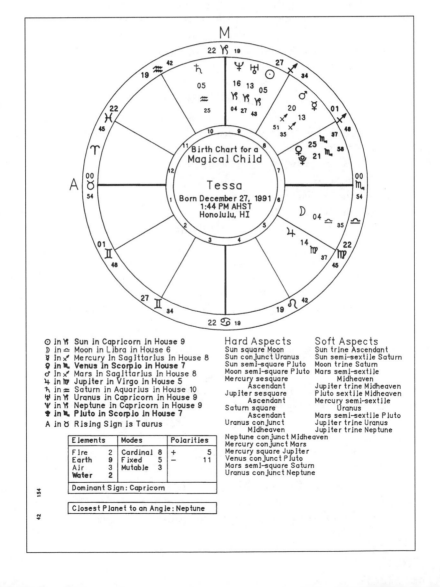

Birth Chart for a
Magical Child

Tessa
Born December 27, 1991
1:44 PM AHST
Honolulu, HI

☉ in ♑ Sun in Capricorn in House 9
☽ in ♎ Moon in Libra in House 6
☿ in ♐ Mercury in Sagittarius in House 8
♀ in ♏ Venus in Scorpio in House 7
♂ in ♐ Mars in Sagittarius in House 8
♃ in ♍ Jupiter in Virgo in House 5
♄ in ♒ Saturn in Aquarius in House 10
♅ in ♑ Uranus in Capricorn in House 9
♆ in ♑ Neptune in Capricorn in House 9
♇ in ♏ Pluto in Scorpio in House 7
A in ♉ Rising Sign is Taurus

Hard Aspects
Sun square Moon
Sun conjunct Uranus
Sun semi-square Pluto
Moon semi-square Pluto
Mercury sesquare
  Ascendant
Jupiter sesquare
  Ascendant
Saturn square
  Ascendant
Uranus conjunct
  Midheaven
Neptune conjunct Midheaven
Mercury conjunct Mars
Mercury square Jupiter
Venus conjunct Pluto
Mars semi-square Saturn
Uranus conjunct Neptune

Soft Aspects
Sun trine Ascendant
Sun semi-sextile Saturn
Moon trine Saturn
Mars semi-sextile
  Midheaven
Jupiter trine Midheaven
Pluto sextile Midheaven
Mercury semi-sextile
  Uranus
Mars semi-sextile Pluto
Jupiter trine Uranus
Jupiter trine Neptune

Elements		Modes		Polarities	
Fire	2	Cardinal	8	+	5
Earth	9	Fixed	5	−	11
Air	3	Mutable	3		
Water	**2**				

Dominant Sign: Capricorn

Closest Planet to an Angle: Neptune

154

42

glyphs. The numbers are degrees and minutes of the Great Circle of the celestial ecliptic. The ecliptic is divided into 12 equal 30° sections. These are the astrological signs. The 12 signs and their glyphs are listed in the column on the left of the next page, just above the chart.

The Sun, Moon and each planet also have glyphs, and these are listed in the right column.

The 12 sections into which the chart wheel is divided are NOT signs. They are Houses. Unlike the signs, houses are unequal. At the dividing line between each house you will see a sign glyph and numbers. The glyph tells you which sign is on the cusp (beginning) of each House. The bolder number (in the outer ring) is the degree of the ecliptic at which that House begins; the other number is the minutes ("minutes" means part of a degree: one degree has 60 minutes). The houses are numbered in counter-clockwise direction, beginning with House One which starts at the line on the left of the wheel marked A (for Ascendant).

For example, at the line which begins the 10th house of Tessa's chart, you see 22 ♑ 19. That means the 10th house cusp is 22 degrees and 19 minutes of the sign of Capricorn.

Houses are determined by location of birth. Remember, they are NOT signs, so please don't confuse them. Houses are increasingly unequal the further the location is from the equator. Sometimes the same sign will appear on the cusp of two consecutive houses, and another sign will not be on any cusp. Don't worry. The sign is still there. It's just entirely enclosed within that House.

For example, on Tessa's chart you can see that 22° ♓ (Pisces) begins House 12, the entire sign of ♈ (Aries) is within the 12th House (indicated by the glyph with no number, and 0° ♉ (Taurus) begins the 1st House. Both the 2nd and 3rd Houses begin in the sign of ♊ (Gemini).

Inside some of the sections that mark the 12 houses, you can see the symbols for the planets. Next to each planet's glyph is the glyph for the sign the planet is "in" and the numbers of the degrees and minutes. For example: Tessa's House 6 section contains ☽ 04 ♎ 35. That means Moon is in 4 degrees and 35 minutes of the sign of Libra.

What Does it Mean?

There are three basic tools that an astrologer uses in interpreting a birth chart, and you've been introduced to how all three appear on that chart—signs, planets and houses. The **planets** are the most important.

When astrologers refer to "the planets," they are generally referring to the list given on page 45: Sun, Moon, Mercury, Venus, Mars, Jupiter, Saturn, Neptune and Pluto. Of course, the Sun is not a planet at all. It is a star. The Moon is not a planet, rather it is a satellite of Earth. Some astrology texts call the Sun and Moon "the lights," but most often they will just be lumped in with "the planets." It's just for convenience, the same reason why a lot of things are said in shorthand.

The Earth isn't "in" the most common type of astrological chart, because the chart is a map of the sky that we are viewing from wherever we are **on** Earth. This form of astrology is officially called "geocentric," meaning Earth-centered. Yes, of course astrologers know that Earth orbits the Sun. However, all things are relative to the perspective from which they are viewed. In that sense, it is valid for each individual to feel as though he or she is at the center of a personal Universe— "my reality is as I perceive it to be, and my perceptions may change as I learn and grow."

Planets in Signs

Planets symbolize: basic energies, drives or motivations
Signs symbolize: the manner or style in which the energy is expresssed

In describing why a planet is the most important factor, over signs or houses, I'll use a couple of analogies. The planet is like a noun or verb: the **ball bounces**. The sign modifies it, like an adjective or adverb: the **red** ball bounces **quickly**. The house tells you where: the red ball bounces quickly **off the wall**.

Here's another one: consider a stained glass window with light shining through its various colors and reflecting on the floor. The planet is the "light." The color it picks up as it shines through the glass is like the sign. It "modifies" the light by giving it a slightly different coloration (or shall we say, style), but the light is still light! **Where** the light is shining is the "house."

Sign styles and planets may be contradictory to each other. For example, no matter what sign Mercury is in, Mercury symbolizes how we think and communicate. No matter what sign Mars is in, Mars symbolizes how we act. Aries is quick; Taurus takes its time. A child with Mercury in Aries and Mars in Taurus might speak up quickly, be quick to come up with new ideas, but be slow in actually acting on them, or won't act at all. With Mercury in Taurus and Mars in Aries, the reverse might be true. The child might take a long time thinking through and planning just what to do, but having finally decided, would then be quick and direct in taking action.

According to astrological tradition, each planet has a sign or signs that it is said to "rule." That reflects the fact that the planet is more important than the sign. It also indicates that some sign "styles" are more closely compatible with the basic energy drive associated with the planet. Their interpretive themes are similar. Also, each house symbolizes an area of life in which a particular energy "style" seems to be expressed most in keeping with its basic nature—again a somewhat similar theme. Astrologers refer to this line-up of corresponding planets, signs and houses as the "natural" chart. Here are the planets, signs and houses that "go together" according to that tradition:

House 1	Aries	Mars
House 2	Taurus	Venus
House 3	Gemini	Mercury
House 4	Cancer	Moon
House 5	Leo	Sun
House 6	Virgo	Mercury
House 7	Libra	Venus
House 8	Scorpio	Pluto
House 9	Sagittarius	Jupiter
House 10	Capricorn	Saturn
House 11	Aquarius	Uranus
House 12	Pisces	Neptune

Planets in Houses

Houses symbolize: areas of life in which the planets and signs are expressed

In the following chapters you will find interpretations for each **personal** planet in each sign, followed by an italicized reference to that planet in the house whose theme is similar to that sign. This is so that if you have a fully calculated chart for your child, you can read the interpretations corresponding to your child's planets in houses, too. Generally, there is not a great difference, in the case of the personal planets, between interpreting the expression of a planet in its sign, or the planet in the house that has the "naturally" similar theme. The main nuance is in understanding the house as the **area of life** in which a planet is expressed, rather than as the general style in which that planet is expressed in all areas of life.

In Chapter 7, however, which is about the **outer** planets (Jupiter, Saturn, Uranus, Neptune, Pluto), you will find specific interpretations of the planets in the houses, in addition to interpretations of the planets in signs. The outer planets move very slowly, such that the sign alone may not "show" in an individually significant manner. Every child in your child's play group is likely to have the planet in the same sign. Obviously, they are not all going to behave the same way. For the outer planets in signs, I'll give you some of my thoughts and observations of how entire age groups, as a collective mass, precipitate social changes in reflection of the outer planets' movements. Though you might find it interesting to see even yourself and your parents in these collective groups, and how one generation differs from another, it isn't of much help to you in understanding one uniquely individual child. However, the house an outer planet is in (houses being based on exact moment of birth plus place) does tell us something about individual behavior, so my outer planet house interpretations will be more personal.

Here are the houses listed according to the area of life, as this might apply to a little child:

House 1   Who I am; how I show myself to you (appearance, behavior)

House 2   What I have—me and mine; what makes me comfortable

House 3   How I talk and listen to my brothers and sisters and my neighbors; my school; short trips I take

House 4   My home; my parent(s) when they are caring and understanding

House 5   Things that are fun; what I love; my hobbies; being creative

House 6   My chores and daily habits; my health; my pets

House 7   My best friend; the person I'm trying to beat (competing with)

House 8   Sharing with others; secrets I tell or am told; mysteries we figure out together

House 9   What I believe; my ideals; my teacher; places far away

House 10   The outside world; doing something everybody knows me for; my parent(s) when they are making rules and making me follow them

House 11   My friends; clubs I belong to; the hopes and wishes they inspire in me

House 12   My inner private world; my secrets that I won't tell anyone

What if there's no planet in a house? Is nothing happening there?

This is a common question. Yes, there is something to "read" about every house, and all the signs are there. The sign characteristics tell us something about the area of life symbolized by the "empty" house, and each sign has its "ruler" (as listed in the "natural" correspondences). These methods are a bit beyond the scope of this book, but there are other basic texts listed in the bibliography, if you are interested in further exploration.

Aspects

Listed below your Magical Child chart wheel, you will find two columns: one is headed "hard aspects," the other is headed "soft aspects." You should read every paragraph in chapters 8 or 9 that is headed with a combination on that list.

Do not be confused by the fact that the chart lists names for aspects, such as Sun **conjunct** Uranus, but in the chapter interpretations you will only find a paragraph headed Sun-Uranus. Such words as conjunction, square, trine, etc. denote types of aspects, and nuances of astrological interpretations differentiate only slightly between them. By far the most significant thing is that the two planets in aspect have a **blended theme**. The fact that they are together means that one modifies the other. You can't accurately interpret one of them without considering the other one.

You may want to learn more about evaluating different types of aspects later (see Chapter 12) but for now I just want you to be aware of the two basic types: hard and soft. **The hard aspects are stronger** and more active than the soft ones. Soft aspects are more passive, and though they may reflect ease, or even a talent, you will probably be so busy noticing the traits listed in the hard aspects that you could miss the soft ones! More about this in the beginning of chapter 8—but Grandma knows that you may just skip over those introductions and go right to the personal paragraphs. So forgive me if I repeat myself once in a while. Now go! Time to read all about your **own** magical child!

Chapter Five
The Sun, Moon and Rising Sign

As you read through the sign interpretations for your child's chart, you may notice a marked similarity in some of the things that are said about different planets in the same sign. If, indeed, you took the time to read all of the planets in the sign of your child's Sun sign, for example, you'd get a somewhat broader run-down on that **sign** than is given under the Sun paragraph, alone. Even so, be sure to notice that there is a distinction in the way the sign is handled for each planet.

Remember: the planet is more important than the sign. For example: Mercury symbolizes how we think and communicate. Shannon, with Mercury in Sagittarius, is idealistic and quite direct in expressing her opinions. Tessa, also with Mercury in Sag, shows signs already about being just as articulate as her mother. Molly, with Mercury in Capricorn, is more likely to keep her thoughts to herself until she has seriously thought them through, or until she's fairly sure of others' potential reaction. Liz, with Mercury in Libra, weighs pros and cons and considers what is fair to all. I dig and probe until I figure out what I want (Mercury in Scorpio), then I may or may not tell you about it. But regardless of the differences, we are still showing how we think and communicate!

You're sure to encounter some contradictions in reading the various paragraphs about your child. Well, I could just say that we all have some contradictions in our personalities. What is important, here, is that you keep in mind **what** the planet symbolizes. In blending and making sense out of apparent contradictions in your child's sign interpretations, look for repeated themes. You will probably find that some similar traits are mentioned in regard to more than one planet. Themes that are repeated over and over are strong. Ideas mentioned only once may not be significant. Be sure to read the introductions to each planet, so you'll understand its basic function, before you read the specific paragraph that applies to your child.

The personal planets are divided into two chapters primarily because putting them all in one just made too long a chapter. This chapter covers the three factors that are considered primary personal points in an astrological chart. Most individual's personalities can be at least broadly outlined by understanding the signs of these three—that is if they are older. In the case of a very small child, you may find that you will see the themes associated with Mercury, Venus and Mars (in the next chapter) more readily than you will observe the Sun sign type. It seems to me that children "grow into" their Sun, as their earlier instinctive behavior is gradually replaced by a more directed effort to "shine." Still, the Sun sign is the basic astrological typing most widely understood by the general public, because it is tied to a birthday whose sign association can be easily identified. The Sun sign, indeed, is how most people identify "the signs." For this reason, I've given you the most complete general sign interpretation for each Sun type, and I encourage you to read them all. This will give you a general overview of the signs. You may find that a Sun sign interpretation will enhance your understanding of other planets your child has in that same sign.

The "Big Three"

In general, the most obvious expressions of zodiac sign personality characteristics for most people will be seen in one, or a combination of, the "big three" — **Sun, Moon and Rising Sign.** This could be modified if the chart has a stellium, which means three or more planets in the same sign, or one planet that is singularly in very strong focus because of its aspects.

In a small child, you may be more likely to notice the Moon and Rising Signs most prominently in the emerging personality. This has certainly been my experience with all of my children. I am going to introduce all of the "big three" together — Sun, followed by Moon, followed by Rising Sign — so you will understand how each of them are distinct from the others, before I give you the look-up paragraphs for each one of them in each sign.

The Sun

Just about everyone, even if nothing else is known about astrology, can answer the question, "What's my sign?" Every newsstand provides dozens of publications in which Sun Sign columns appear, with a message for the day, linked to the date of birth, which sometimes seems to apply to what is going on in a reader's life, but more often is pretty meaningless. After all, there are only 12 signs, and millions of people in the world born "under" each of them. How on Earth can any short blurb of a sentence or two truly address all of those different lives? The popularity of Sun signs, and the ignorance of all of the complexities of astrological interpretation, lay astrology open to continued vulnerability to being the brunt of cartoons and dismissal as "entertainment." Just what is a Sun sign, after all?

Some 2000 or so years ago, ancient Greek scientists were developing the system of astrology that was to become most prevalent in Western culture. They chose to begin their measurement of the celestial ecliptic (the Great Circle that is the Earth's orbit around the Sun, or from Earth's perspective, the apparent path of the Sun around us) with the point of the Vernal Equinox, which is the intersection of the ecliptic with the celestial equator. This "intersection" happens when the apparent path of the Sun crosses the equator at a northward inclination. This is the first day of Spring in the seasonal cycle of the northern hemisphere. The Greeks then decided to divide up the ecliptic circle into 12 equal sections, which they chose to name for the constellations that lay approximately in each sector at that time. Although the images associated with the constellations were a "kick-off" for the development of the interpretation of the signs, a great deal of the interpretive material that has "grown up" around the signs comes from the seasonal cycle itself. Measurements along the ecliptic clearly delineate the seasons.

Unfortunately, those ancient astrologer/astronomers lacked the foresight to see how awkward naming the sign sectors the same as the constellations would become 2000 years later, when self-styled "scientific" skeptics would insist on bothering astrologers with the challenge, "You don't even know where the signs are anymore!" Believe me, we do know. Just in case your interest in astrology should draw that kind of ignorant sneer, this is how it really is:

Signs and constellations are not the same thing. Signs are equal sectors of the ecliptic. The constellations of the zodiac are 12 decidedly unequal groupings of stars that can be seen beyond the ecliptic. Due to the precession of the equinoxes, the zodiac of signs and the zodiac of constellations are now nearly one whole sign out-of-sync.

Western astrology, which uses the signs on the ecliptic, is essentially an astrology of the solar system, primarily interpreting the planets in the solar system, as their positions are measured in those signs. Contrary to "pop" imagery about what's in your "stars," the only actual star that is used in basic astrological interpretation is our Sun. The rest of the primary factors interpreted are planets, or mathematical points of intersection with the ecliptic, one of which is the Ascendant, more popularly known as Rising Sign.

So... What Does it Mean?

The most concise explanation I can think of to tell you what a Sun sign means is that **the Sun in your child's birth chart symbolizes how that child likes to shine** — and it offers strong hints of how he or she will always like to shine at any age. The Sun symbolizes vitality and the outward personality. Because how a person feels about Self is so very important in whether that self will shine at all, or hide from full potential, the Sun sign gives you insight into what feeds your child's self-esteem and sense of pride.

Remember, although the Sun sign is very important, it is only one of many other factors in the astrological profile. These Sun sign descriptions are of "pure" types. In some ways your child will almost undoubtedly show the Sun sign characteristics, but the Sun may not be the most dominant factor in his or her personality. If enough other planets or aspects point to very different characteristics, the Sun sign may not be expressed as overtly as these descriptions suggest. Whether dominant or not, though, you should derive hints from these paragraphs about areas in which success and appreciation are very likely to help your child glow with good feelings and self-esteem.

In applying knowledge of this or any other factor to your parenting role, it is important to keep two things in mind:

1. Your role is **not to push** the child into areas suggested by the astrological chart, but rather to **offer** exposure to activities, **be alert** to any expressions of interest, and then **provide resources**, as best you can, for the child to pursue those interests in a positive manner.

2. Your role is also to **understand** and **accept** ways in which your child's style and interests differ from your own. Guide, of course, but also follow the child's lead. You'll find many more easy opportunities to give encouraging and supportive feedback that way, and in so doing, nurture self esteem and happiness — in both of you!

About the Astro Kid Illustrations

Before you plunge into the Sun sign "look ups," I think a little explanation is in order about the "Astro Kid zodiac pets" that illustrate the Sun signs, because some of them are decidedly non-standard in comparison to the usual zodiac symbols.

I designed the kid zodiac so that color pictures (or pehaps someday, toys) could be made for people who wanted to give them as gifts.[*]

One of my goals in designing Astro Kids was to make every character child-like and appealing, and to avoid having them be gender-specific. Most of the zodiac symbols are animal characters, which makes the boy or girl question easy! However, a few of them — Gemini, Virgo, Aquarius — are human images, and Sagittarius is a centaur — half man, half horse. I could imagine an older and more articulate boy on whose wall one of my pictures might have been hung in babyhood saying things like: "Virgo! U-u-gh. That's a girl. I'm not a girl! I don't want to be a Virgo." Or a little girl saying, "I love the horsey, but why does its head have to be a boy? I'm not a boy. I don't want that sign."

Of course, I could have designed alternate characters for each of the zodiac symbols that usually include people, but let's face it. I'm a

---

[*] See page 289 for information on ordering personalized AstroKid products.

businesswoman. It would complicate the possibility of creating spin-offs. So... I've taken just a few little liberties with the zodiac. May those distant ancestors who saw star pictures around the constellations forgive me. I think my kid pictures fit the generally accepted meanings of the signs, and that's what counts.

The Moon

If the Sun is the strongest outward symbol of the personality, the Moon is the equally strong symbol of the inner self, for it tells us about our emotions. **Here is an important clue to what your child needs to feel secure**, and what you need to provide in order for him or her to feel nurtured, and to know that you can be depended upon. If the needs of the Moon are fulfilled in early childhood, the inner strength to cope with all aspects of later life is greatly enhanced.

If the basic characteristics of Sun sign and Moon sign are similar, they are supported and enhanced, and you are more likely to recognize your child's personality needs as a less-complicated, integrated whole. If they are very different, then understanding your child will be more complex. There may be inner conflicts between what the child **wants** to do or feel, and what that child **thinks** he or she **ought** to do or feel. This will be challenging for your child to integrate, and even more challenging for you to guide. Remember that while the Sun gives you hints about ways in which your child can best "shine," the Moon shows the areas in which he or she needs to feel sufficiently secure in order to be willing to step out there in the world and "shine."

As said before, in my observation young children are, if anything, **more** apt to display their Moon sign characteristics than those of the Sun sign. If this is so (and I can certainly see evidence of it in my own children), it is probably because childlike behavior is more instinctive, and guided by feelings, rather than logic. Indeed, it is not uncommon to say of an adult who is behaving impulsively or emotionally, that the behavior is "childish." Sun sign characteristics will "show," but the child may have to "grow into" the ability to express them to the fullest. Meanwhile, in childhood and in adulthood, when the emotions are at stake, it is the Moon that is likely to be most visible.

The Rising Sign, or Ascendant

The Rising Sign is not a planet. It is the sign that is "rising" or "ascending" at the exact moment of your child's birth, as seen from the exact location of birth. When we say Ascendant, this implies not just the sign that is rising, but also the exact degree of that sign, as well. Because the earth's daily movement causes a different degree on the ecliptic to rise about every four minutes, the Ascendant is a very personal factor in your child's chart. It may indicate differences between people who are born on the same day and in the same place, but only hours or even minutes apart from each other. Even the Rising Sign, alone, without knowing the degree, offers you information about your child's one-to-one relationships, and about how his or her surface personality (first impression) is likely to be received by others.

The Rising Sign is more likely to symbolize the outward personality—how we show ourselves to others—than our basic energy (Sun) or how we really feel inside (Moon). It is also likely to reveal something of how we mirror our environment. Perhaps because of this, it has also been observed that young children often tend to be perceived as behaving according to the Rising Sign type more than that of the Sun sign type.

Unless your child's chart has a stellium (three or more planets in one sign), his personality will more than likely be most clearly defined by a composite of Sun sign, Moon sign and Rising Sign characteristics. If any two of them are in the SAME sign, the individual is said to be a "double" whatever that sign is, and the sign characteristics will be very prominent in the personality. If the sign types are in conflict with each other, look for similar themes for the strongest characteristics, and remember, in attempting to sort out what's what: the Sun represents basic energy, the Moon tells us about feelings and the Rising Sign is more symbolic of outward, surface personality than of the inner self.

Nearly everyone's behavior is at some times contradictory. There are very few "pure" stereotypes of any kind. Whether we are considering astrological characteristics, or studies based on the behavior of oldest children in a family, middle children, the "baby," or those who are very tall, very short, very thin, very fat, or what have you, the information thus derived is for guidance only. Such information is intended to help you be alert to ways you can encourage your child, and to ways in which understanding and acceptance of a style that differs from your own is called for.

The "Big Three" Sign Cookbook

For the convenience of not having to do the "his and her" or "s/he" stuff, and also for equality, the gender pronouns for boy and girl are alternated in each sign. I'm deliberately starting with girl for Aries, because that will ensure that the characteristics that patriarchal culture has most typically defined as "masculine" or "feminine" will have a role reversal for the Sun. Just to make sure you don't get stuck in that, the male gender pronouns will start the Moon look-ups. I'll continue to alternate in this manner through all the planets.

I think "typically" masculine or feminine stereotypes are more a product of environment than anything else, and gender stereotyping has damaged kids who just didn't fit the mold. Yes, I know most of you are more enlightened than that, these days. But watch yourself and others in how the tiniest infant girl is greeted, held, talked to, in contrast to the infant boy. Gender-related expectations are deeply programmed. Even if you try not to impose them on your kids, others undoubtedly will. Sign characteristics may be expressed somewhat differently in girls or boys because of this.

If your child is the opposite sex from the gender pronouns used in any paragraph, just mentally substitute.

Planets in Houses

Following each planet in sign heading is an italicized reference to the planet in the house whose "natural" meaning is similar to that sign. This is for the possible added insight of those of you who know the houses your child's planets are in. Remember, houses refer to particular areas of life, while signs reflect a more general style. Consider the sign interpretation as a theme in which the basic function of the planet espresses within the particular area of life defined by the house. (Review pages 47 through 49° of Chapter 4 for more information on the houses.) To get you started, I'll follow each planet in sign interpretation with a short italicized example of how the same theme might be applied to interpreting the planet in the corresponding house. Keep in mind these basic key words for how planets function: as the **Sun shines**, so the **Moon feels** (needs to feel secure), **Mercury thinks** and communicates, **Venus loves**, **Mars acts**.

The Sun in Each Sign of the Zodiac

Following are interpretations of each Sun sign, with introductory paragraphs keyed to the Astro Kid "zodiac pets." This will be the most complete explanation of the basic sign types—I encourage you to read them all, no matter what your child's "sign" is.

Sun in Aries or Sun in House 1

"Charge," says I, your Aries Ram,
"Look out, world! Here I am!
I'll get there first,
With fiery zest.
Don't ever doubt, I'll be the best!"

Just like the lively, little Ram in the picture, your Aries child likes to charge ahead. This kid shines by being first, by being brave — and sometimes by taking chances that will raise the hair on the back of your neck! Unless many other things in the chart show a very different theme, Aries will be a natural leader, who likes to take charge. She will be outgoing and impulsive and shine with confidence. Your little "ball of fire" has more energy and spirit than any adult can expect to keep up with, even if you are an Aries, too!

Nearly always in motion, little Aries' attention span is likely to be shorter than most, so unless other factors in the chart indicate a steadier theme, you might well consider early schooling choices that allow for an open-classroom, independent approach, rather than sit-in-your-desk traditions. Getting started will be lots easier for this child than following through to your satisfaction. It probably won't do you any good to nag. Trying to point out a new aspect of the project, thus reviving interest, would be a better approach. Patience is not a virtue for Aries!

Impatience may be a problem when your child is working with other children. This quick starter doesn't like to wait for slower people to get finished. For that reason working independently might best be encouraged, unless others are willing to follow Aries' lead. Young Miss Initiative will also be impatient in having to wait for you — which is a good thing for you to keep in mind when considering whether or not to take her along on a boring adult visit or shopping excursion.

You may have concerns that your child seems selfish beyond the "normal" child development stages discussed in Chapter 3. It's not really that — no harm is intended at all. Little Aries just naturally feels like "number one." You may have to tactfully point out the advantages of being considerate. Understand that while Aries may be quick to anger, the "blow up" seldom lasts very long. It passes and is forgotten. Still, your child will need to learn that others do not let go so easily, and can be hurt much more than she ever intended. Try to teach some techniques and language for expressing anger in nonhurtful ways (directing the anger toward an inanimate — and nonbreakable! — thing — or the words of anger at the situation rather than another person, *e.g.*: "I really hate it when I can't..." instead of "I hate you for..."). AND, set a good example — this cannot be overemphasized, for this or any personality type! Children always learn more from what their parents DO, than from anything they say.

See that your Aries child has opportunities for active sports and competitive games, and provide places to be active and noisy. Music lessons on trumpet or percussion might be better received than piano or cello. Independence and freedom are important. Allow your little Aries to make mistakes (unless the hole she's about to jump into seems too dangerously deep). More profound learning will come from those mistakes than from anything you could have said in warning.

Be open to the energy charge of this fiery little character, and you'll be kept young, too, as the child within you is stimulated and delighted by one new adventure after another!

*The Aries interpretation may also apply to children who have the **Sun in House 1** (no matter what sign the Sun is in), in regard to their outward expression of "who I am." Even if her Sun sign theme is of a more passive type than Aries, for example, she shines when she is noticed, and is likely to be quite assertive, if she's not.*

Sun in Taurus or Sun in House 2

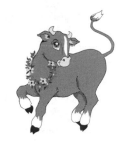

I move through my meadow,
Smelling the flowers
And munching sweet tastes as I go.
Don't try to rush me.
I'll do this job MY way.
A Taurus IS stubborn, you know!

The contented little bovine munching flowers, like your usually contented little Taurus, thrives on being comfortable. This child can't be cuddled too much. His basic nature is very tactile and aware of the senses . Little Taurus loves the feel of your skin, the aroma of your cologne, the gentleness of your voice or the soft music you play. From the earliest babyhood, surround your child with soothing sounds, pretty but soft colors, soft fabrics and plushy, feely toys. Adopt an attitude of calm, and this baby (unless several other factors in the chart contradict) will be an "easy" baby, and you'll be the envy of other parents whose children are more high strung.

It is unlikely that you will have trouble getting this child to eat. If anything, a tendency to overeat might be the case. Best not to start on sweets too soon. When you do, let little Taurus learn to savor the natural sweetness of fruits. The sugary or fatty ones will be discovered soon enough, without any help from you — trust me!

As your child grows you'll find that he shines best when allowed to take plenty of time and do whatever is being done very thoroughly and at his own pace. "Don't try to rush me," as the Astro Kid verse says. If you do, you'll find this little Bull to be a very stubborn little engine, who seems to run constantly with the brakes on. If Taurus is lagging behind when you are in a hurry, nagging won't help. "No" is likely to be one of the first and most favorite words — beyond the normal toddler "no" stage. If you must move, quietly taking this child by the hand, or even up in your arms to carry, will be easier on your nerves. If you have a moment to spare, try just slowly walking away, telling little Taurus, "I'm going now" — once — and then go. Since this kid hates to feel insecure, he will probably come along. If that doesn't work, go back to "plan A," firm and quiet force!

Taurus will shine through patience and persistence, and will develop pride in the ability to finish a job and do it well. Great satisfaction will be derived from being thorough and dependable. And your child probably WILL be quite dependable. You will be more likely to bring out the best in the Taurus Sun by trusting that this child will accomplish what he sets out to do, than to worry or "check up" too often. Remember, that just being a bit more careful than the average child goes right along with wanting to do the job "just right." And when anyone is really enjoying doing something, that person is savoring every moment and wants to make it last. Taurus is just likely to savor longer!

Your child will enjoy collections of things, and will be easy to teach how to save part of an allowance, taking great pride in watching the savings grow. He will thrive on arts and crafts of a sensual nature, such as clay sculpture or fabric weaving. Here you are more than likely to see the stick-to-itiveness and interest necessary to master the piano or other complex musical instrument. You may also discover that he enjoys singing, and he may even have a good singing voice. Quick competitive sports are not a natural bent; sports that require endurance are better choices.

Allow your Taurus' own style to prevail, and give lots and lots of cuddling. You have a steady, down-to-earth child whom you can nearly always trust to do the right thing — all in good time, of course. Don't rush!

No matter what his Sun sign, this interpretation may also fit your child with **Sun in House 2**, *in regard to his possessions, what he considers "mine," and what he considers comfortable. He is proud of what he has.*

Sun in Gemini or Sun in House 3

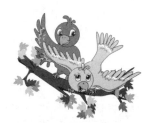

You may think I'm ONE bright Bird
But quite surprised you'll be,
When my Gemini thoughts take flight and change
And I'm twins — or maybe three!
Quick as you are, you won't catch me!

Take a good look at those two little "twin" birds. See how one seems rather wise, but the other is very sassy and spirited? Well, with your little Gemini you may often feel that you have at least two kids in one, and both — or all — of them are like little birds that fly through the air, too quickly to catch and hold. Just when you think you know which way they're going to go, they'll dart in the opposite direction! Well, at least life with Gemini will never be boring! Prepare to be stimulated, to move quickly, and to develop a very good ear for listening. This little one will be always busy, almost never still and will have more to say to you than you may sometimes want to hear! But at least you won't have to worry about what's on her mind. As soon as the "explosion into speech" begins (which will likely be early), she will let you know it... and know it... and know it!

Unless several other planetary placements indicate a strong bent in another direction, Gemini will be lively, noisy, sharp-witted and bright. Provide plenty of room to move and lots to keep this child busy. Don't expect stick-to-it-iveness to one project very long though. Patience is not Gemini's strong suit (unless perhaps a few other planets are in Taurus), and boredom can set in easily. Most Gemini kids are versatile and multiskilled, however, so your child will probably develop the ability to do several things at once. This busy character probably really can follow a TV show, listen to music, read a book, carry on a conversation and toss a ball for the dog all at the same time, and not miss a beat — even though it may set your nerves on edge. Patience may have to be YOUR strong suit!

Gemini could become the "jack-of-all-trades but master of none," however, if allowed to be too scattered. You may have to become skilled at pointing out a new twist on an existing task or lagging interest in order to keep your child at work on it long enough to make it worth while.

If your life and your child's environment become unsettled, she will be able to handle it well. In fact, Gemini likely thrives on change, adapts quite easily to new situations, and should also make new friends readily.

Give your bright little Bird-child a bright mobile over the crib, and plenty of plastic toys with moveable parts that encourage early use of her hands, for as she grows, hand skills can easily develop into strong mechanical abilities. Provide plenty of books and a variety of activities to keep Gemini's mind busy and help satisfy a very lively curiosity to know anything and everything.

Don't count on this child remembering what she promised to do or when to come in. You might try corralling the tyke long enough to tie a bright, yellow string around one of her little fingers as a reminder, or leave strategically placed notes — when Gemini is old enough to read them (which will probably be very early, if you give her half-a-chance).

Consider your little Gemini child like a breath of fresh air who's blown into your life. Let it blow freely and lift you along for the ride. You'll laugh a lot and learn a lot together!

*Your child with **Sun in House 3** may seek to shine through talking, through reading, through being "smart" or through being very adept at doing a variety of things with her hands.*

Sun in Cancer *or Sun in House 4*

My Crab shell is tough, yet deep inside
My soft and loving feelings hide.
Don't worry if my mood seems blue,
For surely you must know
That always you belong to me
And I'll never let you go.

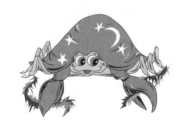

Consider a crab: a little hard-shelled creature that, when discovered, scurries quickly sideways across the sand to hide. Or at another time, reaches out to clamp onto its prey and hang on tightly. Now, take a look at that little Astro Kid version of the crab with trusting big eyes looking up at you. Your little Cancerian is a very sensitive child who may sometimes hide behind what seems like a hard exterior in order to hide his hurts or insecurities. But never doubt the deep emotions that this child feels inside.

Right from the beginning, baby Cancer will pick up and react to feelings. As an infant he needs lots and lots of cuddling and private time with a nurturing parent-figure. The Cancerian is likely to be especially close to Mom (or the primary nurturing caregiver) and may be resistant to being cared for by others. Security is very important — security in being cared for, in being fed when hungry.

Yet also, right from the beginning, you may sense that your little Crab is also taking care of you! He intuitively picks up YOUR feelings, too, and the feelings of others in his environment, and will personalize them. If you are angry, for example, even if you do not overtly express it, your child will feel it and may think you are angry at him. Be open in talking about feelings with this child. Reassure him that everyone has feelings, but those feelings often have nothing to do with him. Your Cancerian needs the security of knowing what is going on. Moodiness, "crabbiness," withdrawn behavior or misbehavior are all likely to be signs of insecurity and/or misinterpretation of feelings picked up from others.

Your child will be great about mimicking your characteristics. This will be fun in some ways, and perhaps uncomfortable in others, if what he is mirroring is something you don't like about yourself! Your little Crab may need reassurance that it is OK to be different from you, to have different feelings. He needs to have warm, positive contacts with other adults, so that he won't identify too exclusively with you. Such contacts will expand his confidence.

Home and family and tradition are important to Cancer. This child will love all of your family celebrations, parties, reunions, and will remember them forever.

Your little Cancerian needs a safe and private place in your home that belongs just to him. There he is likely to collect more things than you might like! Saving things is part of the Cancerian drive for security. The acquisitive Crab will be good at saving money, too — this is generally one of the thriftiest of all zodiac signs. Be aware, though, that accumulating things is an outward symbol of the inner need for emotional security. This child needs plenty of approval, reassurance and calm security in his environment. Your reward: an exceptionally loving, affectionate and unselfish child, who will retain close bonds with you throughout your life. *For your child with **Sun in House 4**, home and family are very important in the development of his self-confidence. He may express deep caring in being able to help take care of you, too, and pride in his home.*

Sun in Leo or Sun in House 5

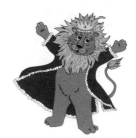

Look at me! See me shine!
The radiance of the Sun is mine.
Whatever I create will be
Most worthy of my royalty,
'Tis Leo's right divine!

See the happy little lion with arms and heart wide open? That's your kid! But also note the crowned head. The Leo child is ruler of all she surveys — or at least needs, in some way, to feel like it. Pride, self-confidence, optimism, dignity and honor — all of these traits may seem inborn. Leo thrives on being the center of attention, and shines brightest in the spotlight. Yet her "subjects" are rewarded with lots of warm affection and much generosity. Little Leo simply likes to do nice things for others and give them little gifts.

The Lion has a strong personality with a flair for the dramatic. If Leo has no opportunities to be "center stage" this natural actress can become the showoff in a manner that could be annoying. Be aware of this if you find that your child is bidding too strongly for your attention at inappropriate times or places. Provide times and opportunities where you (or others) can be an appreciative audience, and your lessons about when a considerate-and well-behaved child must stay willingly "behind the scenes" will be much better received.

Do not be dishonest with this child. Honesty and integrity are very important to Leo, as is a sense of fairness. This little royal personage will set high standards for her own behavior and achievement of goals, and you will generally be able to count on her to do the "right" thing, and to tell you the truth.

Recognition and approval are important for this natural leader. The Lion strives to win the respect of others — and will probably be worthy of it, for self-respect is equally important, and she will want to feel deserving of the recognition received. This kid is strong willed, and has the ability to persistently stick to a chosen goal, working hard until it is achieved. However, persistence on types of work that will remain "behind the scenes" will not be nearly so interesting as persistence on types of work that will result in a chance to show off the achievement.

Provide your little Lion early opportunities to interact with other kids and other adults. Look for opportunities for her to develop skills in areas that will provide a spotlight in which to shine. Encourage creativity and a natural flair for drama — you'll find that "dress up" and role playing games will be favorite playtime activities. If your own wardrobe doesn't offer a bag of interesting costumes, visit a thrift shop and acquire some extra garments and accessories. Try to frequently make it possible for one or two friends to come and play, too, for Leo will love to host a little party. Explore the possibilities of dancing lessons or junior theater experiences that might be offered in your community.

Know always that praise and incentives to achieve will work much better in guiding this child than criticism. When criticism must be given, strive to do so in such a way that you are also offering encouragement and conveying your belief in your child's good intent and ability to rise to (or beyond) what is required.

Leo's fire is definitely not a "flash in the pan." This little "royal" has great persistence to stick to a goal, once her mind is set on it. Your Lion wants to be a leader, or a person who is recognized for some important role, and will work very hard to achieve that. This child will want to earn that recognition honestly, because it is important for her to feel worthy of "royalty" and respect.

*With **Sun in House 5**, your child's ways of expressing her personal creativity, and what she considers fun, may be similar to Sun in Leo. Admiration is important in developing her self-confidence.*

Sun in Virgo or Sun in House 6

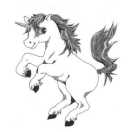

The wild and mystic Unicorn
Comes tamely to the Virgo born.
That's because my heart is pure,
My thoughts are clear — so carefully sure —
My manner calm and quite demure!

Your kid's special pet is the happy little Unicorn, which as legend has it, can only be tamed by the gentle hand and pure heart of a Virgin. The verse hints at the basic character of little Virgo as modest, somewhat shy by nature, analytical and careful in thinking, and generally quite reliable — even though deep in his heart somewhere, he may long for that mystical Unicorn.

Organization and neatness should come easily to little Virgo, with any effort at all on your part to provide him with the means to order his surroundings. You may not even have to try. You might even find that this kid will close YOUR drawers that are left open, stack your magazines or papers, or tidy a table top. Virgo is likely to keep little collections of belongings in organized and labeled compartments. You might do well to offer your old shoe boxes, or better yet, one of those metal or plastic boxes with little pull-out drawers or compartments. It is possible, though, that your child's curious, inquiring mind may acquire more paraphernalia than there is space available to keep it properly categorized, and a surface appearance of clutter may result. Take care in disturbing what may seem to you like a mess. Little Virgo probably knows exactly what is there and where everything is, and he will be quite upset if you DISorganize his "organization." If it MUST be moved, insist that HE do it.

The development of skills will be very important to your Virgo. This child is a natural perfectionist and the prime "workaholic" of the zodiac. He will work hard and patiently to achieve whatever goal is set, and will pay close attention to all of the details. That goal, however, must be seen as having a practical, useful purpose. The fact that YOU would like it done may not fit the criterion of your child, unless the CHILD sees and agrees to the purpose, and sees himself as having the ability to accomplish it. Virgos are said to be critical and that may be true, but they are often MOST critical of self. If your child believes that he will not be able to do a thing well, you may receive a firm refusal to do it at all. Self-confidence does not come easily and needs your encouragement.

Virgo prefers to be clean, and may be concerned with matters of personal hygiene and health. Pickiness in diet is likely, and this is for good reason, because a well-balanced diet will help to alleviate some of the mental tension that is often characteristic of this sign. Little Virgo can be a little worrier!

Your child could be one of those kids that have very decided food preferences, and prefers that the food not be "mixed up." He will be reluctant to try new foods — until one day you may be suddenly told that a particular food is great and why don't YOU serve it! THIS from the same kid that you were unable to get to even taste that same food the last time you offered it? Probably it is the day after your little Virgo visited a friend's house where the food was served. Your considerate child was much too polite to offend his hosts, so "suffering in silence," he tasted it, and found that he liked it after all!

This child will like to shine by helping others, taking care of them, being of service. Find ways to encourage this, even when he is very young. You will find that his ability to competently help exceeds your expectations, and is well worth your own efforts in patiently teaching him how to do a task correctly. Care of a small pet would be good for your Virgo child.

Individualized sports will probably be more enjoyable than team sports. Your child should greatly enjoy reading–so encourage that by reading to him frequently until he learns to read alone. Little Virgo will enjoy leisure activities that involve making things with his hands — crafts, model building, etc. You will most likely find this child to be conservative and thrifty with money.

The characteristics just described may also fit your child with **Sun in House 6**, *particularly in the area of daily routines. Self esteem will be enhanced as his ability to be competent and skillful grows.*

Sun in Libra or Sun in House 7

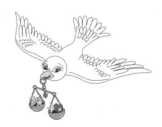

A Dove of peace my pet shall be
For harmony is ALL to me.
Make beauty my life
And save me from strife.
The scales MUST be balanced, you see?

The little white dove carries the Libran scales of balance, and tells us that peace and harmony are all-important. Your child hates discord, upsets, strife of any kind and will go to great lengths to avoid it — sometimes tending to compromise or "give in" too much, rather than standing up for her rights or own point of view. Don't underestimate that as weakness, however. It is only tact. If Libra's strong sense of justice is offended, however, you will see how strong-minded and able to fight this sign can be! Libra types have been known to be diplomats — but also top-notch generals!

Yet, as a child — or teenager — your Libra is not likely to openly argue with you on any issue of marginal importance to her. This kid will politely listen, and may even go along and do what you want done for a time, so long as it does not seriously infringe on her own preferences. But little Libra is thinking quite individual thoughts and forming her own opinions, so don't be too surprised if sometimes this sweet child whom you thought agreed with you eventually chooses to think or do a different way.

The concept of fairness is very important. Like the Scales that are Libra's symbol imply, your child believes in equality and in following the rules of the game or the laws of the land. If Libra is party or witness to a conflict, she will try to mediate, and may be quite good at that role, with a natural ability to see both sides of the issue and look for a point of balance. Don't expect her to take your side if "your side" is not scrupulously fair.

The seeking of balance can come out in a particular brand of indecisiveness when it is necessary to choose between two options that both have merit. Your Libra child wants to "have her cake and eat it, too." This kid can "ride the fence" until your patience is worn to a frazzle. For a very small child, frustration can be avoided by not requiring too many unnecessary choices. Wait to see if a singly offered choice is accepted happily rather than confusing the issue by offering two preferences. Your school age child may be more likely to catch the school bus if you insist that before she goes to bed at night, she selects and lays out the outfit to be worn to school the next day. If she asks your opinion between two choices, pick one. (She may then choose the other, but that's OK. You may have at least cut her frustration time of trying to decide — trust me.)

And speaking of outfits, appearances are important. Libra is naturally refined and concerned with aesthetics. Your child will want to look well and be surrounded by things of beauty. For this reason, saving allowances won't come easy, if there's something pretty around to buy. The taste for beauty also means that Libra will enjoy artistic activities. You should encourage this child in all manner of art and musical activities, for she is more than likely to "take to" one or more of them and develop strong skills as well as a refined appreciation.

Friends will always be important. Generally, Libra prefers not to be alone. Your child is likely to have a stronger than average need to be with other people, to be part of the crowd, and to have a special friend or two to do nearly everything with. Libra is the sign of partnership, and those who have Libra strong in their charts are unlikely to want to do very many things for long without a partner.

This is a child you'll probably especially enjoy taking places with you, or being taken along by her in future years. Your Libra will be cordial, mannerly, charming, look attractive and appropriate, and probably be well-liked by people of all ages.

*Libran characteristics may also be expressed by your child with **Sun in House 7**, especially in the area of her one-to-one relationships. What her "best friend" thinks matters a great deal. Self-confidence wavers or builds as she relates to others.*

Sun in Scorpio *or Sun in House 8*

Don't be afraid of Scorpio's sting
Or of secrets just for me.
I need to deeply search alone
'Till my own truth I see,
Then I'll soar high on Eagle's wings,
My spirit strong and free!

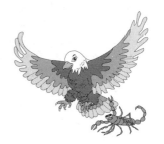

"I'll do it myself!" may be one of the first sentences you will hear when this kid begins to talk. Don't argue — or get in the way. Unless, of course, what he is trying to do is really dangerous. Skinned knees are not fatal, and a little frustrated struggle can be good for the soul. The Scorpion, a more commonly known symbol for Scorpio, has been unfairly feared for its sting, but the Scorpio type is much more likely to sting himself than anyone else, and all in the process of self-discovery. Most modern astrologers prefer the more ancient symbol for this sign, the Eagle, for it symbolizes soaring above the depths of the sting toward the self-mastery that Scorpio so strives to achieve.

Like the verse beside the little eagle says, your Scorpio kid needs to find his own truth — and the intensity with which this zodiac type is capable of probing, digging, persisting and trying until whatever he wants is achieved, is likely to constantly amaze you — from his early childhood on into his adulthood. Intensity is a prime keyword for this sign with good reason. Your Scorpio is a natural skeptic, who won't take your word for it, or anyone else's. This type must draw his own conclusions.

Unless a very outgoing fire or air sign is rising, your little Scorpio is likely to be known as "a quiet type" and/or a "loner." Even IF a lively sign is on the Ascendant, there will be some part of this child that will always be quiet and will never let you know all that he is thinking. Some secret part of Scorpio will always be kept inside. Privacy is very important, and you must especially respect that with this child. Provide a room of his own if possible, or if not, be sure there is a trunk with a lock in which your child may keep things hidden away from prying siblings, or even from you. Give your Scorpio a diary with a lock, and don't EVER be tempted to read it!

Yet don't ever think that you are likely to keep very many secrets from your Scorpio kid. Here you will see the proverbial "sixth sense" at work — the ability to pick up on something outside the norm, and if your child is worried about it, he won't rest until whatever is unusual or hidden is figured out — and don't doubt that Scorpio WILL figure it out!

In likes and dislikes, little Scorpio is not inclined to deal in shades of gray, only in black or white. This kid either likes it or doesn't like it, in no uncertain terms. Scorpio is a creature of extremes — there are no halfway measures. Depending on your level of agreement, this child's strong will can bring you joy or frustration. There's a nursery rhyme about a little girl who had a little curl right in the middle of her forehead. When she was good she was very, very good and when she was bad she was horrid. That rhyme was probably written about a Scorpio. This is NOT intended to scare you —just to make a point of the necessity for you to respect the determination and deep feelings of this child. Your child loves deeply and is very loyal. Anyone who lets little Scorpio down in a way that is perceived as betrayal may never again regain his trust.

Your child thrives on challenge, and may be attracted to risk or activities that promise adventure. He will be quite independent and is rarely ever held back by fear. He may do well at physical and/or competitive sports that involve strategy, or because of his privacy and independent needs, he may prefer sports that are more geared to the development of individualized skills, such as swimming or diving.

Scorpio is likely to love to read, particularly that which involves mystery. He is a natural detective, skeptical and shrewd, ready to dig and probe until he proves or disproves whatever he sets out to investigate. A mystery begs to be unveiled, what is hidden must be found, problems must be solved. Darkness is intrigue, not something to be feared. These qualities mean that your child is likely to be quite successful at studies, and at later career fields, that involve research. Whatever this child chooses to do, he will pursue with intensity and passion.

*Your child with **Sun in House 8** may be quite intense about sharing—who gets what and when—but he will be proud of the self-control he develops as he learns how to give and take with grace.*

Sun in Sagittarius or Sun in House 9

Like the Archer's arrow all aflame,
And a winged horse with flying mane,
I'll seek my dreams, the highest star.
I believe! I can get there!
No matter how far!

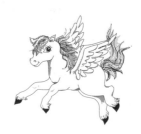

The little winged horse, chosen for your Astro Kid's pet over the usual Sagittarian centaur (so that we wouldn't have to choose between a boy or girl image) tells us several things about your child's personality potential. First, there is the strong desire to be as free as the breeze, to take off and explore the world and reach for the stars. Little Sag is a romantic to the core, idealistic and adventurous, with all the faith of Don Quixote that her "impossible dreams" can become reality. No clinging to Mom's apron strings for this kid. Give her the chance to fly and she will take off without a backward glance. But don't let that break your heart. She is just independent and free-spirited, and needs a wider world in which to test her wings. Your happy Sag loves you — in fact you are probably one of the ideals that she most believes in. So keep that in mind, if you're thinking of stepping off your pedestal. Your child will probably forgive you, and may even put you back on it, in her wish to uphold the ideal — but perhaps not before she has let you know what she thinks about your transgression.

Sagittarius is likely to be quite outspoken. In fact, she may blurt out the truth, even when it hurts. Tact is not her strong suit. This is the basic archetype about whom the adage "open mouth, insert foot" was written. You should try to teach her to think before she speaks, but don't count on it being an easy lesson. Little Sag intends no malice, mind you. It's just that the truth, as she sees it, tends to spontaneously come out.

This kid has an enthusiastic, expansive, optimistic zest for life that will lead her to faraway places and unusual experiences, even if she hasn't left her own back yard. If she can't go in body, the mind will do, helped by reading and by fantasy play. Feed your Sag's imagination by providing old clothes and accessories from attic or thrift shop for dress-up and role-playing games. Give her books of mystical and magical adventure.

Sagittarius will be concerned about broad issues and ideals, and even at an early age, may express articulate opinions about affairs of the world or philosophical issues. (This is the image of the archer shooting his "arrows" of ideas at whomever will listen.) Yet this curious, natural explorer may be pretty sloppy where details are concerned. She will tend to jump to conclusions before all the facts are known, and still express those conclusions quite dogmatically.

Details may also escape this child in regard to the difference between your version and hers as to what constitutes a clean room or finished homework. It's not so much that she is irresponsible, it's just that she thrives on change and hates to be confined. Be patient — little Sag isn't. You may get the job done better if you are willing to have it done in small doses (one task or directive at a time), with some variety in between. Making a fantasy game of the task might help, too.

Most Sag kids will like and excel at some sport, though they may prefer individualized ones to team sports. They need lots of physical activity so give your child opportunities to try various sports and see what "takes." Like her "pet" would suggest, your Sag is likely to LOVE horses (winged or not!) and anything to do with them. Coordination is likely to be quite good, although since she's always in a hurry to get somewhere, little Sag might also often trip over her feet in haste, or because her head is in the clouds instead of watching where she is going!

Sun in Sag traits may also be expressed by your child with **Sun in House 9**, *especially where her ideals and beliefs are at stake. Her dreams may be always hitched to a star. Proud of her big ideas, she may seek to convince you of them.*

Sun in Capricorn or Sun in House 10

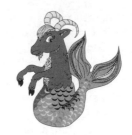

Out of the depths to the mountain top
I'll steadily climb and never stop.
I'll fret until my work is done,
I'm a leader born, who's old when young,
Yet I've a quick, dry wit to spark your fun.

The little Seagoat conjures images of whimsical fantasy, and that can be a part of the nature of your little Capricorn, although this side of his personality is usually quite hidden behind a more dominant serious tone. His rather unusual sense of humor is probably a release from a strongly and unusually disciplined maturity. Wry jokes are more often directed at himself rather than at others. This child is truly a little adult, who relates well to adults from a very early age. He will always seem old for his age... until he really IS old. Older Caps often retain their youth and that sense of humor long after others of similar age have lost it. Perhaps it's because by then they've achieved what they set out to do, and feel they have earned the right to play!

In any case, you are unlikely to have to work at teaching your little Capricorn to be responsible, for duty, dependability, discipline and a strong sense of honor will probably come naturally, as if inborn. You might, at times, be more concerned about how to make him "loosen up" and have fun. This kid will always have a mountain to climb — ambition and determination to accomplish something and be recognized for it will be evident from an early age. Capricorn will get there or else! He will persist in a goal, and succeed where peers may not simply because he will refuse to give up.

Another keyword for Capricorn is "practical." Frivolity will not appeal. If your child is going to do something, he had better understand the reason why and see a practical purpose for doing it. Therefore he will have the ability to work hard and do well in school, but will do best when he can see a practical use for the knowledge gained. Abstractions may seem useless, but ambition/status drives might induce a serious effort at an "A" even in a subject that would otherwise seem pointless.

Security is very important to your child. This means emotional security and acceptance, so be sure you don't begin to take his normally good behavior for granted and forget to give frequent acknowledgment and praise. This also translates to material security. Economy will come naturally. If this kid turns out to be extravagant, careless or wasteful, it's not the Capricorn facet of his personality — look to see if some of the other planets might be in the adjacent sign of Sagittarius. Little Cap will want to save for a rainy day and accumulate enough wealth to get something really worthwhile.

On the downside, all this seriousness breeds worry and a tendency to look at things pessimistically. You may have to often show your Capricorn where the cloud has a silver lining. Though his ability for athletics may be good, he might have some trouble meshing with the team as one of the "guys." Individualized sports could be preferred.

On the plus side, this is a child that you'll probably be able to take anywhere and count on his model behavior and good manners.

Your child with **Sun in House 10** *may express a serious, Capricorn-type approach to following rules. Confidence is gained through being thought responsible—especially by those who make the rules.*

Sun in Aquarius or Sun in House 11

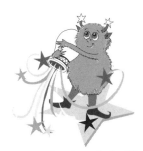

You might often think I'm "way out there,"
Alien to your point of view.
I'll rebel against tradition,
Always searching for what's new,
But I'll shower you with waves of light
And be your friend most true!

Here we have NOT a cute and recognizable little animal, bird or fish, like all the other signs, but a cute, fuzzy little character from another planet. So don't be surprised if your little "star baby" seems just a little different than all the others, right from the beginning. And maybe just a little weird. Or let's be more intellectual than that. After all, Aquarius is an air sign, air symbolizing the conscious mind and the function of thinking. Call this kid eccentric. Ahead of her time! But don't call her an "airhead," at least not if you've made a reasonable attempt to understand her. She is not "flaky," just a natural nonconformist, with plenty of stubborn stick-to-itiveness to make her ideas come into reality.

If YOU are a bit of a free spirit yourself, you and your child should do fine. But if you tend toward conservatism and tradition, be prepared for some upsets. Aquarius is not likely to uphold your traditions unless she sees a very good reason for them — and merely pleasing you or even avoiding punishment will not be a good reason. This kid is an Individual, with a capital "I" and she will want to do her "own thing" even if it means defying your opinions about propriety.

"Why?" is a question you'll hear often, and you'd better be prepared to give a better reason than "because I said so." Or even "because it's a rule." Even a young child will be more cooperative if she understands a logical reason why something must be. Appeal to her sense of honesty (which should be very strong) and to her humanitarian feelings (which will also be very strong). Little Aquarius can be taught to respect the opinions and ideas of others so long as she is not expected to agree with them. Your child will have an innate sense of equality and universality of all people, and of tolerance for others' beliefs and ideas. She will respect the right of others to be different, too, so long as they don't infringe on her individuality. You may do well to think about which areas of behavior are most important to you, and why. You may get better cooperation on major issues if you allow free expression on less important ones. For example, a weird haircut may be a worthwhile trade-off for the good grades in school that will put your little reformer in a better educational position to bring her ideas for social change into reality. Get the idea? Aquarians are good at thinking ahead.

Little Aquarius may give you quick "warm fuzzies" for greetings on occasion, but don't expect undue sentiment and feelings where personal relationships are concerned. This is the most emotionally detached of signs, and unless several other planets are in much more feeling-oriented signs, this child's attitudes will be generally impersonal. Aquarius is friendly and open with everyone, but seldom lets anyone get too close. She may greet you with a big hug, but when she is gone, you're "out of sight, out of mind." Yet she is very concerned with humanitarian issues, and will be unselfish about helping others if she sees a need. So this is a child who is unlikely to cling to Mom, or to express a lot of emotion within the family, but may be found, as a young teen, volunteering to help out at an old people's home or at a soup kitchen for the poor. This kid may not see your reasoning at all to pick up her room ("Just close the door!"), but may walk along the beach or through the park cleaning up litter and collecting items for recycling.

The new and different will always have the most appeal — in ideas, in fashion, in technology. Get the kid a computer, if you can — or steer her in that direction at school. Science will probably appeal. Try free art forms, modern dance. And astrology! Get the kid some books. Let her do YOUR chart!

The new and different will also appeal to your child with **Sun in House 11**. *She may be attracted to people who are unusual and innovative, and be inspired by them. Let her know that you appreciate ways in which she expresses uniqueness and originality, for this builds her self-esteem.*

Sun in Pisces or Sun in House 12

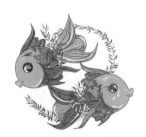

Two fish in one sea of feelings deep,
For romance I'll dream,
Or for suffering, weep.
If you hurt, I'll care for you.
My Pisces heart is always true.

See the little fish swimming in two different directions? One is happy, the other shedding a tear. Your little Pisces is a very sensitive and emotional soul, who may often seem to be quite uncertain just which way to turn. One of the reasons for this is his innate ability to pick up signals — moods, emotions — from everyone around, almost as if he was a little sea sponge. Some of those signals are mixed. Life is full of conflicts, and Pisces does not deal well with conflict. If others are sad or angry or unhappy, your child will find it hard to not feel that way, too. His own feelings are easily hurt, too, and when they are, tears come easily, no matter how hard he may try to hold them back.

Now, if you are a more detached type, your little Pisces' sensitivity may not be easy for you to handle, but understand, it is NOT bad. It is EMPATHY, an exceptional understanding of the needs of others. You may have to gradually help this child learn to develop some techniques of detachment — how to separate his feelings from those of others, and to understand that he is not responsible for them. Pisces will care very much about being of help to others. In fact he may need to feel needed for his own feeling of personal worth.

"Aha!, A mother's helper!" you may be thinking. Well, maybe, if he feels that you really NEED it. More likely you will be asked to assist with baby birds that have fallen from the nest, hurt pets, or a much less privileged little friend from school that your Pisces will adopt as his special friend. Your child is compassionate, charitable and always interested in being of help. He is likely to be particularly attracted to a spiritual path and may be very religious. If you support these very positive traits, your Pisces may be on his way to a future career in the health/helping professions. Or even if he turns out to be a CEO or a military officer, he will be known and respected for his caring treatment of subordinates.

A possible downside of all this empathy is that Pisces may be so self-sacrificing that he could feel like a martyr at times, as if he is carrying an unfair burden that others do not understand. Or, if he is exposed to a great deal of negativity, he may pick up feelings that distort his own personality into negativity and pessimism. Your child will need to learn to avoid unpleasant situations and to find constructive methods of escaping them. You will need to be attuned to this. Escape into a fantasy world can be destructive if carried too far, but if directed into art or music, for example, it can lead to great creativity and very positive accomplishments. There is tremendous hidden strength in this child's depth of feeling and compassion.

Expose your little Pisces to music lessons, to dance, to drama and to arts and crafts. Give him beautifully illustrated books of fantasy and fairy tale. Encourage "dress-up" and role-playing games — and let him have time to daydream. Sometimes he really needs some private time alone.

Don't push too hard if your Pisces seems shy. He needs to know people and develop some trust first. Be sensitive with this child, and take time to point out the wonders and the beauty of the world. "Smell the roses" with him, and you'll be well on the way to bringing out the best in both of you.

*Your child with **Sun in House 12** may also express Piscean traits in terms of his inner, private self. Allow privacy and time to dream. Soft music soothes, art and beauty inspire.*

The Moon in Each Sign of the Zodiac

Moon in Aries or Moon in House 1

> *I need to do it my way,*
> *I need to do it fast,*
> *I didn't mean to hurt you,*
> *It upsets me to be last!*

Aries' emotional responses are likely to be immediate and impulsive, with quick temper flare-ups that can be just as quickly over. Because of that, your child could say something that hurts, something that he really doesn't mean at all, and truly not be able to remember, only a few minutes later, that he ever said it. Obviously it would be best for you to learn not to take such outbursts too personally! Remember, you are the adult. You won't help either yourself or the emotional security of this child, if you match his flare-up with temper of your own. So take a deep breath and try to remain calm. You have an obligation to help your little fireball realize that others may not be so understanding. Try explaining that fact, after calm returns. But don't go on and on, for this child's attention span is short. Acknowledge his feelings: "I hear that you are very angry/upset about..." Say how you feel, without assigning blame: "It hurts/upsets me a lot when you..." Then, perhaps: "Others who don't love you as much as I do could be pretty mad if you blew up at them like that. You wouldn't want to lose a friend. When you feel yourself getting upset, try taking a deep breath and counting to three before you say anything, then maybe you can make your point in a way that won't be hurtful." Then let it go. Aries won't hold on to the bad feelings; you shouldn't either. If actual discipline is necessary, sending the child to a room alone to calm down is far better than fighting. You want to teach your child how to handle emotions, NOT how to aggravate them.

Little Aries Moon will be a high-spirited child, spontaneous and curious, with an eye for adventure. Give him plenty of room for action and encourage independence. He will feel most loving and most secure when allowed to do things his own way, to make his own mistakes, to express courage and self-reliance. Of course you CAN'T let the kid run into the street! But just keep in mind that emotionally confining behavior on your part is not an appropriate way to nurture this child.

Let Aries Moon be himself as much as you possibly can, and your reward will be a peppy, energetic and usually happy little leader who will often lift your spirits and give you much joy in life.

*The Aries interpretation may also apply to children who have the **Moon in House 1** (no matter what sign the Moon is in), in regard to their outward expression of "who I am." Even if his Moon sign theme is of a more passive type than Aries, for example, he needs, in some way, to be "number one." His feelings are right out front —he "wears his heart on his sleeve." Or, he may* *be quite moody—alternately emotional or withdrawn. Family influences are especially important to his sense of personal identity.*

Moon in Taurus or Moon in House 2

> *Leave my things right in their place.*
> *Don't try to push me past my pace.*
> *Don't surprise me, let me know*
> *When you'll return, if you must go.*

Of all the signs, Moon in Taurus is the most likely to require a sense of security. In order to feel emotionally "together," this child needs to know that there are certain things she can depend upon. You, for instance. She needs a parent who is a "Rock of Gibraltar" — always there, and meeting expectations. If you are undependable or unpredictable you could rattle her normally steady self. Lack of security in her relationships or within the environment could provoke her to some form of security compensation, such as perhaps overeating, too much attention on the acquisition of material things, or other forms of over-sensuality. Nearly all little tykes go through the "blanky" stage, but this one may have blanky, plus two or three other notable forms of comforting herself, as well. (Remember, I told you in Chapter 3 about toddler Molly's blanky, her finger sucking and hair knotting.) You try to move away too fast, she is likely to cling. Or perhaps withdraw to pout "you don't love me."

Take your time with this child. Don't rush her unless you absolutely have to. Give her a schedule or routine that she can expect you both will stick to. Let her know well in advance if you have to be away, and how her needs will be provided for. Try not to spring too many surprises, unless you're sure they are happy ones. Cuddle her lots and often in infancy. As she grows, try to set aside a special time before bedtime when you can curl up together with a book. If you work, and your time with little Taurus Moon is limited, be sure she knows what to expect, where you are, when you will be back. Quality time is more important than quantity. When you are with her, try to pace yourself to her pace.

Your child will more than reward you for your affection, calm, trust and dependability by being a loving, affectionate and loyal child whom you can depend upon.

*No matter what her Moon sign, this interpretation may also fit your child if she has her **Moon in House 2**. More than other children, she may be emotionally involved with her possessions and what she considers "mine." It will be hard for her to let go of possessions—the stage of learning to share may be a challenge. She has a real need to feel secure and comfortable. She thrives when she feels safe.*

Moon in Gemini or Moon in House 3

Don't expect me to be still
I need to move! I need to trill!
Listen to me! Tell me why!
And when I want to, let me fly!

Changeable is the word for Gemini. Your little bird can fly through the air one minute and hit the ground like a thud on the next. Emotional reactions are quick and varied, and based as much or more on what he is thinking than what he is feeling (or at least that is what HE thinks). And you won't have to wonder what the problem might be either, for this kid will tell you. He is much better than most about verbalizing how he is reacting to situations or people. In responding, you'll do better to use logic and reason in helping him to process through whatever is bothering him.

This child finds security in knowing, in satisfying his very lively and almost insatiable curiosity. He thrives on variety, and could be nervous, upset or just bored if left alone too much, or confined to an area where movement is restricted. He needs to be with people. As a baby he will fuss a lot less if you keep him where you are, to watch you move around at your tasks. Keep up a running conversation with him!

Expose your Gemini Moon to other people early. He will like getting to know your neighbors, friends and relatives. Lots of people in his circle will contribute to his sense of belonging and therefore his security. Form a play group with other parents, so your child can have little friends, too. A lively pre-school with lots to do would be a good idea.

This child may not want to sit still for too much cuddling. Quick hugs on the run are more his style. Yet every child needs some physical nurturing. Best way to cuddle with this one is to curl up with a good bedtime story. Don't just read it — talk about it. Ask questions, repeat words, put those repeated words into phrases, adding a new word here and there — and be prepared to define it when he asks. Point things out and encourage questions. Soon he is likely to be reading to you, and the close contact achieved through these sessions will help greatly to assure a strong emotional foundation for your special child.

Don't try to confine your child emotionally — or physically either, any more than is absolutely necessary. You might as well try to hold onto the wind, or catch a butterfly. This child needs a parent who nurtures his inquisitiveness, appreciates his quickness, adapts to his mood swings without undue upset, and laughs with him in delight at the infinite variety of life.

*Your child with **Moon in House 3** may talk your ear off when he is feeling safe and good, or clam up tight when he's not. His capacity for objectivity fails when his feelings are involved. Your influence will be especially important on his ability to think, learn and communicate. Read again that* *last paragraph above on Moon in Gemini. Same thing applies here for what the child with Moon in House 3 needs from his parents.*

Moon in Cancer or Moon in House 4

> *I feel so much that I can't explain,*
> *And my moods are seldom just the same.*
> *I need a safe and cozy place*
> *Before the big, wide world I face.*

Whether boy or girl, your little Cancer Moon is a real "mommy" or "daddy." She will want to take care of you, forlorn friends, small pets or anything and anyone else that she perceives is in need of nurturing. She will be very intuitive about all the moods and feelings going on around her, and is likely to feel personally responsible for them. Guard against provoking guilt feelings in this child — she will have enough of those on her own. Instead, strive to teach her that everyone has feelings, and is responsible for dealing with his or her own feelings. Most importantly, convince your little Moon-child that those feelings expressed by others often have nothing to do with her.

Talking about feelings will not come easily for this child. She may know perfectly well how she feels, but be unable to articulate it. The result: moodiness, withdrawal into her "shell," or perhaps, misbehavior. You can help your child learn to articulate feelings in a healthy manner by being calmly open, honest and non-blaming in articulating yours. Cancerian types are especially prone to mimic the behavior of their parents.

Like the very changeable phases of the Moon, your child may show many moods, from the extremes of joy to the extremes of gloom. Yet, the Moon is most "at home" in Cancer, the sign it is said by astrologers to "rule." If this child receives a nurturing, secure emotional foundation in child-hood, she will handle emotions especially well as an adult, calm in crisis, able to be strong for others. This child is an exceptionally sensitive person, strong in empathy, capable of considerable patience.

Home and family are especially important to Cancerian types. The emotional attachment to Mom is very strong, and is an important model for her sense of vulnerability, caring and being cared for. Home is a haven of safety and comfort, so you should provide her with a cozy space within it where she can keep the myriad of mementos and special things she is saving, and where she can entertain friends. Your child may prefer having friends play in her home, rather than to go to theirs, and she will appreciate your willingness to make this possible. Playing house — role-playing as parents with dolls for babies, dressing up in old clothes, etc., will be favorite activities, and ones that are worthwhile encouraging, for they develop creativity and imagination, as well as providing a forum for the expression and articulation of feelings.

*For your child with **Moon in House 4**, home and family are very important to her sense of emotional security. She needs a warm and supportive home environment. If there's stress around her, she's likely to pick it up like a little sea sponge. She may prefer to stay at home and have friends come to play, rather than go out. She may express deep caring in being able to help take care of others—even you!*

Moon in Leo or Moon in House 5

> *Pay attention! Look and see!*
> *I need to know that you like me!*
> *If you don't tell me, I won't know.*
> *Cheer me on, then watch me go!*

This child really needs a spotlight. He is the happiest and most secure when he is the center of attention. Applause, approval, admiration and compliments spur His Majesty on to greater accomplishments. You will always win more easily with this child with praise than with punishment. When you have to discipline, keep that in mind. Keep the criticism to a minimum, directed at the specific behavior and not at the child's character, and encourage him with additional words of praise. It is important to your child to feel worthy of your approval, so if your criticism is constructive and your basic respect of the child and his potential to succeed is evident, you will bring out the best in him. He has the will and the stick-to-itiveness to accomplish whatever goal he sets out to attain.

It is important to understand however, that so great is this child's need for attention, that if approving attention is not forthcoming, a bid for negative attention may be made. The Leo "showman" can easily become the "show-off" if that is the only way to get noticed. Little Leo is one type that you absolutely must not take for granted. He can learn when to take center stage and when it is more appropriate to give the stage to someone else and support from behind the scenes, but he will not be content to stay behind the scenes for very long. Yet if while all eyes are on him, he "blows his lines," he may be so embarrassed that it will take a great deal of encouragement to try again. Remember, it is the FEELINGS that are at issue here.

You must provide this child with plenty of feedback and reassurance, as well as love, in order to give him the secure foundation he needs to shine his very best. Give him opportunities to find a particular stage on which he feels comfortable. Find ways to get him out among other kids. Form a play group with other parents. Look into pre-schools. Look for early age programs in dance, drama, creative play. Visit a thrift store or two and collect a costume box of old clothes and accessories and encourage your child to invite friends over to play dress-up and make up their own little plays. Find time yourself to play with him, making up stories, playing games, participating in sports. Your Leo Moon child is a natural people-person who needs to be doing things with others.

*With **Moon in House 5**, your child's ways of expressing her personal creativity, and what she considers fun, may be similar to Moon in Leo. She needs to be admired, recognized—to have some special way of being "center stage." This is very important to her emotional security.*

Moon in Virgo or Moon in House 6

> *Let me help you keep things neat*
> *For me, to serve you is a treat.*
> *I need to know what I can do*
> *To be of use to me and you.*

The child with Moon in Virgo really needs to feel useful. One of the best ways you can nurture this child is to give her your time and patience, even when she is very young, to learn the skills necessary to help. Teach her how to do all the little daily things that need to be done. Make it a game, but let her know that she is helping you even when the thing that she has learned to do is primarily for her own benefit, such as fixing her own breakfast, making her bed, etc.

It can be emotionally upsetting for this child to live in a disorderly environment, or to be dirty. If your style is "lived in," you may find your little Virgo Moon picking up after you! Sloppy or stained clothing will be avoided. You won't have to chase her to take a bath — she will be eager. If at all possible, give your child a space of her own, rather than a shared room with a sibling, so that she can keep her things the way she wants them. She needs organization and order. Even if perhaps her order may look like disorder to someone else, this child knows where everything is and may be quite upset if it is disarranged. She will appreciate being given things to help organize, such as a tackle box or other container with little compartments.

To nurture the development of skill so important to your Virgo Moon's sense of well-being, provide her with the space and materials to make things — crafts, models, etc. She likes to do things with her hands, and she will work carefully. She is a bit shy, and a perfectionist, so let her do things at her own pace, with a minimum of interference.

Your child will be more concerned about health than the average child. Personal hygiene and good eating habits will be easy to teach. But she could be more sensitive to "not feeling good" than some, and even worried about it. Or disorder and mess could be enough to cause "not feeling good." Yet she is much more practical than emotional, and a reasonable, realistic approach to a problem will appeal. If something needs fixing, you fix it, she feels. Even a mess, an illness or something broken or dirty can be dealt with calmly and efficiently if you just proceed with "let's fix it!"

The characteristics just described may also fit your child with **Moon in House 6**, *particularly in the area of daily routines. Her sense of security and safety will grow with her ability to feel competent and skillful. Teach her to do things for herself from a very early age, and be patient. Emotional insecurity may bring tummy upsets. Good nutrition is important, and as she grows older, she may take the lead on this and teach you about what is and what is not good for you to eat!*

Moon in Libra or Moon in House 7

> *Don't leave me alone!*
> *I need to be*
> *Friendly, sharing,*
> *Just you and me!*

Little Moon in Libra really needs someone to play with. He will seldom be content to be alone for very long. Relationships — friends — can be everything to him. When there's no one to relate to, this kid often just plain doesn't know what to do! When there's no one to react to what he does or says, he's bored — and he is going to come to you for the feedback he needs. Doing whatever he's doing is just no fun when there's nobody else to share it with. Understand that! Too many brush-offs with "go read a story" or "watch TV" or "you've got a room full of toys, how can you be bored?" just will not meet this child's needs at all.

You will find that you will get lots more done yourself if you find your child a friend to play with, even if that means inviting the friend to play at your house. So long as the friend is reasonably like your child in basic personality, you should not have to worry about trusting them to play nicely. Little Libra prefers everything to be pleasant and peaceful. He won't, by his own initiative, go in for rowdy play and will prefer not to argue. Although he is generally sociable and charming to everyone, and can mix well in a group, he will tend to pick one special friend, or do best when having one friend at a time over to play. If there are three friends playing together, and a conflict arises, your child is likely to be the mediator, for he will want to restore peace and will instinctively be able to see both sides of the issue and how to compromise.

However, this child can exhibit a particular brand of Libran indecisiveness when faced with two alternatives of possibly equal merit. He wants them both, or he doesn't want to give one up, so he argues the pros and cons until he drives you nuts. Don't ask this child to make too many trivial decisions — it will help keep the peace for both of you if you just say, "Wear this, it looks so pretty," instead of "What do you want to wear?" or "Let's have a great chocolate ice cream!" instead of "Do you want chocolate or strawberry." If he has a decided preference, he will probably tell you, but if you ask him to choose between things upon which he has no clear preference, it may take a long time!

*Libran characteristics may also be expressed by your child with **Moon in House 7**, in the area of his one-to-one relationships. Having a "best friend" is an important issue of emotional security. If he feels insecure, he may be too compromising in relating to others, too dependent on what they think. He is happiest in an environment that is peaceful; he is upset when he thinks something is unfair.*

Moon in Scorpio or Moon in House 8

> *I need to feel that I'm in charge*
> *Of everything inside,*
> *And I have deep and secret thoughts*
> *I'd really rather hide.*

Your Scorpio Moon child has deep and intense feelings that are so complicated at times that even she doesn't understand them, so don't be surprised if you can't either! But know that whatever it is that she is feeling, it is not felt lightly, nor can it be trivialized. It MATTERS — a whole lot! Yet don't worry too much. This child can handle those feelings, even if you can't. She LIKES to brood, and probe around inside her brain, and confront the dark corners in there. Give her some space. Allow her a large measure of privacy. Let her have a secret hiding place or two or three that you — absolutely! mind you! — do not violate. What do you think she is going to do anyway? Do you HAVE to know? OK, there are some things a parent has to be aware of — especially when an older child might be tempted to try something self-destructive like drugs. But then you should be able to observe symptoms. Just don't feel that it is your right to do routine snooping. Unfair! Your child has a right to her personal thoughts, even if you don't agree with them, and to some personal tokens, writings, drawings or such that she can keep secret until she feels like revealing them. Which may be never. Accept it. This kid feels most secure when she is in control of things. She may trust you, but ultimately, she trusts herself most! So don't try to control everything she does or thinks. It won't work — unless maybe you, yourself, are a DOUBLE Scorpio — and even then, you are in for a major power struggle.

Although this child feels very deeply, her emotions may not show. She is likely to keep them hidden much of the time. That doesn't mean she has forgotten about something that upset her deeply. Quite the contrary. She is capable of continuing to brood over it for a very, very long time. Scorpio has difficulty letting go of emotions. She may not talk about what she is feeling, but inside she is processing it to pieces, examining it from every angle. Yet if you ask her if something is bothering her, you're most likely to get "No, I'm just fine." Of course, she holds onto good feelings, too, thus is very loyal to those she cares about. But she is also possessive, and may tend toward jealousy if she feels any reason to mistrust that someone is loyal in return.

Do not expect to have much success in keeping secrets from this kid. She may not let you know everything she is feeling, but she is an expert at ferreting out the secrets of others. This is a major strength if she involves herself in any kind of work that requires investigation, research and the ability to focus and concentrate until she discovers what she is after. She is a natural at picking up nonverbal messages, and is good at figuring out subtle ways of motivating others to do things her way. This a very powerful personality — complex, but very strong. No matter what, a survivor!

Your child with **Moon in House 8** *may be very emotionally intense about sharing—about who gets what and when. Her sense of security will grow as she develops control of her emotions and learns how to give and take with grace. She has a strong need for privacy, which needs to be respected.*

Moon in Sagittarius or Moon in House 9

> *I need to be free!*
> *Let me go! Let me fly!*
> *I need to have faith,*
> *I need goals that are high!*

In order to make this kid feel safe with your love, you must truly let him go! Yes, you can catch a firefly and keep it in a jar, but after awhile its light won't flicker anymore. Your child needs to have adventure, if not physically, then with the mind. Nurture him by seeing that he has plenty of opportunity to explore and expand. His mind craves stimulation and adventure. The new and the foreign will appeal. Travel will be fun and expose him to lots of new ideas — but if actual physical travel is not possible, he can travel through the mind. See that he has access to lots of books. Consider ways in which you might expose him to contacts with people/playmates of different cultures, for he will likely learn much of value from them.

Unless many other planets are in very different signs, your Sagittarius Moon is basically an optimist, preferring to look on the bright side of any issue. He is outgoing, friendly and very enthusiastic about life in general, and about whatever is his interest of the moment. Very idealistic in his outlook, he expects the best of everyone and expects the world to be wonderful. That, of course, means that at least sometimes, and maybe often, he is going to be pretty disappointed. But he won't stay "down" long. Your little Archer will shoot another flaming arrow into the sky and find a new light to chase.

When a grand idea lights up your child's own special sky, he will want to share it with everyone. That's when the little Archer starts shooting the arrows of his ideas into you and anyone else who will listen. Since he believes so strongly and idealistically, he is likely to be very dogmatic and convincing — so long as the object of his faith does not let him down.

This kid is generally happy, friendly to all, confident and fun. He is inquisitive, and is likely to ask you a LOT of questions about subjects that may seem deep for his age, such as about God and various ethical or philosophical issues. Be prepared!

Moon in Sagittarius traits may also be expressed by your child with **Moon in House 9**, *regardless of what sign the Moon is in, especially when his ideals and beliefs are at stake. He may be very emotional in his expression. This child thrives on adventure. Feed his sense of security with as many opportunities for learning as you can.*

Moon in Capricorn or Moon in House 10

> *Don't try to kid me,*
> *Tell me the facts*
> *I deal with what's real*
> *I stay on my tracks.*

This is a kid that lives in the real world, in spades. Her feet are firmly on the ground, with the toes digging in. She is serious, cautious and very much in control. That is what makes her feel secure. What she needs is to understand what is going on, where her place is within it, and where she is going from there — preferably "up." She will select her "track" on which to climb up her own particular mountain, and then move steadily along it.

Your child with Moon in Capricorn is ambitious and craves status and leadership roles. Because it is a sign of upward progress, appearances will matter. She is likely to care more than some kids about looking "right," having her home and things look "right," and having you look "right."

Little Capricorn is very much a pragmatist. Given choices, she will consider them in an orderly way and then do the practical thing or make the most useful decision. Not a dreamer, this child. If she seems to be daydreaming, she is probably only brooding on a practical solution to some issue. Brooding is possible — the "real" world has lots of problems, and your child will be more aware of them than the average child. Seriousness and caution easily translate into worry and pessimism. You may have to be the one to find the "silver lining" on occasion, when your child seems stuck on only seeing a cloudy sky.

This is a little person who is likely to seem mature for her age right from the start. You might wonder if you have a gnome-adult sometimes, instead of a tot. She will not be overtly emotional, and indeed may seem more than a little emotionally inhibited. After all, it is not seemly to wear one's heart on one's sleeve, you see. Capricorn Moon is not cold; she cares. She just does not feel that it is appropriate to be effusive about it.

Your child with **Moon in House 10** *may express a serious, Capricorn-type approach to achievement. Her sense of security is fed through organization and structure. She needs to feel responsible, and that she is perceived as being responsible by those who make the rules.*

Moon in Aquarius or Moon in House 11

> *Hey! I like you!*
> *But don't hold me tight.*
> *I need my freedom*
> *To seek my own light!*

The Aquarian emotions tend to be cool and detached. Yet your Moon in Aquarius child may be open and friendly to everyone he meets. He loves the world, loves his friends, loves you... but don't ANY of you get TOO close. You are scrunching his aura, cutting off his air. He is suffocating. Coolness sets in — or he is just gone, off to seek some other friends. He will come back later, probably with a big hug and happy greeting, and stay — until you crowd him again. The point? Don't be possessive, and don't try to impose too many of your own standards or conventions on this child. Likely he will simply "tune you out."

This is an individual who needs to be his own special self — unique, and not what others expect him to be. That's no fun! This kid needs to have a forum in which to be unconventional. It may be in his way of dressing, in the activities he chooses, or in the ideas or philosophies he espouses. Whatever the expectation is, your child will enjoy doing some part of it a different way. If you understand that, and allow him space for it, you'll be a lot more comfortable — and you will be doing what you need to do to best foster security in your child's feelings for you, and for his own emotional foundation for meeting the world.

Aquarius Moon needs to feel a sense of openness from those he loves the most. There's a bit of the rebel in every Aquarian personality. Let him rebel against something else, not you. Of course, there are some standards that you will need to expect him to uphold. But you will do better with the things that are most important if you can give ground on other things that are not so major. Eccentricity in dress, for example, is only superficial. Skipping school is major.

You will more successfully appeal to your child with a rational, intellectual approach than with an emotional one. He is uncomfortable with emotional displays. That doesn't mean he hides his feelings. He's likely to come right out and tell you how he "feels," meaning "thinks." But he may be impatient with those who lose control. Be cool!

*Your child with **Moon in House 11** needs to feel that he is unique and independent. Feed his emotional security by encouraging his individuality. Try to trust, and give him his space. Try to keep your cool—emotional upset on your part won't move him. Objectivity and logic might.*

Moon in Pisces or Moon in House 12

> *Deep inside I feel that I*
> *Am safe when I can see*
> *A world of beauty, peace and light*
> *That won't hurt you or me.*

This is a very sensitive soul, your little Pisces Moon child. She cares deeply and compassionately about others, and is likely to present you with a succession of little "causes" from a very young age. There may be the bird that fell out of the nest, or hurt its wing. Or the sick pet, or the neighborhood or school waif who for one reason or another has stirred your child's sympathy. She will always want to be helping somebody. She needs to feel needed.

But that does not at all necessarily mean to clean her room or help with the dishes. This is not a Virgo type, it is the opposition sign. Little Pisces is not characteristically a neatnik. To the contrary, her mind could be so focused on some "larger issue" that disorder around her won't matter or even be noticed. "Helping somebody" is more likely to be caring for the sick, being empathic with someone who is sad, or it could be a social or religious cause. This is a child who might be attracted to larger issues at a younger age than you might expect. She could become very interested in whatever religious group she is exposed to, and want to do things through it to help others. She may adopt a cause such as animal activism, or helping the homeless, etc. Whatever she feels that it is within her capability to do, at any stage of her life, to make the world a better place, she is likely to try to do it, even if it means self-sacrifice.

Moon in Pisces has a very vivid imagination, and especially if she is hurt or disappointed with the world, will be inclined to retreat into daydreaming or fantasy. Because she is so sensitive, she is easily hurt and may overpersonalize things that are trivial. She is most unlikely to be assertive in a conflict, and indeed may not stand her ground at all, therefore she can be bullied or taken advantage of. You may have to try to help her develop a "thicker skin" and some self-defensive techniques. When she's upset, soft classical music may be very soothing.

If other planets, especially the Sun, are in more assertive signs, a Pisces Moon child can well grow up to be a real fighter, but she will always have a soft spot and be a soft touch for someone who needs her. Be glad. It might be you, someday.

*Your child with **Moon in House 12** may also express Piscean traits in terms of her most inner, private, secret feelings. She is moved by beauty, art, music, romantic fantasy. She needs privacy and some time to dream for emotional equilibrium. Moon in House 12 may mean more than normal intuition, even if the Moon is not in a sign that is usually thought to be intuitive.*

The Twelve Rising Signs

Aries Rising

> *My color is red,*
> *I glow like a flame,*
> *I want to win*
> *In every game!*

You may hear others describe this child as "a fiery personality," "always has to get there first," "a real leader," "impulsive," "rash," "adventurous." Life won't be dull with little Aries around. You'll have to move fast to keep up with her! So get set for a joy ride, with some hair-raising scares along the way likely. See that she has a safe place to be physically active and noisy. If such activity is not "your thing," do consider an early play-oriented pre-school.

Your child has a shorter attention span than most (unless other planetary placements in the chart are steadier). She will be good at getting things started, but may lose interest long before they are finished. Try to make "pick-ups" and other little chores fun, encourage her to take the lead (maybe you could race!), do things his or her own way as much as possible, and be ready to point out something new about a project if interest seems ready to lag.

Try not to take this child along when it will be necessary for her to be quiet for very long, but if you must, take along a big bag with an interesting variety of little things for her to do, and be prepared for the fact that you will have to pay fairly close attention. You may have learned to live with this little "ball of fire," but other adults may not be ready to deal with her. You are the one who must be considerate. It's not fair to expect the child to be, at least at a young age. It's her basic outer nature to be very active and busy and, let's face it, quite self-centered.

At play with other kids, this kid will be a natural leader, happiest when she is in the center of activity. She will be competitive, which may lead to conflicts. Help her to respect the rights of others, without assigning blame. Look for ways in which you can encourage appropriate competitive games, and ways in which Aries Rising can develop her sense of independence and skill.

Taurus Rising

> *Here I sit*
> *Content as can be,*
> *Comfortably doing*
> *What pleases me.*

Other's may describe your Taurus Rising child with such words as calm, quiet, slow and steady. As he grows, he may be noted for being "down-to-earth," practical and dependable. A Taurus Rising personality sometimes seems to be almost physically more solid than others, as if rooted to the earth on which he stands. Sometimes, when you are in a hurry, you'll believe that he actually does have roots. Prepare to be patient. On the other hand, there will be times when you will appreciate the calm and patience with which this child handles a situation that would upset others.

It may be difficult to get this kid started, but once he gets going, you can depend on his follow-through. He will be quiet and probably undemanding. Unless other chart placements strongly suggest a more active personality, this is a child that you can most likely teach to come along with you for adult occasions and behave properly. He may really enjoy a concert, the theater, a nice dinner out. If he isn't particularly interested in your adult affair, he may be content to quietly play alone, if you have provided appropriate toys.

At play with other children, your Taurus Rising may be quieter than others and less likely to stick up for his own rights — unless he is pushed into a very uncomfortable situation. Then, watch out. "Stubborn as a bull" is another apt description for this sign! And remember, the bull may munch calmly in the meadow, until provoked into "seeing red," and thus to charge with strong will and persistence.

You will find that your child likes what he likes — in comfort, food, places to go, clothes to wear, whatever — and that's that. He will want it that way and may be reluctant, or refuse outright, to try something new. If he doesn't like something, then it's no way. You may as will give up because your stubborn little bull won't! Eventually he may try something new, in his own good time, when he is ready. Not before.

Gemini Rising

> *I'm bright and quick*
> *As I flit and fly,*
> *First here, then there*
> *All things I'll try.*

Others are likely to describe this colorful little bird as quick, lively and curious, one who always has a question, is a "will-o'-the-wisp," an intellectual (when she is older), outgoing, sociable and friendly. She also might be seen as "scattered" or a bit "high-strung." Nervous energy, lots of hand motions when talking and a wiry build are also likely to be characteristics of this child.

This kid is a bundle of energy and seldom sits still. You'll need to provide an environment where she will be able to move freely and safely, or her restlessness will fray your nerves to a frazzle. Her lively curiosity will mean she is into everything. Child-proofing your home has extra meaning for this child! If you're not prepared to watch her every minute, you'd better put anything dangerous well out-of-reach.

The attention span is short, and interests can flit from one thing to the next. Your Gemini Rising child will literally run circles around most other people. This one won't be poking along behind. She will dash ahead, and you may have to run to keep up with her! And be prepared to suddenly change direction as something you failed to notice catches her eye and interest. Your child will need plenty of exercise and stimulation, but she needs rest, too, and relaxation often doesn't come easily. Settling her down for nap time or bedtime will probably go easier if you start with a "wind-down" time over a good storybook. Read to her at first, and when she is older allow her to read for a while before lights out. She needs the transition time from rush to rest.

Children with Gemini Ascendants are usually good at anything requiring manual dexterity. Provide your child with things to do with her hands. Fingers may fly easily over piano keys, but the teacher will need to be versatile, flexible and lively to sustain this kid's interest, and you won't have much luck with anything but short practice sessions. So don't nag — just catch her "on the run," but frequently.

Your child will thrive on an environment full of variety, change and mental stimulation. Take her on trips. Go for walks. Fly kites. Be with people, but in an active setting. Don't expect her to sit still while you visit with other adults.

Little Gemini Rising will make friends easily and probably have lots of them. She is a natural salesperson, so she can also "sell" herself. Yet she may not be too close or emotionally involved with any of her friends. She needs the stimulation of a variety of relationships, with lots to talk about and lots to do. Freedom in relationships is very important. Those who attempt to confine this child with possessiveness are likely to send her off like the wind to seek a new interest.

Cancer Rising

> *I might laugh*
> *Or I might cry*
> *From moment to moment,*
> *Don't ask me why.*

You generally won't have to wonder about what your Cancer Rising child is feeling. It will be right out on the surface, obvious. Your little "crab" is a creature of moods, and the moods can swing from extremes of joy to the depths of despair. (This may be modified if some planets are in less emotional signs, but even then, the Cancer Ascendant child will not hide feelings well. Even in a quiet way, those feelings will show.) Yours is a very sensitive child, and this will often be expressed as caring and compassion for others. He will like to take care of people — may especially enjoy helping you prepare food for family or guests. Cancer Rising can be a good, sympathetic listener, is protective of friends and family, and is very loyal.

Do not expect this child to be especially interested in athletics — competitive sports in particular — unless the Sun or Moon are in assertive, competitive signs. Cancer is reserved, non-aggressive, even shy. It may be difficult to lose in a competition without feeling somehow rejected. The body type is likely to be rather soft and rounded. Of course, everyone needs physical activity, but you would do well to point your child in the direction of noncompetitive sports. Swimming would be a good choice — water is Cancer's natural element. Choose individual sports where one's skill is measured against oneself and games are played as games. Dance is a good expression of your child's creativity and sensitivity. Don't push for competitive team sports unless the child takes the lead. Cancer kids usually are quite responsible about school work, but may not speak up easily in class unless very confident of the right answer. Approval is needed; criticism is hard to take.

Your child will probably be quite good at handling money and can be trusted with an allowance early. Saving will come quite naturally — Cancer's need for security calls for something tucked away for that "rainy day." Expect also to provide space for many collections. This child is a saver of just about anything he thinks just might be needed sometime in the future. You'll also need space to save the arts and crafts projects that you should encourage, for Cancer Rising is likely to have a natural flair for such creativity.

Leo Rising

> *I shine like the Sun*
> *My outlook is bright*
> *I do things with style*
> *And I do them right!*

Looking for your Leo Rising kid? Find a group, a stage, a circle of admirers, and that's where she will be, right in the middle. Others are likely to describe her as outgoing, dramatic and exciting, with lots of energy. She can sell anything. This child can be a natural showman or show-off, depending upon one's point of view and how hard she must work for attention. The kid has charisma — "it!" Don't try to fight it. Find her a stage. If she has an appropriate outlet for all this creative energy and style, she will be happy, develop it constructively, and not need to bid for attention at times and places when it may be annoying to you or others.

Whatever your child sets out to do, she will probably approach it with lots of enthusiasm and do it with flair. She is a "people person" and will usually want to have others to relate to, who will give her feedback and approval on what she is doing, how she looks, etc. Approval is not just desirable; it may be necessary to keep that sunny disposition shining. But she isn't all take — far from it. She is generous to a fault and will look for ways to spread her benevolence on others, and enjoy making them happy with the same zest she does everything else.

Give your child plenty of opportunities to be with others. Form a play group, find a pre-school, look into junior theater programs in your community. Give her a costume box of old clothes and accessories (thrift shops are a good source) and art materials, including large papers, old boxes and such. Encourage her to take the lead to organize the neighborhood kids into putting on little plays. Do all you can to encourage her creativity, admire the results and just watch her shine! (The Sun "rules" the sign of Leo, so Leo Rising, too, is a ray of sunshine, even if the Sun sign is a less showy one!)

Virgo Rising

> *I'd rather not speak up*
> *Until I'm sure that I am right*
> *Each detail must be known to me*
> *I can't trust what's not in sight.*

This child is likely to be known among your friends as a "quiet child." He may be shy, is usually calm in temperament, and prefers not to be in the spotlight unless he is quite confident about what he is doing. He may be willing to speak up or perform, but it is not likely that he will do so spontaneously. Only after he has practiced and knows he can do it well.

Your child tends to be a perfectionist about what he does. Virgo types are said to be critical, and that is true. But Virgo Rising may be most likely to be "hard on" self. If he really wants to do something, though, he will work until he gets it right. He is not afraid to work hard and long until what he is doing measures up to his high standards.

Additionally, this kid prefers to do his work in his own way. After all, he can plainly see that most people are not nearly so conscientious as he about paying attention to the details. He can count on doing it to his satisfaction if HE does it. He is not so sure about you!

Expect that your Virgo Rising will be meticulous about his appearance. He may play in a manner in which he gets dirty, but he won't want to stay that way for long. This is a kid with whom you shouldn't have to fight to get him in the bath tub. He will probably just love it, from babyhood on. Later on he will probably take a daily bath or shower on his own, and wash his hair to boot. Expect to have a lot of damp towels. Show him how to do the laundry early! He will tend to pay more attention to good health habits than the average child, and may be fussy about what he eats as well. He could insist on foods being separated from each other, could be very reluctant to try something new, or perhaps, like my Elizabeth could even become a vegetarian at a young age.

Libra Rising

I am nice and I am calm.
You will like me, come and see!
We can play and sing and dance,
Have lots of fun, just you and me.

This Ascendant is more than likely to belong to an attractive child. And whatever natural physical attractiveness she has will usually be enhanced by refined and mannerly behavior, and a natural grace and charm. So charming is she, that you may all too often start out to say "no" and then "wake up" sometime later, realizing that you really gave her her way and are not sure when and how that happened.

Libra is the sign of the zodiac most associated with relationships, and this child will be very concerned about having friends and wanting to do things with them and to be liked. This is a child who will always want "somebody to play with" and is unlikely to be content to play alone very often. If there is no one to play with, she is going to want to play with you. So if you want some time to think your own thoughts, you'll quickly find that the easiest thing to do is invite one of her little friends over to play. Artistic activities will have great appeal, so it would be a good idea to look into dance, music or art classes.

Your Libra Rising child likes everything to be nice and peaceful. She is willing to be competitive in a game she likes, but unpleasant conflicts and strife upset her equilibrium. Libra needs to balance the scales. If others are disagreeing, she may become the mediator, trying to suggest a way to reconcile the issue. If she is in conflict with someone, she is more likely to give in, or try to find a compromise. At best, she is a natural diplomat; at worst, she can be taken advantage of because she would rather given in than stand her ground.

The urge to balance leads to a particular brand of Libran indecisiveness. It is not that she doesn't know what she wants, but that more than one alternative seems so equal that she just can't decide which. She can get really "stuck" while your patience wears thin. The school bus could go by while she ponders which color of socks goes best with her outfit. Do both of you a favor. Don't ask her to make trivial decisions like that. If she is stuck, tell her what you think is in best taste. Let her save weighing the pros and cons for her major decisions.

Scorpio Rising

I have a secret
Maybe I'll tell you
And maybe I won't.
If you think you can make me,
In a word — DON'T!

Scorpio Rising may be one that others will describe as a "loner." He tends to be quiet and deep, and no one will ever know for sure what is going on inside. He likes it that way. It's not that he has any deep, dark secrets — probably not. He just likes to feel in control of the situation, and that is more likely if he doesn't give away all his moves ahead of time.

This child is likely to have striking eyes that seem to see far and deeply. Intensity shows, and you will learn to know a fierce determination in his approach to anything that really matters to him. This is a powerful personality, with a relentless drive. When this kid wants to do something he will go after it with a strong will and great persistence.

If your child wants to learn something he will probe and dig until he finds out what he needs to know. You may not know everything that is going on in his head, but don't kid yourself that you will be able to keep any secrets from him for very long. He will have a way of pulling it out of you, one way or another, if he has any reason to think there's something he ought to know. He is a natural detective.

Respect this child's need to often be alone. Privacy is very important to him, and he needs the time and space to think his own thoughts. Try, if at all possible, to provide a room of his own, or at least a private trunk with a lock. And then stay out — or knock before entering. Don't snoop. If you really need to know something, it would be far better to ask direct questions and observe behavior. This kid is resourceful and wants to do well. Mutual trust will foster great loyalty and the wish to please you. Mistrust may never be forgotten.

Encourage challenging activities that call for investigation, examination, and research. Whatever catches your child's interest, be it sport, art or science, will be pursued intensely.

Sagittarius Rising

Wow! Let's go!
Let's fly to a star.
Life is great
And I'm going far!

Little Sag Rising is most likely to be outgoing and characteristically self-confident with lots of energy. She is usually quite optimistic, expecting the best of people and situations. Naïve? Yes, that she can be. She is so idealistic that she is bound to be disappointed at times, but if one goal doesn't work out she won't be "down" for long. This little Archer will soon find another star to shoot her arrows at, and new hopes on which to pin her dreams. If a person lets her down, she will most likely forgive and forget. She is very friendly and upbeat most of the time, and there is not much of anything that will dampen her spirit and zest for life for very long.

There are two expressions of Sagittarius Rising that are notable. Your child may notably demonstrate one or both of them. One is the athletic, peppy, lover of the outdoors. She may be exceptionally well-coordinated (except when she is in too big a hurry, which may be often, and she trips over her own feet). If you think, from observing your tot, that she might be this type of Sag, you might try her out on kiddy acrobatic dancing or gymnastics classes and see if it "takes." She might also excel at early swim lessons, and she will probably absolutely love horses and anything to do with them. The athletic expression is more likely to be the case if your child's Sun or Moon signs are also outgoing and extroverted. If other things in the horoscope suggest a more introverted type, she may still enjoy and do well in some individualized sport, but may avoid competitive ones.

The other notable expression of Sagittarius Rising is the philosopher and the seeker of higher truth. Your child will likely show at an early age, and continue throughout her life, an exceptional quest for higher knowledge. As a young person this may first take the form of gung-ho enthusiasm for the youth activities of whatever religion your family belongs to. But it will have to live up to her ideas. If she is ever let down by it, or detects hypocrisy, watch out. She will be off in search of another, higher truth in which to place her faith. What she believes in, this outspoken Sag is likely to "preach," sometimes dogmatically. She will most likely be eager to pursue higher education. Even when she is young, be prepared to have good answers for frequent "whys!"

Capricorn Rising

I will do the best I can
But there are rules to mind
With honor I will work to climb
The path that I shall find.

This kid is a realist. He will probably exhibit, from a very early age, a clearly practical point of view on just what is possible and what is not. Since he tends more toward pessimism (life is very serious) than optimism (life is full of wonder), he will tend to set his own limits to a sufficiently large enough extent that he won't need many more from you or from his environment. Too much limitation, in fact, could breed considerable frustration and a tendency to give up: "I can't do it." It will be his instinct to figure out what the rules are, and then honor them. With this type of child, you should be primarily gearing your mind to how you are going to encourage and provide opportunities, rather than how you are going to child-proof and corral. If you tell your child not to do or touch something, he is more likely than the average child to obey. Responsible behavior comes easily.

As your Capricorn Rising child develops his skills to do almost anything, you will see the strong, hardworking side of this personality. The hardy little Seagoat has his eye on that mountain over there, and is very determined to get to the top. There's an instinctive will to achieve, to "get there," to attain status. But he has to see that the direction he is going is possible. He is too practical to waste time on an activity in which he does not feel competent. That's where you must do a little reality check, and assess when you should back off and when you should step in with some encouragement and perhaps a little help — not too much! — if you can see that your child really does have potential in an activity and is only suffering a momentary block.

It will be very important to this child to succeed in something, and to be recognized as being an expert in it. Ultimately, he will be the one to decide just what area that will be. You can guide, but don't choose for him. Respect his preferences, for you will most likely be well able to depend on him to take a responsible direction, play within the rules, and work hard to achieve.

Aquarius Rising

> *Do I shock you? Good!*
> *I like to be unique.*
> *As freely I must live my life*
> *And my own truth I speak.*

Throughout her life, the Aquarian child is one that you can count on to find something to do, wear or be that will set her apart from the crowd. This kid is an individual — unique and very independent. She likes to be different, needs to have freedom, and may even like to shock people a little. She is not at all impressed with traditions and not particularly impressed with rules, either. If YOU are very concerned about issues of "what will people think," be prepared for a little breath of fresh air in your life and a possible shake-up in your own attitudes. This child is probably quite open and tolerant about your beliefs and preferences, as well as anyone else's, so long as you don't impose them on her. The word is "live and let live."

Are you uncomfortable with the prospect of a little rebel? Some standards MUST be followed... of course, they must! This is an intelligent child, and the intellect can be reached with reason. She is a child of the future, and can understand the logic of trade-off for future benefit. Just don't think that "do it because it's a rule" or "because I say so" are necessarily going to work. Emotional appeals won't be effective either. Aquarius is the most emotionally detached of all signs, so you will do best to approach her with reason. Your best bet is to provide opportunities for her to express her creativity and uniqueness — group activities in which individuality is an asset.

Be willing to give ground on things that do not really matter all that much, such as arty, unconventional dress, as a trade-off for "working within the system" on the things that do matter. A good record in school, for example, can pave the way toward being able to change society through being in a position to influence trends. That, my friends, is an example of reason.

Pisces Rising

I am dreaming and floating
In a world of my own
Where no one's unhappy
Or sick or alone.

Pisces Rising may be perceived by others as a quiet, ethereal child, with perhaps the aura of a dreamer or mystic. He may seem often to be lost in a world of his own, and in his head that is probably true. There's a special, lovely place inside that little soul, to which he can retreat and escape whenever the real world seems harsh or uncomfortable. There he can stay by the hour, dreaming and fantasizing, creating a world of beauty and love where nobody is in pain.

This is a very sensitive child, who can intuitively sense how others are feeling. Sometimes the "noise" of all those feelings in his environment is just too much to bear, hence the escape. When he tunes in on what is going on, he will want to help and to heal. There is great compassion and willingness to give to others. He will try to save and heal hurt pets, and he will try to comfort others who are upset or worried or ill. All this is most likely to be done with grace and consideration, modestly and with some shyness.

This child may have an exceptional feeling for beauty and for aesthetic pursuits. He may do very well with music and with art, and you should consider various lessons, as well as provide him with materials, from the time he is small. See what appeals to him and encourage it. Music, for example, can provide a constructive and expressive outlet for all the emotion he feels inside. Your child will need a creative outlet, in order to handle those fantasies and function as he needs to do in the everyday world.

It is possible that this child may be drawn to a future career direction in the helping/healing professions. Whatever he does, he is likely to be known as a sympathetic listener to his friends.

Chapter Six

The Personal
Planets in the Signs

Other than the Sun and the Moon, there are three planets that are considered to be personal planets, because they move rapidly enough in their orbits that people born on different days will usually have them in different degrees. These are Mercury, Venus and Mars. Mercury and Venus are "inner planets," meaning that they orbit between Earth and the Sun. Mars is an "outer planet," being the first of the planets that orbit farther out from the Sun than Earth, but since it is also a fast-moving personal planet, it is in this chapter instead of in the next chapter on outer planets.

Again, I am introducing all three first, before the look-up paragraphs, so you will have in mind the basic nature of each planet, by itself, before you filter its "light" through the "colors" of the signs.

Mercury

The placement of the planet Mercury in a birth chart shows how the person thinks and communicates thoughts with others. Mercury, in mythology, was the winged messenger of the gods. This planet is always quite close to the Sun in the chart, often in the same sign, and never farther away than the sign before or after the Sun. If your child's Sun and Mercury signs are the same, everything said about the Sun sign will be emphasized in all of his or her communication activities. If the Mercury sign is not the same as the Sun, then a very different energy is introduced, for adjacent signs contrast sharply from each other.

Here, as an example of how adjacent signs might work, you could have the "boss" (Sun) who likes to be in the lead and take the initiative (Aries), but has a "messenger" (Mercury), who may either lose the initiative by daydreaming after an alternate goal or complement the initiative with a fantastic hunch that works (Pisces). Or the messenger (Mercury in Taurus) may take so long to think through an approach that a competitor wins, or more positively, may take that initiative and follow through with a well thought-out plan for success.

Venus

The placement of **Venus in the birth chart shows how a person expresses affection**. (Venus, in mythology, is the Goddess of love, the Roman equivalent of Aphrodite.) Here we get clues as to what your child seeks in comfort and pleasure, what he or she values (including possessions, the handling of money), and how he or she appreciates beauty. Venus is an important key as to how your child will relate to others.

Venus is never more than two signs away from the Sun sign. If Venus is in the same sign as the Sun, the basic energy and the style of expressing affection will be essentially the same. If Venus is in an adjacent sign to the Sun, the two signs are very different. Two signs away will indicate a style that is somewhat similar to that of the Sun, yet not the same. For example, the intensely passionate Sun in Scorpio type, who has Venus in Libra, may be much more refined in his or her taste than the extremist nature of Scorpio would, by itself, suggest. This is my combination. My Mom has described me as "prissy" as a small child (an example of one of the things Moms say about older kids that they'd rather not hear!)

If the Scorpio's Venus is in Sagittarius, a natural fixed quality and stick-to-it-iveness might, in the area of relationships, be modified with a tendency to be fickle, or on the other hand, to be very idealistic about whom it chooses to associate with. Just one sign past Libra and Sag, on either side of Scorpio, are two "down-to-earth" signs that are more easily compatible with Scorpio's basic energy, even though much less intense. Deeply emotional Scorpio with Venus in Virgo will be analytical in considering what he or she values. With Venus in Capricorn, Scorpio's natural passion might be tempered by what is proper or practical in choices and affections.

The fact that Mercury and Venus are always so close to the Sun is often a reason why some people whose Sun degrees are very near the beginning or end of a sign feel that they relate more to descriptions of the adjacent sign than to their own. They likely have both Mercury and Venus in that adjacent sign, and their communication styles (Mercury) and their relating styles (Venus) are important factors in the sum total of their behavior patterns.

Keep in mind this necessity to blend each factor with the others as you continue to look up your child's planets. Look for repeated themes. The more often a chart tells you something, the more significant it is.

Mars

Mars, mythical god of war, and the "red" planet, is an indicator in the horoscope of how an individual acts. Here you have a key as to the expression of assertiveness and personal power. The placement of Mars helps you understand your child's sense of personal identity, his or her manner of fighting or sticking up for self (or reluctance to do so), and the method of going after what he or she wants in the world.

No matter what sign Mars is in, the principle is still action. The sign tells us about the style of action. Some people get things done by plunging ahead very quickly and directly. Others may get things done better by working slowly and steadily. Still others find a way to get around the task, by getting someone else to do it, or by waiting to see if it will still be necessary to do it — the art of creative procrastination, shall we say? All of these alternatives and more are personal styles of action, and Mars in the birth chart can give us hints as to what that personal style might be. When you understand the style with which your child is most naturally comfortable (and how that might differ from your own favored style), you might also come to understand what you can do to motivate that child. By contrast, you can also learn to better understand which of your attempts to motivate are, instead, likely to cause the child to "put on the brakes" or "act out" — in other words, do just the opposite of what you would like.

Remember, the planets in signs represent "pure" types. The styles of action suggested by Mars in each sign may be substantially modified if Mars is in close relationship (aspect) with another planet whose basic themes are contradictory. Chapter Eight provides a look-up on aspects.

Mercury in Each Sign of the Zodiac

Mercury in Aries *or Mercury in House 1*

> *Let's get to the point,*
> *'Cause I can't wait.*
> *Speak up — or I will*
> *And you're too late!*

Your child thinks and speaks very quickly, which means he may actually talk early (Aries likes to be first!). Mercury in Aries is likely to impulsively speak out before thinking about how the words might "hit" others. He won't "beat around the bush." He will be direct, assertive, and sometimes insensitive. Always in a hurry, he will be quick to rush onward to a new thought. Patience is not his strong suit, and neither are details. You may have to frequently remind him that interrupting another person is not polite. He doesn't mean to be rude. It's just so hard to wait.

This kid will learn more quickly in an active environment, and this is important not only to know now, but to remember when it comes time to consider a day care or pre-school. Don't expect your child to be ready to sit still and methodically study too readily — if ever. Yet given the chance for freedom in self-expression, he will delight you with his curiosity and zest. Later you might well encourage activities such as debate. This kid will learn more by getting into the fray and challenging and being challenged than he will ever learn out of a book. You won't have to encourage him to speak up — just try to channel that talent into an appropriate form of expression!

*With **Mercury in House 1**, "who I am" for your kid is likely to mean he'll tell you...and tell you...and talk your ear off about everything else, too. He'll be curious, eager to learn, skilled with his hands, and he may be quick in motion, too. Remember that mythological image of Mercury, messenger of the gods, with wings on his feet? There he goes!*

Mercury in Taurus *or Mercury in House 2*

> *Just give me time*
> *To think it through.*
> *Then if I feel like it,*
> *I'll tell you.*

Your Mercury in Taurus child thinks slowly and deliberately. She may not say too much too fast, but when she does, what is said has most likely been thought through very thoroughly. This is a child who may come out with a first sentence, when you had about given up on that first word. She may get stuck in a rut mentally, because she is stubborn about changing her views, so be prepared to be patient. On the other hand, when you need her attention, you'll appreciate that she has a longer attention span than most children.

Your child may want the same bedtime story a zillion times — and she will have it memorized so you won't be able to get away with skipping parts. Her memory is strong, so if it takes her a little longer to learn something, she will be more likely to retain it than many other types.

In school, your child will thrive more on a calm and somewhat structured routine than on a too-busy environment, but allowances for independent work should be made, because she will work better at her own pace. She may not be too quick to speak up in class, but she will have the ability to stick to an assignment until it is finished, be thorough in its preparation, and remember what she has learned.

This child will probably enjoy singing, and is likely to have a nice voice. Learning can be augmented by an appeal to the tactile senses.

*For this **Mercury in House 2** kid, take a logical approach to saving those pennies for something special. She'll think it through and understand. Then point her in the direction of a bookstore! She probably can't be pushed, though. She likes to be comfortable and will learn at her own pace.*

Mercury in Gemini *or Mercury in House 3*

> *So much to see!*
> *So much to know!*
> *I'll do it all!*
> *Quick! Let's go!*

This clever, inquisitive, intelligent, bright mind needs lots of mental stimulation. Give him lots of books and lots of space, freedom and variety to feed his insatiable curiosity. Verbal abilities are very strong. Gemini Mercury is likely to talk early, and if exposed to multiple languages, will be easily able to pick them all up at once. This could be an advantage in later life, so don't suppress an opportunity for him to be around someone who speaks another language. Your child's interests will be many, and could be scattered. Because there are so many interesting things to do and see and know, he might have trouble deciding which way to go next.

He will learn quickly in school, but will have to be helped to acquire the self-discipline to stick with any subject long enough to learn it thoroughly. Pointing out new aspects of the subject may renew interest. A logical reason for doing it may convince. Repetitive tasks will bore him to distraction. If there's a short cut, Gemini will find it.

This kid will be quite articulate and never shy about speaking out. Encourage such activities as speech, debate, drama, creative writing.

Whatever you want to get across to this child had better make sense. Emotional appeals won't get you far; reason is much more likely to do the trick.

Mercury in House 3 may mean your child is restless, even scattered, with a short attention span that may not fit well within a structured school setting. On the plus side, he'll likely talk articulately and early, and be eager and quick to learn. He not only adapts easily to change, but may thrive on it. Curiosity plus!

Mercury in Cancer *or Mercury in House 4*

> *I don't think with my mind*
> *I think with my heart*
> *And I'll never forget you*
> *When we're apart.*

This position of Mercury often belongs to people who are described as having a photographic memory. Your child may soak up facts and details like a sponge and remember them forever. Yet "thinking" is not a natural mode — the word is "feeling." This kid thinks, learns and responds on an emotional level. Don't try to figure her out with logic and reason — it just won't work. Logical appeals won't work either; decisions are more likely to be made emotionally. Intuition is strong, perhaps psychic. Your child will know things but not be able to explain why or how. Yet, trust that she does KNOW. Something about what is going on inside her head will always be hidden.

The imagination is vivid, and will flourish through creative activities such as art, dance, drama, creative writing, poetry and lots of books. Encourage it! Your child will probably be quite conscientious about school work, but will not readily speak up unless she feels secure. Creative activities will help build confidence. This child needs to work at her own pace, not competitively. The best learning environment will be one that allows the child to learn through all of the senses — to feel and touch and smell — although the power of memory will aid in subjects where facts and lists are important.

Your child with **Mercury in House 4** *may soak up information like a little sea sponge. Intuitive, even psychic, she thinks what she feels, and feels what she thinks. She may clam up when she's feeling insecure. Stress within her home environment may be felt more than you think, even if you think it's going on out of her hearing range, so be aware. Confidence soars when homelife provides safety and intellectual stimulation.*

Mercury in Leo *or Mercury in House 5*

> *Listen! Have I got*
> *A story for you!*
> *You won't hear another*
> *So grand and so true!*

Exaggeration may be the word and style for this kid. If there is a way of dramatizing the situation, he will find it. Not a fib, mind you. He is honest. Maybe just stretches things a little bit! This is a talent that may find good use. The kid can probably sell anything. And persuade! If he wants something from you, watch out! He can employ humor, compliments — whatever it takes. Words may be accompanied by stagy gestures, facial expressiveness. He may have a natural ability to act whatever role serves the purpose of the moment.

If proper attention is not paid to him, Mercury in Leo may turn up the volume, just to make sure you don't miss the point. His enthusiasm and excitement for the idea he is trying to convey can be contagious at times — or annoying at others, when what YOU need is peace. Then the showman can become the showoff. You will have to help him learn when it is appropriate to "take the stage" and when it is best to yield to someone else.

The best learning environment for Mercury in Leo will be one in which creative expression is encouraged and much positive feedback is given. He needs praise and approval. He thrives on it. The more he feels admired and respected for his thoughts and his communication skills, the harder he will try.

*Tall tales and exaggeration may be an expression of **Mercury in House 5.** This is the house of creative self-expression, after all, and Mercury's function is communication. Expect a little drama, here. Perhaps encourage it and channel it through play-acting. Learning through games might appeal, too. Challenge him and have fun, at the same time as you're feeding his ability to mentally shine.*

Mercury in Virgo *or Mercury in House 6*

> *I think so very carefully*
> *I must know that this is true,*
> *Before I'm satisfied that I*
> *Can share my thoughts with you.*

This is a careful and cautious thinker. Until she knows she is right, your child is most unlikely to speak up or write. When she does, her ideas are built upon a meticulously thorough and logical analysis of all the facts and potentials and options. She will have organized her work carefully, planning each point that she intends to make. If it is written work, it will probably be quite precise and clear, with all the "t"s crossed and all the "i"s dotted. This kid is a perfectionist and a very hard worker. She will have a highly developed critical sense, which could make her an eagle-eyed proofreader of someone else's work, but which will most of all be directed at her own work. She will never be satisfied until it is right.

Little Mercury in Virgo is also likely to be very good at making things with her hands. She may like to work with models or with those little miniature statuettes that one must so carefully paint. She can be good at any very fine detailed work, and is also likely to be good at mechanical, technical skills. She likes to fix things. If her Sun is also in Virgo, she is likely to prefer working alone. Her style is rational and somewhat cool, with good common sense.

Trust her to handle your tools with respect and take care of them.

*With **Mercury in House 6,** this kid's thinking tends to be serious and detail oriented. She may be too hard on herself sometimes, and will need to be helped to look on the bright side. Though she'll not want to call a task complete until it's perfect, she can become bored and frustrated in the process. She might do better with a series of short-term things to do, rather than one long-lasting project. She'll likely be good with her hands, and should be encouraged in crafts.*

Mercury in Libra *or Mercury in House 7*

> *I don't like to argue,*
> *I'd rather agree.*
> *Can't we find a compromise*
> *To please both you and me?*

Libra is the sign most associated with relationships, which may suggest emotional issues, but Libra is an air sign. Your Mercury in Libra child takes an intellectual approach, rather than an emotional one. He will think through a situation with cool objectivity, comparing and contrasting the alternatives from every angle. It is very important to him to resolve any conflict harmoniously. For that reason, he will sometimes get "stuck" between the pros and cons, and have great difficulty making up his mind, because he has been unable to find the balance point where everyone can be satisfied. If it is possible, he will end up with a compromise position that allows him to stay in the middle, to some measure "having the cake and eating it, too." In a conflict between others, your child may be a good mediator. He is not likely to say anything to upset things, if he can possibly avoid it. He greatly dislikes strife. Therefore he is sometimes prone to tell others what they want to hear, even if he privately does not agree with it. His style of communication is refined. He is mannerly and cordial, even charming, and very fair — one who might be described as a born diplomat. He will work well in a team or within a group, will most likely prefer that to working alone. This child will learn best in a harmonious, pleasant environment.

Your child with **Mercury in House 7** *will look for intellectual stimulation from his close one-to-one relationships. He's a communicator, likely to develop good "people skills." He'll be very interested in fairness, and may be quite a little diplomat in mediating disputes. Encourage interests in public speaking and debate, as he moves up in school.*

Mercury in Scorpio *or Mercury in House 8*

> *Some things I'll tell you*
> *But others I'll hide*
> *You'll never know*
> *What I keep deep inside.*

Mercury in Scorpio will want to cut through the superficialities and get down to business. "Tell it like it is!" she might say to others. Or if she does not feel like she is getting a complete picture, she will probe and dig until she finds out what she wants to know. Yet, this child may not be so direct with you. She will never let others know all she knows. A few things will be kept back, just in case, just to make sure, just to use if needed.

In this little one you may see signs of a budding researcher or investigator, or perhaps a lawyer or politician, too, if her emotions are controlled. Her mind is deep and incisive, skeptical and shrewd. Her manner of expression can be very forceful and persuasive and passionately convincing. Sometimes the emotions get in the way of the thinking, however, when she gets upset, and then the expression might turn to sarcasm and cutting comments. This child won't dodge a confrontation, and in fact may meet it head-on, if the issue really matters. Self-control, particularly of the emotions, will need to be developed.

Your child is likely to learn best in an environment that permits independent study, and a considerable amount of privacy. She needs access to a library, and teachers who are willing to let her take things apart and examine them. Debate could be a good activity to encourage when she is older. It will help her develop control.

Mercury in House 8 suggests an intuitive mind, curious and probing. Don't think you'll easily keep secrets from this kid! If, on the other hand, she wants to keep something from you, you'll have a hard time prying it out of her. She needs a good deal of privacy and space to think her own thoughts. She may have psychic ability. When she's really interested in something, she'll study it intensely.

Mercury in Sagittarius *or Mercury in House 9*

> *What an awesome idea!*
> *Exciting! So true!*
> *I believe it. I'll tell you,*
> *And you'll think so, too!*

This is a curious, inquisitive mind who will probably ask you more "whys" than you ever thought anyone could. Many of the questions will be tough ones to answer, because they will be on complex subjects like God and ethics and what makes things the way they are. Pat answers won't satisfy, they'll just breed more questions. That something "IS" does NOT answer "why." This child needs a learning environment where he is free to ask any question, discuss any issue. Rigid, conformist schools and teachers would be terribly stifling to his spirit.

One possible problem with this child's manner of thinking is that he is prone to jump to conclusions. A new idea will catch his fancy and the Archer's little arrow will pierce right through to the center and pull him along, just like a string was attached. He has made a leap of faith, and is just sure that "this is it" and may even immediately rush to convert everyone who will listen. The details? The possible other side? Lost in the rush. Though this kid is likely to be a quick, bright student, who will pick up concepts with a minimum of study, he may be prone to mistakes because of the tendency to rush ahead.

Honesty and truth are all-important. And your child is more than likely to let you know what is on his mind — bluntly. Sag is sometimes described by the saying, "open mouth, insert foot." In other words, sometimes he speaks before he thinks. You may need to help him learn the art of diplomacy.

*With **Mercury in House 9,** the mind focuses on the entire "forest" rather than the individual "tree." This kid thinks big, with optimism. He is eager to learn, and is likely to be especially interested in ideas, people and places* outside of his normal environment. *A lively, outgoing communicator, he may be prone to jump to conclusions, to speak before he thinks. He'll do best when home and school stimulate ideas, experimentation and a sense of adventure.*

Mercury in Capricorn *or Mercury in House 10*

> *In all seriousness, now,*
> *If I know that I know it,*
> *I might even structure*
> *My thoughts as a poet!*

This is a very practical, down-to-earth, let's-stick-to-business, manner of thinking. This kid is careful, making sure she is right before she speaks or writes. She will not speak up quickly, and when she does, she is most often serious and polite and respectful, choosing her words with care. Yet she may have a wry sense of humor that will surprise you at times! Often she is especially deft at self-directed humor. It is perhaps a release from all that seriousness.

Don't expect your child to devote much interest to any subject for which she does not see a practical value in the "real world" in which she lives, or expects to live. Abstractions do not appeal. If she does not see how she will use it, she may refuse to try at all — unless her sense of status has focused on being on the honor role, in which case she may study the subject, just to get the grade. She will care about getting ahead.

This child will learn best in an organized, structured environment. Even if she is a creative artist, she will be more productive with deadlines to meet, and project outlines to work within. When she has an assignment, she will approach it with thoroughness and a strong ability to concentrate. Early inhibitions in expression are best broken down with increases in skill. The more she knows, the greater will be her confidence. But spontaneous she will seldom be — unless perhaps Sun is in Sagittarius. Even then, she will be a cautious, practical thinker. Fanciful dreams she may weave, but she'll find a way to weave them into usefulness.

The manner of thinking for **Mercury in House 10** *is serious and pragmatic. Since this house represents parental authority, your example will be especially important as to whether "serious" will mean an overly timid and self-critical little person, or a good organizer whose ability to think realistically becomes a major asset in school, and later, in her career. It will be most natural for her to study hard, and follow the rules. When she lacks confidence, she may clam up. When she knows her topic she can be very articulate.*

Mercury in Aquarius *or Mercury in House 11*

> *Just when you think*
> *You might know what I'll say*
> *I'll be off on a new thought*
> *And tell you MY way!*

This kid will surprise, and hopefully delight, you with his original and inventive thoughts. But if you are a traditionalist, be prepared to have a few of your ideas challenged by this unconventional thinker. Your Mercury in Aquarius is likely to be attracted to the new, the unusual, the offbeat, the fantastic and the futuristic. The mind is bright, and grasps new ideas quickly, sometimes with flashes of insight. The fact that the new idea may be considered inappropriate or uncomfortable for parents or teachers will not particularly impress your child. Indeed, he may enjoy shocking you a little with it! And he will let you know what he thinks, rather outspokenly. Some ideas may be put out just to try the wind, and see what reaction he gets.

You'd be best off to develop an attitude of tolerant interest and bounce some ideas back, without emotion. An emotional reaction to an uncomfortable idea is more likely to impress its virtue even more strongly on your free-thinker's mind, and then he will defend it to the bitter end. His mind is fixed and stubborn when he wants to be. He is not impressed by emotion, and in fact is quite detached and dispassionate. Logic and reason may convince, but not emotion, and not any statement about standards of what others may deem proper. But consider this, when challenging and questioning authority, your child is learning, in what is probably the best way for him to learn. Provide a learning environment where intellectual freedom is encouraged, where new technologies are explored, and where teachers are open-minded and sharp.

Your child with **Mercury in House 11** *is likely to be quite sociable, and attracted to friends and groups who are original and perhaps even rebellious in their thinking. Don't expect him—them—to agree with your more conventional ideas. Best to not make an issue of it, unless his safety is involved. (Letting some things pass with openness gives you more leverage in matters that are really serious.) Healthy interests might be stimulated through exposure to computers, or to groups involved in helping/healing causes.*

Mercury in Pisces *or Mercury in House 12*

> *I'm not sure how to put in words*
> *The things I feel down deep.*
> *Perhaps I can tell you through art or song*
> *Or a dream that I'll send when you sleep.*

Astrologers have been known to describe this placement of Mercury as one in which the student may learn as much by sleeping with the book under her pillow as by reading it. Well, that may be an exaggeration — or maybe not. In any case, this child is very sensitive and intuitive, and learns like a sponge, soaking up elements from her environment and processing them in nonverbal ways. She absorbs information in whole gulps rather than in separate steps or details. At memorizing lists and dates she may have problems, but at understanding whole underlying concepts, she may be quite good — although she may have difficulty putting into words what she actually understands quite well.

The imagination is very rich and vivid, and it can and should be constructively channeled into poetry, art and music. Your child has deep feelings and a talent for images that need an outlet for expression. She may have natural ability for acting or singing. She is likely to be very creative in the arts. Mercury in Pisces will probably not be interested in abstract or detailed studies like math or science, and she is not by nature particularly practical or logical. She will be attracted to the spiritual and the romantic, or to things that are shrouded in mystery. Give her a learning environment that allows reign for her imagination and creativity, and stimulates the expression of her deep feelings. Empathy for others may alternatively lead her into a helping/healing direction.

*With **Mercury in House 12**, your child has a very vivid imagination and may be empathic. She may need your help and understanding in sorting out what is logical from her fantasies, in reconciling bad things she may see in the real world with her ideas of the way things should be, or in separating what she really feels from what she is picking up from those around her. Expose her to opportunities in music and the arts.*

Venus in Each Sign of the Zodiac

Venus in Aries *or Venus in House 1*

> *I like excitement*
> *Sparkling bright*
> *I live in the "Now"*
> *With love and light!*

The child with Venus in Aries is attracted to energy, initiative, independence and lots of action. She may "take to" a new friend very quickly, especially if that person has some "sparkle." But the friend will have to keep "sparkling" or your child may move on to someone else.

The "Now" has great appeal; the future is too far off to bear. Money, therefore, is likely to "burn a hole in the pocket." Don't expect this kid to be very good at saving part of an allowance! The term "impulse buyer" was probably coined with an Aries type in mind.

The expression of affection comes naturally to your Venus in Aries child. Quick, enthusiastic hugs will come easy and often — you'll want to give them as well as receive them, with energy and joy.

Art forms that are bright, quick and free will appeal, and encourage creativity. Try your tot at a painting easel with big brushes and bright jars of tempera paint — and a big, old shirt for a smock, with an even bigger plastic drop to cover the floor! Try dance lessons. Choose a peppy, free-spirited teacher. Try books that have accompanying musical/game audio-cassettes.

*With **Venus in House 1**, your child's sense of "who I am" is to be closely tied to how she looks and to what she has (her possessions). Most likely she is naturally attractive and graceful, and craves pretty things to enhance those attributes. She may express affection directly, openly and easily. She may have artistic talent, and should be given the opportunity to try visual arts, music and dance.*

Venus in Taurus *or Venus in House 2*

> *My love is loyal*
> *My heart is true*
> *In comfort I'll savor*
> *My life with you.*

Pleasure and enjoyment can come from all things sensual. Your child is attracted by romantic music (and may have a pleasant voice and like to sing), by the feel of fabrics and textures (try encouraging sculpture—Play-Dough for a tot—weaving or other crafts), by good tastes (especially sweets, which may bear some watching). When he is little, allow him to touch many different textures, for this will help him learn better than just seeing or hearing — and he'll enjoy the process a lot more, too. But take along a packet of those moist/wipes, because whatever he touches is also likely to be tasted soon after!

Your Venus in Taurus child prefers relaxed, calm and comfortable relationships, with cuddling and warm affection. He will be very loyal to you and to his friends, so long as his interactions are basically comfortable. Rowdiness, quick handling and loudness will not appeal.

Venus in Taurus can likely be counted upon to handle money and other possessions carefully and responsibly. An allowance with encouragement to save part of it will probably work at an early age with this child. He will enjoy various collections of things. Provide a space for them. This child will most likely enjoy and be able to take proper responsibility for a small, soft pet, and this would be a good outlet for expression of affection.

*Your child with **Venus in House 2** has a strong desire to be comfortable. An easy-going personality, he prefers calm handling and a peaceful environment. He may be quite a collector, because his sense of security is fed by having things—and money—tucked away. Teaching the prudent handling* *of an allowance should be easy with this kid. He'll like giving and receiving hugs, too!*

Venus in Gemini *or Venus in House 3*

> *I'm not really fickle,*
> *There's just so much to do.*
> *Don't expect me to stick*
> *Too close to you.*

This kid thoroughly enjoys learning. Satisfying her insatiable curiosity about life, people and everything within reach gives much pleasure. She will be playful and flirtatious in expressing affection, but may seem a bit superficial or fickle. It's only her need for variety and a lighter touch. Don't try to confine this "will-o'-the-wisp!"

Talking and all forms of communication are important in all of her relationships. She is attracted to bright minds and quick wit. Your Venus in Gemini will probably be sociable, kind and sympathetic — and she likes to receive the same from others. But she is too detached and "in the head" for sentiment and "mush." Keep it light. Express closeness and affection through talking and listening. Curl up together and share a book, or even a video. But don't just read or watch it — talk about it. Trade opinions, ask questions, stimulate ideas.

Art and beauty in a variety of forms and colors will appeal, so long as it can be done quickly. Try free painting, even finger-painting, and lively dance and singing (a pleasant voice is likely). In the handling of money and possessions, objectivity and reasonableness prevails; possessions of a mental nature (books, as an obvious example) will be prized.

*With **Venus in House 3**, your child likes to communicate with grace and beauty. She might express herself through singing, or perhaps through writing poetry or prose. She probably won't push too hard in school, though—she prefers to take it easy. Ease in her social contacts is important to her, too. Naturally tactful, she's likely to say whatever is necessary to keep the peace.*

Venus in Cancer *or Venus in House 4*

> *I love to be cozy*
> *Right here with you.*
> *Cuddle me close,*
> *I'll take care of you, too.*

Emotional warmth and feelings of closeness within the family are very important for your child in order for him to enjoy life. Some kids can't wait to get out and explore the world; this one will genuinely like being at home, doing things with you and other family members. You might have to give him a nudge to get him out of the nest! It is essential to his sense of comfort to feel part of a family. A strong foundation in family relationships will contribute considerably to his success in life outside the family.

When disciplining this child, make sure he knows that although the behavior may be unacceptable, you do love him. Insecurities about feeling loved are likely to result in shyness, overprotectiveness, excessive possessiveness or forming dependency attachments to others outside the immediate homelife. Your child is by nature quite affectionate, protective and nurturing, and will appreciate receiving such expressions of affection from you, too.

Venus in Cancer is a faithful friend, more likely to choose a few very close relationships, rather than many friends. Whether boy or girl, such a child, when small, will especially like to have special dolls or stuffed animals to love, and would probably also greatly benefit from taking care of a small pet. He is likely to handle money cautiously and well, so it should be fairly easy to teach him how to handle an allowance.

Your child with **Venus in House 4** *finds security in a comfortable, attractive and stable home. The emotional warmth you, as a nurturing parent, provide becomes a highly significant role model for his future relationships. He may nurture any insecure feelings with food, or by holding onto possessions, never wanting to throw anything away. Give him lots of affection.*

Venus in Leo *or Venus in House 5*

> *I love life!*
> *I love you!*
> *With passion! With drama!*
> *Please love me, too!*

This kid will want to be in the center of whatever excitement is going on. She is a "people person" and will rarely ever be content to stay on the sidelines for long. She craves excitement and drama in her life, and she thrives on attention and approval from others. For friends, she will tend to be attracted to the most popular and fun-loving group, because that is where the spotlight is. And she is likely to have enough charisma to hold her own within that crowd.

Venus in Leo's innate sense of honor and fairness means that she will not be so influenced by her friends that she will go along with behavior that is dishonorable. Also, it would be well to teach her to seek the good qualities of the kids that are not so much in the spotlight. Whatever friends she chooses, she is likely to want to be a leader and gain their admiration and respect. This is a child to whom you may have to gently teach the potential advantages of letting others have their way sometimes. Appeal to her natural warmth and generosity.

Your child will be enthusiastic and even passionate in expressing her affection. Give her lots of big hugs back. The more love and approval she feels as a tot, the greater will be her growing confidence.

Encourage her creative zest with opportunities for dramatic self-expression. Role-playing games with costumes (old clothes for dress-up play) and fantasy will be lots of fun. Perhaps there's a community junior theater where she could take classes, or a neighborhood dance studio. Get large rolls of plain wrapping paper and some tempera paints, spread it across the yard and let her invite some friends to paint a large, gay mural.

*This child, with **Venus in House 5**, is more than likely to express herself through some creative talent. She craves the spotlight, thrives on approval, and may have a natural charisma and a flair for the dramatic. How she looks and what she has are very important to her self-esteem and her sense of security—she wants to be proud of both appearance and possessions.*

Venus in Virgo *or Venus in House 6*

> *Do you have a problem?*
> *What can I do?*
> *Is it broken? I'll fix it!*
> *I love to help you!*

Your Venus in Virgo child will tend to be most comfortable in expressing affection by doing nice things for you and for others whom he likes. He is not naturally demonstrative, and indeed he may be rather shy. Probably depending upon other things in the chart as well, sometimes this Venus placement denotes a person who is reserved about physical contact, and at other times it belongs to one who is quite earthy and sensual. The former type may be rather cool about cuddling, while the latter may crave it. Even the earthy one, though, is unlikely to be overt about it or take much initiative unless he feels safe. Either way, little Virgo tends to be modest. You'll know which style your child prefers by how closely he snuggles when you read him bedtime stories. If you have a snuggler, he will be happiest with frequent hugs!

There's nothing that this child enjoys more than feeling competent and needed. So one of the best things you can do for him is provide opportunities for the development of skills. Teach him to do the practical little things that need to be done and then let him help you. Provide craft materials and tools so he can make things, or fix things that are broken. You'll be able to easily teach him how to do things carefully and neatly.

Your child is most likely to seek dependability in others. He has innate common sense, and will tend to expect that quality in friends as well.

Venus in House 6 *means that this child's sense of security is very tied up with his feelings of competence in what he does. At the same time, he likes his work to be easy and enjoyable. Start at a very early age to teach him how* to do little daily tasks for himself. Make a game of it! He may also thrive on the development of arts and crafts skills.

Venus in Libra *or Venus in House 7*

> *I want everything nice*
> *And pretty, too.*
> *If you're kind and polite*
> *Then I'll like you.*

Venus in Libra is a seeker of beauty. She is attracted to that which is harmonious, peaceful, balanced, serene, refined and aesthetically pleasing. Not only is she attracted to these things, but she actually requires this kind of environment in order to be comfortable. She also needs to feel attractive and "put together" in her own appearance in order to feel at ease. This is NOT to say she is a super neatnik. Artful disorder is more than possible, especially the state in which she may leave her room after a flurry of deciding what to wear and getting ready to go somewhere. She, however, will emerge from the mess looking terrific — everything coordinated and every hair in place.

In your child's associates she will also tend to choose refinement. Rowdiness, crudity and sloppiness are major turn-offs. She generally greets others with politeness, even charm, and she shows that she likes them by being nice and considerate. This child is most apt to defer to her companions' preferences, unless her own preference really matters a great deal. One thing she will insist upon is that things are fair. She will defer and she will be nice — but she will probably not be imposed upon, at least not for long.

This child will have great appreciation for the arts, and quite probably talent in one or more art forms. See that she has plenty of opportunities to try various kinds — painting, drawing, crafts, dance, vocal and instrumental music. Take her to concerts, art museums, the theater.

*With **Venus in House 7**, your child's sense of security may be very tied up in her close one-to-one relationships: her best friend, and in later life, her choice of partner. With her natural charm and diplomacy, she'll most likely be attracted to refinement and charm, and disdain rowdiness. Fair play is important to her—she'll insist on it.*

Venus in Scorpio *or Venus in House 8*

> *My love is so strong*
> *As deep as the sea,*
> *Words can't express*
> *What you mean to me!*

In expression of affection, for your Venus in Scorpio child, it's likely to be all or nothing. Scorpio is a sign associated with extremes and great emotional intensity. If he loves you, he loves you fiercely and deeply. If you give him reason to doubt you, he may at first try possessiveness or even jealousy. But if he feels really betrayed, he may detach from you completely on an emotional level — forever. Once emotionally detached, Scorpio may be cordial, even friendly, but the passion toward the former love is gone.

This child will probably not form a great many friendships. He is not interested in superficialities. Friends with whom he can feel a deep connection and strong mutual trust will be the only ones he considers to be worth having. His few close friends are likely to remain friends forever, and he will be very loyal to them. Because his friends are few, he may be inclined to be possessive of them, which in some cases might, of course, cause problems if the chosen friend is a type who does not wish to be possessed. Your child may have to learn a few hard lessons in the area of control vs. freedom.

There could be a magnetic, seductive type of attractiveness in this child, with perhaps an aura of mystery. He may cultivate such qualities, because he enjoys having secrets and the sense of power they give him.

In art forms, Venus in Scorpio will also be attracted to power and intensity. His outlet might be expressionistic painting, deeply emotional music, interpretive dance or drama. Expose him to opportunities to find such an outlet for the expression of his deep feelings. He may have trouble verbalizing them, if they are very intense. But he needs to get them out.

*For your child with **Venus in House 8,** sharing is very important. He will tend to be very intense and possessive about his few close friendships. Before he learns to balance his needs for closeness with the rights and preferences of his little friends, you may have to witness and mediate a series of power struggles. An artistic outlet may help provide an outlet for him to express his deep feelings.*

Venus in Sagittarius *or Venus in House 9*

> *Isn't life wonderful!*
> *Isn't it great!*
> *We're perfect together,*
> *It's gotta be fate!*

That little verse may be one you hear just days or hours before that object of your child's affections is history and she is off in search of a new ideal. With this kid the affections are likely to be an open book. Her preferences are seldom, if ever, hidden. She is friendly and outgoing — if she likes you, you know it. She doesn't, and you're probably just not there any more. She is busy with someone else.

Don't ever try to fence her in. She needs freedom, and if you try to tie her down too much, the relationship — be it parent/child, friend, or lover — has little chance of lasting. That doesn't mean she can't be loyal or have a long-standing relationship. She is VERY conscious of fairness, ethics, honesty and honor. She will just not be able to understand NOT being trusted, and NOT having you understand that she is ONLY being friendly with those others.

For those your child cares about, nothing is too good. She is generous, sometimes grandly so. (Watch that allowance — it's likely to burn a hole in her pocket if she sees something that would please a special friend.)

Your Venus in Sagittarius child likes excitement; she likes to have fun. The great outdoors is hers to explore. She is out for adventure and is probably willing to take some risks to have it. She is eager to learn, generally optimistic and very idealistic about life. She expects the best of people… and consequently is sometimes disappointed. But she won't be "down" for long. There's too much to do and see. Nature will likely be a major source of inspiration for her if she is an artist.

*Your **Venus in House 9** child may have a real love of learning. She'll especially enjoy people and places that are different from her normal environment. Read to her about them from when she's a tot. She'll be adventurous and idealistic, enthusiastic and fun-loving. She may put her "best friends" on a pedestal and be disappointed if they don't live up to her ideal. Ethics, honor and trust are very important to her.*

Venus in Capricorn *or Venus in House 10*

> *Did I forget to mention,*
> *How much you mean to me?*
> *By working hard, I honor you,*
> *I would think that you could see.*

Reserved is a word you might use to describe your Venus in Capricorn child. He keeps his emotions under control. No hearts worn on this sleeve. He is most likely to express his love for you by being responsible, both in attending to whatever duties he feels he owes you, and by working hard for success in his own areas of interest, thereby to increase his status, which will reflect well on you. You're not likely to get many big hugs and "I love yous" from this child, but hey — the trade-off may well be less worry than most parents have. This kid really enjoys being responsible. He will probably even enjoy the company of you old folks, and be quite respectful of what you can teach him about life and love. It's important that you very frequently show him that you love him—cuddle your tot, and be generous with hugs, smiles and affectionate pats on the shoulder as he gets older. He may have a hard time showing his affection unless he feels very sure of being loved—but he cares. This position of Venus usually reflects a quite sensible and stable love nature, one who is mature and faithful.

A possible downside: status and achievement are so important there could be an inclination to choose friends for status, or what they can do for him. Some may feel this is just smart, but if your child does not get beneath the surface with his friends, he could miss the more intangible riches that nurture the soul. Help him to look for inner gold in others.

In arts and pleasures, the practical will have the most appeal, therefore handicrafts that have a useful purpose may be the best choice to suggest.

Your child with **Venus in House 10** *takes pleasure in being responsible and in being recognized for his achievements. He may not be especially inclined to work hard, if he can think of an easier way, but he will work hard if necessary, to gain that recognition he seeks. Your pride in him will inspire. He may show talent in the arts and should be exposed to opportunities to develop his creative abilities.*

Venus in Aquarius *or Venus in House 11*

> *I'm a little offbeat,*
> *And I must be free!*
> *If you're like that, too,*
> *Then friends we'll be!*

Venus in Aquarius is very gregarious, friendly, open and quick to give hugs... but DON'T get too close! Closeness crowds her, possessiveness is scary. This kid needs lots of space and freedom. She likes being liked, and wants lots of friends, so long as no one demands that she be anything other than unique, original and one-of-a-kind. She may be inclined not to choose "best friends," but rather to be as happy to play with one friend as another, so long as what they are doing is "fun," meaning new and interesting. Aquarius tends to be afraid that becoming too closely attached may result in loss of freedom.

Your child is very tolerant of others who are different, and in fact, tends to be attracted to those who are different, unusual, unconventional — perhaps even those who are somewhat bizarre, in the opinion of the mainstream. Her affections are not really fickle; she has the stick-to-itiveness to be loyal if she chooses. But the relationship will have to remain exciting and open, with an element of freedom. She will work well with others in groups and on teams, unless her goals do not coincide with the groups', in which case she will either attempt to reform the group to her tastes, or will leave and find another group.

In arts, too, this child is more likely to like the new and unconventional, that which is nontraditional. However, this does not necessarily mean you are doomed to experience the most extreme trends of teen-age music and dress—unless you make it attractive to use that form of rebellion against your tastes. If the peer group is too conformist in its nonconformity, your kid could just as well decide it expresses her individuality to love opera or the symphony! Be cool!

Your child with **Venus in House 11** *loves to be with friends and enjoys clubs and group activities. She may be attracted to groups that are a bit off-*

beat and eccentric, or groups that are involved in the arts. She likes her freedom, though. She has lots of friends, rather than "best friends." Since she likes to be easy-going, and tends to be emotionally detached, she may be one who can mediate little disputes among others.

Venus in Pisces *or Venus in House 12*

> *Magical music*
> *Through my dreams I see*
> *Singing deep in my soul*
> *That my true love loves me!*

Your Venus in Pisces may be a dreamy child, and a romantic to his very soul. So great is his sense of idealism that he may be inclined to spin fantasies around the ones he loves and place them on pedestals. He will be very unselfish about wanting to help others. Put these things together and you have the potential of one who could go overboard in "doing for" someone who is really not worthy of all the affection and attention he is giving. He will continue to see them as he wants to see them, or as he is sure they will be with just a little more help. Your child is inclined to be rather gentle and sensitive, and/or he will be attracted to that kind of person. Rowdy, loud or crude people will intimidate him.

Little Venus in Pisces has a very vivid and creative imagination, which will be of great help if he is steered in an artistic direction. You would do well to encourage his dreams, fantasies and imaginings to be expressed in music, dance, art or creative writing. No way will you be able to stop the dreaming, yet used productively, he may become an accomplished artist. Play to it! Read him fairy and fantasy tales when he is a tot, and as he grows, provide opportunities for his sampling of various artist pursuits to see which ones appeal the most. Your child may well find his best means of communicating through art or music, and being able to express his feelings this way will greatly enrich his life, no matter what career he ends up pursuing — and his imaginative expressions will probably enrich your life, as well.

Your child with **Venus in House 12** *may be quite a dreamer. His private world is beautiful and romantic—the real world can't compete. He may escape into his own secret inner place to avoid conflicts. You won't stop him from dreaming, so provide a healthy channel for him to express his feelings through creating beauty in art or music activities.*

Mars in Each Sign of the Zodiac

Mars in Aries *or Mars in House 1*

> *I just have to be active*
> *I don't want to be bad*
> *But if you make me sit here*
> *I'll be restless or mad!*

Mars is the natural planetary "ruler" of Aries, so in this sign the assertive energy is stronger than in any other. This child needs plenty of space and freedom to be active. You won't have to encourage the little Ram — just find a safe area to let it happen! This fiery style of action has competitive instincts that are strong, so early opportunities to develop skill in some competitive sport would be very good.

A small child with Mars in Aries will be especially restless if asked to sit still too long. Keep that in mind when considering your choice of day care or school programs, as well as your own comfort in taking your child places where other adults will not like being distracted by a very active little "ball of fire!" You'll need to have plenty of things to keep this one busy.

Your child, unless several other things in the chart contradict, will be a natural leader. He will want to get there first and do it in his own way. Provide plenty of opportunities where this child can be spontaneous, take the initiative, try new things. He will be better at starting things than finishing them, so short term projects will work best, will be the happiest for both of you, and the most encouraging for your child's success.

Energy repressed could pop out in angry flare-ups, or if very suppressed, even in sudden fevers. Understand that the child must have ways to release excess energy and anger. Trying to put the clamps on him may give you momentary peace, but at a greater cost at another time. Instead, you should think about what can be provided within your environment to permit his constructive release of energy. Teach this child ways of working off his anger in some nondestructive but physically active manner.

Your child with **Mars in House 1** *has a fiery energy that is right out front. Be prepared! He'll hit the floor running as soon as he can walk, and you'll need to be in good shape, yourself, to keep up with him! He has plenty of initiative—but may jump before he thinks. Temper flare-ups are usually quickly over. Channel this ball-of-fire into constructive physical activities, perhaps competitive sports. (Remember, even though this paragraph, in my alternating style, says "he," your little girl with Mars in House 1, may be quite a "tomboy." Don't try to suppress that energy. Channel it!)*

Mars in Taurus *or Mars in House 2*

> *Let me take my time*
> *Don't push me so fast*
> *I might do it the best*
> *Even if I'm done last.*

Your Mars in Taurus child may seem to be a quiet type, but it is a quiet strength. Her style of asserting herself is one of steady persistence, never stopping until the goal is achieved. She may be reluctant to start a project, but when other types drop out and falter, this child will doggedly continue until what she has begun is completed.

Your child's energy may not be overt; she is not particularly competitive, but her endurance is strong. Expose her to opportunities for appropriate physical activities, the kind where carefully developed skill, strength and endurance are measures of success, rather than quick action and speed.

Mars in Taurus will be very slow to anger — naturally calm. Yet like the complacent bull who is provoked into "seeing red," there are limits beyond which such an individual just won't be pushed. If provoked to fight, your child will be a tough opponent who won't give up. Or, in a quiet but stubborn style, she may be inclined to follow that old adage, "I don't get mad, I get even."

Try to choose a calm day care or school environment for this child, one where an expected routine is followed, and children are allowed to work at their own pace. Your Mars in Taurus will not perform well for a high-key adult who wants students to move faster or change more quickly than they may be ready for. But she will be an absolute joy to a teacher who appreciates thoroughness and responsibility.

*With **Mars in House 2,** your child will move at her own steady pace, no matter how much that may frustrate you or others who want her to move faster. On the plus side, she has a longer attention span than most kids her age, which will help her settle into early school routines well. She may seem calm and easy-going, but she can be very stubborn at any attempts to push her around. She'll stick up for her own preferences and her own comfort.*

Mars in Gemini *or Mars in House 3*

> *So many things to do and be*
> *How I can I choose just one?*
> *Come and try them all with me,*
> *And we'll have lots of fun!*

This child is able to do a variety of things. Versatility is his basic nature. Mars in Gemini is usually good with the hands, with all manner of manual dexterity. The coordination is good, and excellent motor abilities are likely to develop early. All this should be encouraged.

Your active little Gemini type is quick and clever, and he may be good at sports that require the combination of thought and fast action, such as tennis, fencing, basketball or dancing. He probably won't like rough sports, though.

A bundle of energy, your child will be restless if expected to be still for long. It's different than the restlessness discussed under Mars in Aries. Gemini isn't restless because there's something else he is burning to "get out of here" and go do. Gemini might not know what he wants to do — maybe flit like that butterfly over there, or fly away on the next breeze — it's just too boring to sit here! Provide plenty of time and space for this kid to be "on the go" with safety. Good books might hold the older child still for a while — as the mind takes flight — but for the little one, it's probably best to avoid occasions that necessitate sitting still.

All activities will be some way or another tied to his mental processes. When Mars in Gemini must stick up for his own rights, a spirited and clever verbal defense — or offense — is much more likely to be the favored mode of action than any form of physical fighting.

Because your child likes to do, and is able to do, so many things, it can sometimes be difficult to focus on one. You will need to help him learn both to get started and to follow through on a task. Be aware, though, that successful work for this child will allow for a variety of tasks, or being able to move from one thing to another. Success in motivating him will be best found in matching that style, rather than expecting one thing to be completely finished before he is allowed to start on another. Give him the chance to see if he can "juggle more than one ball" without dropping any of them.

*Your child with **Mars in House 3** is a very independent thinker with a restless energy that is constantly curious and eager to learn anything and everything. He is likely to be noted for his versatility, both mentally and in skills that require good coordination and manual dexterity. He'll be quick to speak up when he has something to say. Later, in school, encourage him in debate and other speech activities.*

Mars in Cancer *or Mars in House 4*

> *I feel so very strongly*
> *Sometimes I let it show*
> *But other times I hold it back*
> *And never let you know.*

Emotions rise to the surface quickly for your Mars in Cancer, which could result in upsetting outbursts. Or it could result in an unhealthy internal holding back and even a tummy ache. You will need to help this child learn how to express her upset or irritation over minor frustrations in an acceptably normal manner. Your example in regard to your own language and actions in expressing upset is, of course, the best teacher — so be aware! Other options that might be suggested: a private punching pillow or a "worry doll" to whom your child can talk. Remember, holding back is not the answer; getting it out acceptably is.

Home and family are very important to this child. She needs to feel protected and secure, and will do best in everything when those needs are met. Like the little Crab hiding in its shell, this type may be more likely to withdraw than to be assertive in regard to personal needs, but, at the same time, is quite capable of being assertive in the protection/defense of those she cares about.

In regard to sports, your Mars in Cancer child is likely to especially enjoy water activities. (One friend delighted her "water babies" by running a hose down their backyard slide.) She might also like miniature golf, badminton or dancing. Activities of a quieter nature are preferable to very physical or competitive ones. It may be difficult for this child to depersonalize losing.

With this highly emotional sign type, feelings are very tied up with actions. Crying is usually a healthier release for hurt feelings or feeling bad about losing, than withdrawal into a shell. The latter could cause premature quitting rather than chance facing further hurt. Alternating gender pronouns for these paragraphs came up with "she" for this one, but remember that the old "little boys don't cry" idea is out-of-style these days and good riddance. With this (or any sign type, for that matter), never belittle your child when he or she is hurt. Listen with empathy and acknowledge your child's feelings as OK. Then express confidence in his or her ability to improve with practice.

This child will greatly enjoy collecting things, and she will probably be imaginative and creative, with a flair for handicrafts.

You, as the nurturing parent and role model, will have strong influence upon how your child with **Mars in House 4** *learns to handle assertiveness—whether she is independent and self-confident in expressing herself, or whether she suppresses and holds back. She identifies with her home and with you, and will be caring and protective. On the other hand, she needs some independence within her home—a space of her own, where she can arrange things as she chooses.*

Mars in Leo *or Mars in House 5*

> *Right there in the center*
> *I must be!*
> *The star! The spotlight*
> *Shines on me!*

The natural place for Mars in Leo to like to do most anything is in the Sun — or in the spotlight. This enthusiastic, usually "sunny" people-person will want to be on the go and in the center of whatever is happening. This Mars type probably has a great deal of energy and vitality, is concerned about how he looks, and will have extra motivation to take good care of his own body. You won't have to encourage this kid to get out of the house and do things. On the contrary, just try keeping little Leo home! No, you may as well just go along and watch the games or play from the sidelines, and be prepared to applaud! Your Mars in Leo child is likely to enjoy team sports, and will strive to be the star. He may also be attracted to drama or any of the performing arts. This kid does not like to lose, however, and will be the "sunniest" if his role is a leading one.

Pride is very strong in your child. Count on this one to want to be honorable and fair and to earn his applause. If Mars in Leo knows you have high expectations, he will try very hard to not only live up to them, but exceed them. This child is not likely to handle any perceived offense to his dignity, though. It is important to treat such a little person honorably and with respect.

Expose your child to various opportunities — sports, drama, art activities, dance — to see what attracts. Then follow the child's lead on what he wants to pursue. Your Mars in Leo will do the best, try the hardest and enjoy the most what he has chosen on his own personal initiative. This kid can be quite fixed about wanting to make his own choices. The harder you try to push your "thing," the more stubbornly this one may resist and in order to pursue his own individual choices.

What your child with **Mars in House 5** *loves is to be on the go, and in the center of activity. He is courageous and competitive, and he thrives on praise and attention. Expose him to opportunities in sports and dramatic activities. Help him to find an area in which he can excel, because he needs to have his place in the Sun—an activity of which he can feel proud. This child may be a natural leader—he's willing to be the initiator, and may also be a risk-taker.*

Mars in Virgo *or Mars in House 6*

> *I do my work*
> *In great detail*
> *I'll do it right*
> *And never fail.*

Your Mars in Virgo child is by nature likely to be quite a perfectionist. She will want to do things in a certain way, according to a system, with a great deal of attention to each and every detail. She will not be satisfied until everything is just right. That which this child chooses to do will almost certainly have a practical purpose. She is not likely to waste much time doing anything "just to be doing it." This practical type has to have a reason, with some expected useful result. She will like to make things, and that often involves tools. Count on her to take care of tools much more carefully than most kids, so you can provide her with good ones with confidence. Provide her with plenty of opportunities, for she could become a good craftsperson or technician.

This Mars placement may indicate a child who is not particularly physically active, one who may be more inclined toward mental activities. Her choices for sports may run toward more individualized ones such as hiking, rock climbing, bike trips, jogging, aerobics or the like. She will be concerned about having a healthy body, so she will not be lazy about getting exercise. However, your little Mars in Virgo just may not be that interested in competitive team sports.

Whatever your child chooses to do, you can probably rely upon her to be responsible and dependable. This conscientious type will also be more likely, without nagging on your part, to finish her homework or assigned tasks before she takes off to play.

*Your **Mars in House 6** child puts a lot of effort into her work, making sure that she does it thoroughly and well. She may do better when working independently, than she does with others, if the others are less conscientious than she— " do it MY way!" It is important to her to feel competent—her basic identity is tied up with what she does. This child might do especially well with taking care of her own pet.*

Mars in Libra *or Mars in House 7*

> *That's not fair*
> *There's got to be*
> *A way to please*
> *Both you and me!*

Whatever your Mars in Libra child likes to do, he will probably prefer doing it with someone else, if given a choice — unless everyone else is doing something very rowdy and dirty, in which case this child may prefer to go off and do something quiet, and quite probably artistic, even if that means he must do it alone.

Though this child tends to work with groups very cooperatively, and is inclined to compromise in order to facilitate the group work and avoid conflict, he is likely to be quite competitive in some areas. People with this Mars placement can seem to be constantly trying to balance the need to relate with the wish to assert themselves. The concept of fair play is very important, and one that your child will assertively insist upon, both in regard to his own interests or in defense of those of others.

Deciding what to do can sometimes impede action that needs to be taken. This kid must always consider both sides of a matter before acting. The inability to resolve things in his mind according to a balanced or "win-win proposition" may mean that by the time he is ready to act it is too late. Mars in Libra will greatly enjoy all kinds of social functions — parties, dances, etc. You should expose him to cultural and artistic activities, and to opportunities to try out various arts, crafts and musical skills. He may become quite good in one of those areas, and derive much enjoyment from it. Plan on the fact that your child will probably opt to invite a friend along whenever he is given the chance.

*With **Mars in House 7**, your child's identity is closely related to best friends, or sometimes also to competitors. He has a lot to learn in life through relating to others, and a big part of it is balancing what he wants with what others want— "my way," give in, or compromise. He may need your help in learning the arts of negotiation and finding "win-win" solutions. He wants to be with others, but wants to do his own thing. Easiest choice: independent projects in a group setting.*

Mars in Scorpio *or Mars in House 8*

> *Never underestimate*
> *The power and the might*
> *That I can draw from deep inside*
> *If I am forced to fight!*

Your little Mars in Scorpio will probably be quite a fighter — energetic, determined, strong and intense about everything she does. If she sets out to accomplish something, she will do it. This one enjoys a challenge, and is generally unafraid of anything. This is a good Mars placement for the rougher, heavier sports. Your child may enjoy physical contact sports, and if she does, she will be a strong competitor. Usually water sports, too, are much enjoyed. This type likes to investigate the unknown, so exploring the underwater world through snorkeling or scuba diving may appeal. Some people with this placement seem almost attracted to danger, so your child may be more inclined to take chances than you might find appropriate to your comfort level.

This kid is unlikely to do anything halfway. If it is not worth doing passionately and intensely, it is generally not worth doing at all. Mars in Scorpio tends not to be neutral about anything. She either likes it a lot or not at all. (A note on blending: Liz, with Sun and Mercury in Libra prefers to keep the peace, and will easily compromise if something really doesn't matter all that much. If she really **cares** to do something, though, her Mars in Scorpio can turn on like a bulldozer. She—and I— get no peace until its accomplished!)

Your child does not anger easily. It takes quite a lot of aggravation before she gets very upset. But if she is pushed far enough, again this is a fighter and she will fight body and soul to the bitter end. And she does not forgive and forget very easily at all. When she is finally pushed to the edge, she is likely to dredge up every past event leading to the "last straw" and become even angrier.

Mars in Scorpio will like to delve into mysteries. The little detective will like to probe and investigate. While she's digging for the facts, she will want to keep some things secret until she has everything figured out to her own satisfaction. Respect her privacy. Sometimes she really needs and prefers to work things through alone.

*With **Mars in House 8**, your child is a strong willed little person who has important lessons to learn in life through pitting that will against the will of others. She wants close involvement with others, but to have them, she'll need to learn to share. She seldom does anything halfway. Whether its a task to complete, a mystery to discover, a game or argument to win, she'll drive, probe and push to accomplish her goal.*

Mars in Sagittarius *or Mars in House 9*

> *I'm out for adventure*
> *To reach for a star*
> *I'll go where it leads me*
> *No matter how far!*

Little Mars in Sagittarius is more than likely to love the great outdoors and all the adventures that are possible there. He is spontaneous, somewhat impulsive, very idealistic and usually exudes self-confidence. Often kids with this Mars placement are natural athletes who love vigorous sports. Often they are especially attracted to horses and any activity that has to do with them. Other outdoorsy activities that may attract are hiking, camping, hunting, archery, etc. This may be a child to whom you should introduce scouting at an early age, for this would be a good combination of enjoyable activities with the idealism and higher purpose that would also appeal to a Sagittarius type.

Freedom is of paramount importance to this child. He will want to make his own choices and do things as much as possible according to his own schedule. He is very idealistic with a strong sense of honor, and this will motivate all of his actions. For this reason, your Mars in Sagittarius will expect that you will trust him. In spite of the freedom that he demands, you are likely to get much more trustworthy behavior if you trust! Idealism may also lead this child to work for some cause that he feels will improve the world.

Details are not this child's strong suit, however. His fiery spirit wants to be on the front lines and in the action. Daily routine stuff is boring and not worth his time. Want the room cleaned up? Well, maybe not all at once. One task at a time, between forays into adventure, might work better!

*Your tyke with **Mars in House 9** has a great sense of adventure and the courage to go with it. He thinks big. When he really believes in something, it's the grandest, the highest, the only truth, and he'll fight for it. This trait could lead him to be a strong competitor in sports, or a strong defender of fair play, justice and whatever else he believes to be true.*

Mars in Capricorn *or Mars in House 10*

I don't waste time on frills,
For time is running out.
Success means sticking to what's real,
Of that I have no doubt.

Little Mars in Capricorn is a pragmatist. Don't expect her to waste much time on that for which she does not see a practical, useful purpose. She wants tangible results. With a realistic goal in mind, this child will work very hard, for she is ambitious and wants the success, recognition and rewards of getting ahead. You are likely to find that this child is quite mature and responsible for her age. From the time she is a tot, you will sense that she seems somehow "older." She is inclined to follow whatever rules are set down, and in fact, will be quite self-disciplined. Even at a young age, you are likely to find yourself talking about what needs to be done to prepare for some future career with this child, and you will see her taking tangible actions toward that goal.

Sometimes your Mars in Capricorn child may seem too serious, or could seem pessimistic or as if she feels blocked or frustrated. It may be best for you to let her set the goals. The practical approach of this child could tempt you to push beyond her own current limits. She needs to feel that the power to achieve is within her. She is likely to be disciplined enough, without been pressured. You may do well to teach her that the way to work through a block is to take a break, and that sometimes recreation is the practical thing to do. One comes back refreshed and with new energy.

Introduce this child to opportunities in music. Often playing a musical instrument proves to be a very valuable outlet and balance for a serious, goal-oriented personality. Try challenging her in board games. She's likely to be good at strategic thinking—an excellent skill to encourage.

*Your child with **Mars in House 10** is likely to be one who feels naturally driven to achieve, and will enthusiastically pursue her goals. The influence of parental authority is very important in how she learns to handle her assertive energies. She'll respect reasonable rules, but she needs space to be independent, too. Too much control and pressure could result in her blocking her own energy and giving up. She identifies with her accomplishment, thrives on recognition for work well done.*

Mars in Aquarius *or Mars in House 11*

There's got to be a better way
To do this, that I know.
I'll think of one, and tell you
Then we'll be set to go.

Your Mars in Aquarius child is likely to be quite inventive and independent in all types of work or activity. He is inclined to be sure, without having tried it, that the accepted way of doing just about anything, cannot be the best way. His way must be better! Sometimes he will be right; sometimes wrong, and time will be wasted. Very creative teachers may be delighted. Structured types won't, and there your child is likely to have trouble. This kid just plain doesn't follow rules or orders very well. But he is VERY creative!

Team sports may not work so well. Again, Aquarius prefers to do it his way, and that is not how teams work best. Physical activity will generally not be as interesting to your child as intellectual activities. Individualized sports may be the best choices for exercise, especially anything that might be considered somewhat unusual for your locale. Your child may work quite well with a group if there is a humanitarian cause attached. He is quite willing to submerge individual preferences to the group purpose if the purpose matters to him. Winning a game, for the sake of winning, is just not as likely to be perceived as a worthwhile purpose.

Technological and futuristic activities may be very attractive to your Mars in Aquarius child. He may become especially proficient at working with your home computer, for example, if given the chance.

*With **Mars in House 11**, your child is likely to identify quite strongly with his friends and club groups. He'll have energy and enthusiasm to fight for a common cause. He's not a follower, though. He's very much an independent individual, though, who won't hesitate to stand against the group if he thinks they're wrong—or to leave if he becomes bored. He needs to be where the action is.*

Mars in Pisces *or Mars in House 12*

> *Let me dance through my dreams*
> *On a rainbow of light*
> *And flow with the tides*
> *In the stars' twinkling light.*

This is not usually a high energy position for Mars. Generally, your child may show very little interest in sports and may tend to avoid them. If she does exhibit interest and ability in physical activity, it will most likely be in water sports, such as swimming or boating, or in sports that have a connection with music, such as dance or figure skating. Sometimes people with highly developed talents in those areas will have Mars in Pisces. (The little Astro Kid poem was written with little Molly in mind, who always had plenty of energy for her dancing, even though she might procrastinate or "wait and see" on less romantic or artistic activities.)

This child has quite a sensitive and dreamy nature in her mode of action. Your best bet may be to encourage her imagination and creativity through artistic activities such as music, dancing, drama, and the visual arts. Look into music lessons early. See if there is a junior theater group in your city. If not, encourage her to put on little plays with neighborhood friends. Mars in Pisces may well enjoy just daydreaming the hours away, and some of that activity should be allowed. But then it should be channeled into the development of creative skills. This type is not a self-starter. You may have to take the initiative to get her out of the house and get her going.

Your child is not likely to be at all assertive with others, and will tend to avoid noisy or pushy people. She will be quite willing to unselfishly help others when she sees the need. But she may not be particularly concerned about being "the best" at anything, or even if she does, may have trouble taking sufficient initiative on her own in order to achieve it. Nurture the talent, but realize that this may be a highly skilled talent who will do best with an agent!

*Your child with **Mars in House 12** is, in some way, seeking perfection in her activities. Ideally she'll put her energy into working for her goals. She can fight hard to succeed, whether in competition or for a cause. Or, if she becomes caught up in the fear of not being able to do well enough, she may dream, but block herself from real accomplishment. She'll work best and excel when she believes in something higher than herself and her own will.*

Chapter Seven
The Outer Planets

The **sign** placement of planets in the solar system outward from Mars — Jupiter, Saturn, Uranus, Neptune and Pluto — are not as important to your child's individual personality as are the signs of the personal planets and the Rising Sign. This is because the outer planets move so slowly that everyone who is born in the same year (or more) as your child is likely to have them in the same sign. The sign placements of the outer planets, then, represent generational tendencies. The aspects that the outer planets make to each other are also shared in common with everyone else in the same age group, so these, too, are not so significant in themselves, other than in defining the characteristics of a generational group.

The significance of Jupiter, Saturn, Uranus, Neptune and Pluto in your child's individual chart are best seen through their aspects to other more personal factors in the child's individual birth chart. The personal planets (Sun, Moon, Mercury, Venus, Mars) change positions relatively quickly around the zodiac, and therefore form patterns that are more unique to one individual. Ascendant and Midheaven, and the houses (which are mathematically derived from them) change even more quickly, so sensitive are they to exact moment of birth, and exact geographical location of birth. For these reasons, the slow-moving outer planets will be most useful to you in understanding your child when you consider where they are in the houses, and what aspects they make to personal planets, Midheaven and Ascendant.

Reading the symbolic meaning of each of the outer planets by itself, first, gives you a foundation for understanding how the planet modifies other planets in the chart when in aspect. The short look-up delineations of each planet-to-planet aspect will give you a few ideas, but can't possibly cover every possibility. Knowing the general theme of each outer planet will offer clues to other potentials. The "modifications" that outer planet aspects give to the personal planets and points is very important. It seems as though the slower a planet moves in its cycle, the "heavier" it "sits" on a faster planet that it aspects. For this reason, the themes of outer planet aspects to personal planets and points may quite likely represent the most dominant characteristics you will notice in your child.

We'll start with the two outer planets that are visible from Earth without a telescope, Jupiter and Saturn. These two cover a lesser number of years per sign, and thus are not truly "generational," but not really personal either, for they are held in common by children of the same ages.

Jupiter

Jupiter is the fastest moving of the outer planet group. It takes about 1 year to move through one sign, so all your child's playmates who are the same age are likely to have Jupiter in the same sign, but those who are a year or so younger or older will probably have it in an adjacent sign.

Since adjacent signs are so different from each other in expression, it could be pretty useful for a teacher, or hostess for a play group, of children all the same age, to be aware of their Jupiter placements, because it could help in knowing what type of environment would best encourage those children. Jupiter, the largest planet in our solar system is appropriately associated with the principles of expansion and growth. It is possible that it will quite literally represent "**how I grow**" in some placements. For example, some astrology books that place emphasis on the Ascendant as representative of physical appearance (which I do **not** think always "works") will say that a person with Jupiter on the Ascendant will be bigger than average, taller and/or heavier. I can't offer you any actual statistics on how often that works — maybe so, maybe not. In fairness to the "theory," though, I do have to say that my daughter Molly, who has Jupiter "on" her Ascendant by only one degree, was always a bit tall for her age as a child. In her early teens she quickly sprang up to her adult height of 5' 9" — quite a few inches taller than her sisters, me, or her grandmothers or aunt, and as taller or nearly as tall as most men in the family.

More generally, "how I grow" can mean many things. Strong Jupiterian themes in a horoscope lend a jovial, upbeat, optimistic note to the personality. This planet was considered the "greater benefic" in ancient astrology, and was considered to be very fortunate. As with everything else, however, modern astrology has found that interpretation to be too simplistic. Nothing is "black or white," or "good or bad." It's a matter of perception. Optimism is generally better than pessimism — unless it causes one to take such a blithe attitude toward things that practicality is thrown out the window and problems result. Too much expansion (overindulgence) in other areas can mean problems for the bank account or problems with the health.

"How I grow" includes that which is associated with higher knowledge — with higher education, philosophy, spirituality, and the gaining of wisdom. Jupiter is also associated with faith and ideals, and as such may give clues as to what a person most idealizes or values. In these areas, how Jupiterian themes are expressed in the individual may be strongly influenced by the cultural and religious background.

Remember that every other child in your child's immediate age group probably has Jupiter in the same sign, and the modifications of expression as will be seen through aspects and house positions are more important than the signs. The signs of Jupiter are most likely to be significant if Jupiter is in the same sign or the opposite sign as Ascendant or Midheaven, or in close aspect to Sun or Moon.

Saturn

In many ways, Saturn will sound to you like just the opposite of Jupiter. Where Jupiter symbolizes expansion, Saturn is contraction. Where Jupiter's theme is "how I grow," Saturn's is "**how I handle my limitations**." Where the Jupiterian placements may show the quest to be what it is most comfortable to be, the Saturnine placements show the necessity to deal with the reality of the situation in which one finds oneself. Jupiter tells us about the ideals; Saturn about the "rules" one has to follow to reach them. Saturn is not the "bad guy" or the "great malefic" that old fashioned astrology books might tell you. It only points out that which needs extra attention in the area of responsibility and discipline, and where the most concrete learning and accomplishments in life may be made, when responsibility is effectively accepted.

Saturn, in a small child's chart, is often perceived through the authority figures in his life. Traditionally, many astrology books link Saturn to the father, but it is well, in these days of increasing single parent families and changing roles for men and women, to not focus too much on that "tradition." Saturn may represent whomever in the child's life is most strongly guiding him to become a civilized person — the disciplinarian, the one whose love may sometimes seem to depend on doing or being that which gains approval. If you see yourself in that role in your child's life, heed any interpretations regarding Saturn well, for you as a role-model may have a very strong influence on the development of your child's own inner Saturn (sense of responsibility), his or her ability to handle and conquer fear, and his or her feelings of self-worth through handling the realities of life.

Saturn's cycle through all the signs takes about 29 1/2 years, so it will be in each sign for about 2 1/2 years. This means that all other children who are at or near the same age as your child will have Saturn in the same sign. Much more important than the sign, then, are the aspects Saturn makes to the personal planets, Midheaven or Ascendant in his or her chart, and the house Saturn is in. As you will see, when you look up the aspects in the next chapter, Saturn modifies with a generally sobering motif.

Keeping in mind that the aspects (to be covered in the next two chapters) are more important, here are a few, brief notes on possible traits associated with the sign placements of Jupiter and Saturn for all children who are at or near your child's age. Following each sign paragraph is an interpretation of the possible expression of the planet in each house of an individual child's birth chart. The signs are most likely to be individually significant in children who have the planet in the same sign, or the opposition sign as Ascendant or Midheaven, or in close aspect to Sun or Moon.

Jupiter in the Signs and Houses of the Zodiac

Jupiter in Aries or in House 1

Jupiter in Aries children grow through bold discovery of who they are, and being themselves. They should be encouraged to express their individualities and to develop self-reliance.

Your child with **Jupiter in House 1** wants everything to be big, romantic and wonderful, and to feel optimistic and lucky about life. When self-confident, he can be a leader—or expecting too much of himself could dampen a normally natural enthusiasm. He can be indignant if his sense of morality is offended—That's not fair! And he chafes when restricted— don't fence him in!

Jupiter in Taurus or in House 2

The **Jupiter in Taurus** age group prefers to grow in a secure environment where they can feel safe, and depend on when and how some things will be. The ideals tend to be practical ones.

Your child with **Jupiter in House 2** is likely to learn and grow especially well through sensual experiences — through sound and sight, touch, smell and taste. (This little one is likely to have quite an appetite!) Physical affection from family is especially important in increasing her sense of security. She'll want to save her pennies, but she might also easily give them away. After all, she feels lucky. There's more coming her way— and she's often right! She has a taste for the best in whatever she considers "hers," and won't compromise easily.

Jupiter in Gemini or in House 3

The approach of **Jupiter in Gemini** to growth and higher ideals is more likely to be intellectual. The quest may be somewhat scattered, because the interests are many. Variety in the learning environment is important for these children.

Give your child with **Jupiter in House 3** the opportunity to grow through the development of versatile skills. Choose a school with lots of stimulation and an open approach. Take him on trips—he'll love learning about people and customs different from his. Expect to (often) give logical and objective answers to a great many "whys" and "hows" from this bright little mind.

Jupiter in Cancer or in House 4

Emotional security is an important foundation for growth for the **Jupiter in Cancer** age group. They especially need to know that family and caregivers really care for them, so warmth and affection will be especially encouraging. The family and other emotional attachments will greatly influence beliefs and ideals. As an outgrowth of that, your child with this placement will develop a generosity that will extend to taking care of others.

Your **Jupiter in House 4** child has home and family on a pedestal—and you know what that means in terms of setting a good example! Your sense of right and wrong will become hers. She'll be happy if she feels free to have friends over often to show off you and her home.

Jupiter in Leo or in House 5

The **Jupiter in Leo** age group idealizes that which is exciting and showy and grand. A teacher or parent with a dramatic flair and a willingness to foster creative, dress-up play will be a winner with these children. Role-models of integrity, whom the child can respect, are important for every sign, but perhaps especially so here, because these children will not respect themselves (and thus grow to their best) if they cannot do so honestly.

Your child with **Jupiter in House 5** is likely to possess a natural self-confidence, pride and enthusiasm. A challenge to the ego may be especially disappointing. He's quite a little actor, when he gets a chance for a stage. What or whom he loves, he may idolize—dramatically! He thrives on admiration, and receiving it spills over into a natural generosity with others.

Jupiter in Virgo or in House 6

Jupiter in Virgo children grow and thrive best through the development of a good work ethic. Their beliefs and ideals are closely related to what they do, by knowing it is useful, and by living up to their responsibilities. They value that which is practical. Let them help. Give them a learning environment that will teach them to do practical things, and to become competent.

Allow your child with **Jupiter in House 6** to help you do things from the time she is a tot—whatever little tasks are appropriate to her age. She thrives on being able to accomplish things. Don't give her too much at once, though. So eager is she to achieve that she may want to take on too much, and then be nervous or unhappy when she can't meet her own expectations. Encourage small goals with small successes that can lead on to the next step. She'll feel wonderful when she knows she's done something well.

Jupiter in Libra or in House 7

Beauty in all things is an all-important ideal for **Jupiter in Libra**. Also, they place a high value on relationships and will grow through relating to others. Concepts of fairness and equality are very important. They will want to be objective about any such issues, to see both sides, and to strike a balance between them that is "fair" to both. This placement does not indicate artistic talent in itself, but it does enhance any other indicators your child has. An environment of refinement fosters growth.

Your child with **Jupiter in House 7** seeks the ideal in his close, significant relationships. He may expect more of his "best friend" than is reasonable, but on the other hand, he's likely to attract fortunate friendships. Shared beliefs are important. He needs to be with people who will share ideas with him, and encourage him to seek his own truths. An aesthetic and refined setting also encourages learning.

Jupiter in Scorpio or in House 8

Children with Jupiter in Scorpio need to dig beneath the surface of things to discover the depths of meaning. Scorpio is the most intense of signs, and these children will grow through probing mysteries and solving them. They may tend to be secretive, and it will not be easy to figure out what is going on in their minds — but they are likely to ask lots of questions in the attempt to probe yours! They can become totally absorbed in anything that has their interest. You won't have much luck in directing their attention toward that which they consider boring.

Your child with **Jupiter in House 8** may be quite intense, when what most inspires her at the moment, be it toy, game or attention must be equally shared with others. A similar determination can show in going after "what's ours" when she teams with others for a goal. She believes that anything worth having is worth whatever it takes to get it, so you may have to help her see when it would be best to let go. Yet when there's a worthy goal to encourage, strong will and intensity combined with optimism and faith can take this little one far.

Jupiter in Sagittarius or in House 9

Big dreams, grand plans, exotic places, high ideals, strong moral principles — these are all keynote possibilities for **Jupiter in Sagittarius**. What these children think is "right" is "right" and they can be downright dogmatic about it. Still, there is a strong value placed on freedom to be what they want to be and do what they want to do in their own way. They will learn through direct experience and chafe under confinement. They need variety and plenty of opportunity to explore.

Your child with **Jupiter in House 9** will have his arrow aimed at a star, and probably the classic "cock-eyed optimist's" faith that he can reach it—and maybe he will someday. He's eager to learn, but may gloss over details and jump to conclusions. He needs strong educational opportunities that offer wide perspectives. He'll be interested in other cultures, and may be quite talented with languages, especially if exposed to them from an early age.

Jupiter in Capricorn or in House 10

Children with **Jupiter in Capricorn** place high value on results. They grow through work, accepting responsibility, and making concrete achievements. They may idealize status and authority figures, and will work to win their approval. They trust that which is real and practical, and they are concerned with being "right." They could be especially hard on themselves if they perceive that they have failed or made a mistake, and may need help in developing a sense of compassion both for self and for others.

With **Jupiter in House 10**, your child's ideals are focused on success in the world, and she may strive hard to win the approval of those she sees as authorities. An authority figure is likely to be a strong role model for her in her sense of what is right and wrong. She tends to have faith in "the rules." She can be a leader who inspires others.

Jupiter in Aquarius or in House 11

For children with **Jupiter in Aquarius**, that which is idealized is likely to be that which is unconventional and progressive. When older, these children could be in the forefront of some humanitarian social cause. When little, they will be seen to place high value on fair play and equality for all. Freedom is also quite important, in an environment that encourages individuality and innovation. They grow through being allowed to experiment, and through stimulation of the intellect.

Your child with **Jupiter in House 11** is most likely a very open and tolerant child, who makes friends from a variety of cultures, backgrounds, races, religions. (This has been true of Liz whenever she's had even half a chance. Now, as a teen, she's eager for any opportunity to visit foreign countries or meet people from them, and seeks educational opportunities that will allow either.) Your child is attracted to and values uniqueness. He is very independent and thrives on freedom.

Jupiter in Pisces or in House 12

Jupiter in Pisces children are truly idealists, with beautiful dreams of a utopia that could be always beyond mortal reach. They are attracted to fairies and fantasy, to all that is beautiful and mystical. A deep empathy for others may result in satisfaction and growth through helping them. Disappointments discourage when reality fails to live up to the romantic ideal. A confusing, bustling environment is difficult; quiet and time alone to reflect is essential.

With **Jupiter in House 12**, your child has a vision of perfection, and a faith in her vision that may know no bounds. With confidence in herself, too, she may make dreams come true. She is likely to want and need some kind of religious or spiritual activity. A learning environment rich in music, art, beauty and fantasy is expansive for her. She's also likely to be a compassionate child, who is interested in helping and healing.

Saturn in the Signs and Houses of the Zodiac

Saturn in Aries or in House 1

The Aries sign theme is that of "doing your own thing," but **Saturn in Aries** may inhibit that through fear of failure. A too-controlling authority figure can increase the inhibition, or provide a role model for over-controlling behavior in the growing child. It is important for these children to be with people who will let them be themselves while encouraging self-reliance, in order to allow the best of this sign placement to manifest.

Your child with **Saturn in House 1** may have a natural reserve about his personality. He is quiet, perhaps shy, and is likely to be seen as mature for his age. He will want to be responsible, and he will like to be given little chores from an early age. Respect how much he wants to do these things right, and be patient with those early attempts. He is likely to feel best if he is allowed to work in his own way, without too much direction from you.

Saturn in Taurus or in House 2

Children with **Saturn in Taurus** have a strong need for security, a strong foundation, and a situation that can be counted upon. The reliability and consistency of the authority figure is also important, but sometimes this placement is associated with the unreliability or absence of that very person or situation in the child's life, which sets up a need to deal with insecurity. Insecurities may manifest as concern with material things, or as a stubborn resistance to necessary change. Lots of support and love from parents will bring out the best of these children.

Your child with **Saturn in House 2** is likely to be a hard worker, but is also one who may need to learn how to relax and enjoy the results of her work. She takes her possessions very seriously, and so may be more responsible about taking care of them than the average child. She should be easy to teach the value of saving money, waiting a bit for the pleasure of using it for something she considers special. Show her by your example and by what you expect of her that it is more important who she is inside, than what she has.

Saturn in Gemini or in House 3

With **Saturn in Gemini,** children may learn best in a systematic, structured environment. Still, the authority figure — teacher — would best be warm and able to combine that structure with fun, for harshness could cause excessive self-doubt within these children, in regard to their mental skills. They are more likely to be interested in ideas and facts that are seen as useful, than in those that are only abstract.

Your child with **Saturn in House 3** may have significant lessons to learn with siblings or in finding his niche in school. He may be shy, or feel self-doubt in comparing his own mental skills to others. He thinks carefully about what he will say before he speaks up. Still, he has a practical mind, capable of strong, concentration. He will learn much from observing you, of how (or how not) to communicate well with others.

Saturn in Cancer or in House 4

Children with **Saturn in Cancer** tend to have a rather tight rein on the emotions, yet a deep need for emotional security. An emotional vulnerability may manifest in pretending that feelings don't matter, or just aren't there, when there may, in fact, be an inner crying out for affection. These children may constantly play parent, through games and actual care of others in the family, or they may reverse the role and play more the baby than they really are, in order to gain attention.

Your child with **Saturn in House 4** may feel personally responsible for matters of home and family, and therefore guilty, if there are tensions in the home. If you are "down" somehow, she could feel that she must take care of you. She probably has a very strong rein on her own feelings, but just because she is reserved, she still needs affection. No matter how busy you are, be sure you spend quality time with this child. Give her lots of hugs, and make sure she knows how much you love her.

Saturn in Leo or in House 5

The natural showiness and flair of the sign is inhibited, with **Saturn in Leo**, and the self-expression of these children may be reserved. There is still likely to be a strong drive for achievement and recognition. They will tend to set high standards for themselves. Authority figures who pay attention to them and set a positive example will be important role models.

Your child with **Saturn in House 5** does not take risks without feeling fairly confident he'll succeed. Because of this, he may sometimes be shy about taking center stage. He may be too hard on himself, in how he perceives he measures up to the competition. Or he may have too much bravado and rush ahead without proper preparation, which may result in the disappointment that makes him hold back the next time. But as he grows older, the discipline and persistence he can apply to his creative expressions can bloom into considerable success.

Saturn in Virgo or in House 6

Saturn in Virgo emphasizes hardworking dedication, a sense of duty and responsibility. These children are likely to be good with details, and are very careful and practical. A problem is in the tendency to be overly self-critical, which can backfire in avoidance of responsibility for fear of making a mistake. Obviously, one in charge of such children would do well to avoid overly controlling what they are doing, while at the same time providing practical activities that lead to tangible results. When truly called for, point out the way to improvement, rather than pointing out the problem.

Your child with **Saturn in House 6** needs a role model of competence and good health habits. She is learning to be productive, herself, but may be inclined to try to do too much, or to be too worried about making mistakes. Minor illnesses could crop up as a relief from that stress. Show her a good balance of effort and dedication to your work, and taking time for your own health needs—proper diet, exercise, and time for leisure.

Saturn in Libra or in House 7

Children with **Saturn in Libra** tend to be very loyal in their relationships, even though they may take a long time in making up their minds to whom they will give that loyalty. Fairness is very, very important, and these children may be quite outraged if they perceive that someone is being unfairly treated by someone else.

Your child with **Saturn in House 7** is looking for security in his close relationships. He needs to learn to balance the other person's needs with his own. He may want to "do" for his friend constantly, taking all of the responsibility for the friendship, or he may choose a very domineering friend, who makes all the decisions. From his authority-parent, he will learn about equality and fairness in relationships—or the lack of it. Show him a balance of respect for others and for yourself.

Saturn in Scorpio or in House 8

Emotions may be very deep in **Saturn in Scorpio** children, but are suppressed. So strong is the need for self-control, that close, intimate connections with others may be inhibited. Or, power struggles could be an issue. Still, relationships are important to learn sharing and trust. Responsibility is accepted with emotional intensity and a strong sense of purpose.

Your child with **Saturn in House 8** has lessons to learn in sharing equally and learning to give and take with grace. She may confront intensely, or she may withdraw and play alone—the silent, stiff upper lip approach. You as authority can help her if you are a good role model for handling strong emotions well, and of sharing power fairly. This is a good placement for her in any work that requires patience and persistence.

Saturn in Sagittarius or in House 9

Children with **Saturn in Sagittarius** may take a very serious attitude toward principles of ethics and morality, toward spiritual ideas or toward any clear goals they set for themselves. Great respect is likely to be given to authority figures. A quite dogmatic attitude may be taken in regard to beliefs.

If you are the authority in your **Saturn in House 9** child's life, you may be right up on his pedestal. But—lest you lose that respect, don't step off that pedestal by betraying your own (and his) high standards. He'll learn his basis for ethics, values and ideals from you. Your child will most likely place his faith in what is orderly and real. He could be dogmatic about what he believes when young. Show him an example of openness and tolerance, and broaden his horizons and yours.

Saturn in Capricorn or in House 10

Saturn in Capricorn children are inclined to be serious and responsible, conservative and traditional. They may need little direction in accepting responsibility, doing their share and working hard. Instead, they may need encouragement to "lighten up" and have some fun. They are likely to seem old for their years, which could cause adults to take advantage of their seriousness by loading on too much. Remember, they also need to be children.

Your child with **Saturn in House 10** learns much from you, as authority figure, about how to handle (or not handle) work, responsiblity and power in the world. She needs a sense of control—within her, not overdone from you. If she feels that all the power is yours (or outside herself), she could cease to try. What she most needs is to feel really good about something she does—efficient, expert, special. As she gains in competence and confidence in her ability, she may become quite a leader!

Saturn in Aquarius or in House 11

Here the sign of the individualist is occupied by the planet of the tradition-alist, and the children who were being born as I wrote much of this book ('92-'93), have **Saturn in Aquarius**. This may be a group who will grow up to give widespread form to ideas that are now called "new age." They will have the Saturnine qualities of responsibility and structure, but their structure will not likely be that which their parents might desire or expect. They won't change things just for the sake of change, but because they have systematically demonstrated the usefulness of a new way of doing something.

Your child with **Saturn in House 11** is testing and learning when it's best to follow the rules and when to stand up and oppose them, if they are unfair or unjust. What his peers think may mean more than the opinions of adults. Or, he may feel responsible for his friends, and try to keep them in line. He might respond to your ideas (as authority figure) best when you treat him as a friend, respect his freedom (and yours), and display an attitude of openness.

Saturn in Pisces or in House 12

Closely following the Saturn in Aquarius group, and being born as this book is published, are the children with **Saturn in Pisces.** Here may be a group of visionaries, who are able to bring their ideals into practical manifestation. Still, this is not an easy mix of themes (structure and reality vs. dreams), and real difficulties could arise for some of them when fantasies refuse to materialize. Integration of faith with reality is an important challenge, which may associate this time period and this generation with changes in long-held religious traditions, which will be augmented with the movement of the transpersonal planets into signs of similar theme.

Your child with **Saturn in House 12** can make her dreams come true—but she tends to be fairly practical about what she dreams for herself. Her realistic visions oculd be influenced by a parent who escaped from reality (played a victim role in some way). She may be inspired toward creating beauty of her own in the world by an authority figure who is artistic, or perhaps a healer—one who flows productively within a strong faith in the Infinite.

The Transpersonal Planets

The astrology of the ancients used only the planets that could be seen from Earth without a telescope. All of them orbit the Sun rather quickly, compared to the planets beyond the orbit of Saturn. In one sense, all of the "visible" planets, could be called "personal planets" in that their place-ments by sign are more indicative of individual traits than the "invisible" planets, which are called "transpersonal." Even Jupiter and Saturn, both visible without telescope under good atmospheric conditions, change signs quickly enough that they indicate only an age group of a three year range or less, rather than a true "generation."

**The truly generational planets are the transpersonal ones —
Uranus, Neptune and Pluto.** It's difficult to recognize sign-associated
characteristics for these planets in an individual, or even in an age group
of children. But the sign that the transpersonal planets are "in" when an
entire generation of children are born will be synchronous with major
social issues of change that will surely be recognized in retrospect, even if
they are not evident in related news stories that "break" at the time.

We can speculate on the generational traits of any planet/sign combination, but of course, the ones most meaningful to you will be those in
which you can place yourselves, your own parents, or actual memories of
events. All of the signs of Uranus could apply, so all are covered here. The
signs of Neptune and Pluto are interpreted only if they apply to age ranges
of your parents, yourselves and your present and potential children.
Although this is probably of marginal help in the main purpose of this book,
it might be useful to you in comparing some of the styles and attitudes of
the various generations to that of your child's generation. We are all
unique individuals, but we do lead our lives within the context of larger
cultural groups.

You are more likely to notice a transpersonal planet's theme in your
child's **houses,** than in the signs. For this reason, **planets in houses** will
come first, in this line-up, with the generational sign interpretations
following. First, the basic meaning of each planet:

Uranus

Uranus is in one sign for about seven years, so obviously it would take
living to about the age of 84 to see it go through an entire cycle of the zodiac.
As an orbiting planet, Uranus is unique and eccentric, rolling along
sideways, "doing its own thing." Synchronous to that, it is symbolically
associated with doing things differently, with innovation, with sudden
change. In signs, it represents areas in which a generation seeks freedom
and expressions that break from the conventions of the past. It can
represent considerable tension in the signs in which it is least compatible,
by nature.

Neptune

With a total cycle around the zodiac of about 164 years, this planet spends
about 13 to 14 years in each sign. Because of that, its sign interpretation
is even less significant for an individual than Jupiter, Saturn or Uranus.
Still, its symbolism for its generation has significance for everyone.

The general symbolism of Neptune is complex and wide-ranging in its
potential expression. I think that one of the best key words for it is
escapism. In its lowest and most unhealthy themes right up to the highest
and best, in one way or another, it represents an escape from the hard
realities of life. At the bottom of the heap, one might escape by blotting out
the world and its worries with drugs or alcohol, and Neptune aspects will
be found to relate to that. A bit higher, but still destructive, we might find
the chronic liar. Similar Neptune themes might point to a less destructive

but still unproductive form of escape through aimless dreaming — building sand castles that are forever washed away by the tides and come to nothing. Climbing the list of possibilities, we come to constructive escape through the development of great skill and the production of great beauty in the arts — music, dance, visual arts, poetry, literature. At perhaps the pinnacle, providing it is truly selfless in its expression, we find high spirituality, the mystic and seer, the "saint" who impersonally and selflessly serves in whatever capacity his or her spiritual path leads.

There are more possibilities, of course, but you get the idea. Neptune themes idealize "whatever," and seek to transcend the muddy, mundane world — escape. As such, Neptune also indicates how a person — or by sign, a generation — creates, romanticizes, glorifies, and serves ideals.

Generational Neptune themes are also associated with change, but not of the rebellious, reforming style of Uranus. Rather, Neptune represents the gradual dissolution of the old order. It just fades away, in the wake of a new romantic ideal.

Pluto

Pluto takes about 248 years to go through all of the signs. Its orbit is considerably more elliptical than the other planets, so its time in each sign varies from about 12 years up to 32. Obviously, entire generations, from parent to child, will have Pluto in the same sign, and the sign symbolism, in itself, is not meaningful in an individual chart. It is interesting, however, to reflect on how you and your children, as individuals, might deal with Pluto's generational transformations.

Transformation is a major keyword for Pluto. Others are control, rebirth and regeneration. In an individual chart, its aspects have to do with power and control issues, and areas of transformative experience, where one probes deeply for meaning and seeks self-mastery. When this planet goes through a sign, mass cultural themes associated with that sign are uprooted, probed, turned upside down and inside out, and reborn in a new way. The upheaval is not pleasant for many, but there does not seem to be any going back. An individual may stubbornly stick to an old way, but the world will change all around, just the same.

Uranus in the Houses and Signs

Uranus in House 1 or in Aries
Your **Uranus in House 1** child's very identity may rest on being different. He is a nonconformist who does not want to be "one of the crowd," and won't like being compared to other kids unless it is in recognition of his uniqueness. In one way or another he will express his individuality. It could take the form of eccentric dress, rebellion against restrictions, or choosing activities that are constructive but very original. Understand this need for free expression and subtly steer him toward ways he can "stand out" that won't get him in trouble! Outlets could be art or drama, but

he may have a scientific or technical interest, too. A tot computer whiz, perhaps?

The last group to have **Uranus in Aries** was born in 1927-1934, and the next children with it will not be born until 2011. With a strong drive for individual freedom, they are disinclined to live (as adults) in the style of their parents. The older generation were children and teens during World War II, during which few lives were not touched, with many torn apart. They will fight for their freedom if necessary, but because the issue affects them personally, rather than because of abstract principle.

Uranus in House 2 or in Taurus

Your **Uranus in House 2** child would benefit from early training with an allowance, because her natural tendency with money (and possessions) may be careless. She may just love something and "have to have it" one day, and not care about it at all the next. What she chooses as favorite things may often seem unusual to you—she's attracted to what's different. Her idea of comfort may be upside down in a chair with feet in the air, or her taste in food may be in weird combinations. Flow with these small expressions of her independence—who knows? She might lead you to a new experience that you'll enjoy, too.

Uranus in Taurus includes some grandparents (like this one) born 1934-1942 . The next births to have this placement will begin in 2018. Uranus is a tense tenant in stable Taurus, especially when it is very prominent in the horoscope. With a tendency to be insecure in regard to material resources, this generation may either be very concerned about building a stable financial base, or they may take the opposite course, and prefer to rid themselves of property and the responsibilities inherent in having it — or they may veer from one style to another at different stages in life.

Uranus in House 3 or in Gemini

Originality for your **Uranus in House 3** child will most likely be noticed in his way of thinking. He'll be curious, and your first challenge may be keeping one step ahead of his ability to figure out how to get into anything. This is the tyke who was born to thwart child-proofing devices. Later, when he talks, he may jump from one idea to another so fast you'll wonder where you got lost in the process. Liz has this placement. She's quiet a lot of the time, as other things in her chart express, but even as a young child she could toss off more crazy jokes than I could ever remember. She read and talked on an unusual variety of subjects. Shannon has it, too. She questioned everything—a zillion whys, with little taken at face value without challenge.

The 1942-1949 **Uranus in Gemini** group is the beginning of the constantly talked-about "baby-boomers." In the sign most associated with thinking and communication, this generation brings uniqueness and innovation — so much for the coincidence of a boom in computer and related technologies that came with their adulthood. It's probably due to the massive influence of the baby boomer that we are constantly bombarded these days with Gemini-like talk and writings about their ideas, desires and styles.

Uranus in House 4 or in Cancer

Uranus in House 4 often reflects a home life that is unusual in some way. It could mean that a parent is very original and different, or it could mean that there are many changes of residence, or that there are lots of activities in the home with people coming and going. It could even express that the parents are not available much of the time, or "not there" for the child. Whatever the individual situation is, the experiences would lead the child to develop an inner sense of independence because she has to rely more on her own inner resources. Uranus in the 4th often reflects a person who grows up to be more detached or objective than most people in regard to family ties.

Last born during 1949-1956, the **Uranus in Cancer** group probably led the parade of mass moving away from home that has led to the breakdown of the family. Born in the overly idealized "50s" of perfect TV sitcom families, many of them were already part of a growing mass migration from small towns to cities, from cities to other cities in Dad's quest for career advancement. Many lacked the stable home environment that would support a strong inner security. This generation, drawing less security from home, may seek freedom from emotional entanglements.

Uranus in House 5 or in Leo

Your **Uranus in House 5** child may be a risk-taker, one who seeks excitement and variety. His self-esteem may be tied up with expressing his freedom. He may sometimes enjoy actually shocking people. Obviously, allowing him acceptable space in which to express himself, in activities in which you can even delight in his accomplishments, will be a lot easier for you than trying to restrain him. Of course, some limitations are necessary, but try not to throw up unnecessary ones. Risk, challenge and inventiveness can be found in sports, in acting, in games…he'll show you where his interest lies. Your job is to expose him to a variety of activities, be alert to what he likes and then share his excitement!

Uranus in Leo, born 1956-1962, was an individualistic group with an eccentric flair. As young people in school, many of them were taught by teachers who came out of colleges during the 60s rebellions and innovations. This encouraged an already generational tendency for individual expression, often at the expense of discipline and academic achievement. This generation also presented a major challenge to previously accepted social mores in the areas of romance, courtship and sex.

Uranus in House 6 or in Virgo

Uranus in House 6 often reflects someone who is entreprenurial, works in an unusual job, or needs to have variety and express independence in work (like me). In a child, you'll likely find that details can be glossed over, or too much routine is stifling. The child will want to do things in her own way, and may express quite a bit of inventiveness in figuring out how to do whatever she is doing—which may not be the way you instructed her to do it. Be patient. She's learning, and her idea of freedom and independence is very tied up with doing her work well, but in her own unique way. Being stuck in a routine she doesn't like can lead to frustration or even illness. Give her the space to be creative, and the freedom to try things her own way.

The **Uranus in Virgo** generation, born in 1962-1968, includes my eldest daughter and her peers. Uranus can represent considerable tension in practical Virgo, but not so much as in the less flexible Taurus. These kids are inclined to seek freedom through becoming competent. They innovate in practical ways that will serve their lives. They are not too happy with routine, unless it's one they have set up for themselves. This may be why so many of them are becoming entrepreneurs these days — starting small businesses in reaction to the impersonality of corporate life.

Uranus in House 7 or in Libra

Your child with **Uranus in House 7** expresses freedom and independence in his interactions with his friends (and in later life, partners), or he may be attracted to a very unusual friend. This could mean erratic relationships—one child is his "best friend" and the next week it's someone else. Or it could just mean that he's more detached about friendships than average, wanting variety and independence rather than a relationship with one close friend. In any of his relationships, fair play will be important. He may express a good deal of openness and tolerance of individual differences in his associations, but when it comes to cooperation and competition, things will have to be "even."

The **Uranus in Libra** group, born in 1968-1975, includes my middle daughter, who like so many of her generation, lives a balancing act between needs for freedom and for close relationships. They were born during a time when the news was breaking frequent stories of nontraditional relationships that have now become fairly commonplace. Libra is also a sign closely associated with art and beauty. Look for these young people to set new and unusual trends in the arts.

Uranus in House 8 or in Scorpio

The 8th house has to do with sharing of resources, and you may experience erratic behavior in your child with **Uranus in House 8,** or more than a few upsets, as she learns to share with others. But she's also capable of being quite detached about things. A toy may be fiercely "mine" one minute, and easily given to another child the next. Help her understand the difference between what is hers, alone, and what is intended for common use with others. She'll be curious about mysteries or secrets, and is capable of being inventive about figuring them out.

The last kids to be born with **Uranus in Scorpio** (including my youngest), were born 1975-1981, and it may be yet a bit too soon to know the full extent of what their generation's cultural reforms might be. Most of them aren't talking about it, at least not to adults. Many of them (especially the less advantaged ones, in inner cities) are acting out their very intense challenge to life with a vengeance. Even the quieter and well-behaved ones, though, are in their own way, probing for meaning and purpose in a culture that seems to have lost it. When they come into their power to effect change, they won't take halfway measures.

Uranus in House 9 or in Sagittarius

Your child with **Uranus in House 9** may be a radical thinker, challenging the norm in ideas and ideals. In a smaller child, you'll probably see a strong need to be unconfined, so he can explore everything. This is how he learns. Don't stick him in a playpen, if you can possibly avoid it. Put what is dangerous out of reach, and let him go. Freedom is really important to him. Later, it would be good if you could find him a school environment of the "open classroom" type, where independent thinking is encouraged. He'll be fascinated with outings to unusual places where he can learn about people, animals, ways of living that are different than his ordinary environment.

Many **Uranus in Sagittarius** children, born 1981-1988, some of whom are now just entering their teens, are likely to seek their freedom through a challenge to the beliefs, traditions and values of their families. Sagittarius is among the most idealistic of signs, and these kids won't buy any mandate because "I say so" or even because "God says so," unless it seems honest, fair and just according to their own perception of reality. They will seek their own path, and then blaze that path for others with great enthusiasm.

Uranus in House 10 or in Capricorn

The little rebel may emerge with **Uranus in House 10**, questioning any and all authority. Or the more authoritarian parent is a role model (plus or minus) for freedom and individuality. That could mean that too much rule-making brings out the rebel. Or it could mean interest and acceptance of the child's unique tastes and talents will help guide the child in positive ways of expressing his individuality. She'll most likely choose an unusual career someday. Even now she'll be happiest when she's able to choose her own style of expression. She wants to be seen as special and will strive to stand out of the crowd. Help her find a way to do so that will also win the respect and approval of others.

Kids born now (1988-1995) have **Uranus in Capricorn**, and it is a time of great tension and change in long-established big-business-type Capricornian institutions — corporations, churches, governments. They will grow up with the many challenges to established authority that are now just beginning, and their generation will probably reinforce and restructure those changes on a practical level. More purposeful and cautious than the previous group, they may seek to return to "the old ways," but will nevertheless effect cultural changes to work within new realities.

Uranus in House 11 or in Aquarius

Your child with **Uranus in House 11** may be attracted to friends and groups that are out of the ordinary in some way, or who have unique goals. He has a streak of the nonconformist himself, and this may show in the groups of other kids that he wants to be with. He's very open, and meets people and makes friends easily (which means, of course, that you'll have to teach him a bit of caution in regard to strangers). On the other hand, while he may be gregarious, he may not be inclined to form close friendships, preferring free-flowing relationships with a variety of other children. Even as a child, he may be attracted to causes, wanting to reform what he sees as unfair in the world.

Kids born 1995-2003 will have **Uranus in Aquarius**, and a few of them might still have living grandparents who were born during the last time of that placement, 1912-1919. In Aquarius, Uranus is "at home," so this group will be quite effective at creating constructive changes for humanitarian social purposes. The older group were young adults who lived through the Great Depression and helped rebuild society after it. Aquarius is more adept at group reform than at individual needs, however, so their changes could sublimate individual freedoms to the "good" of society as a whole.

Uranus in House 12 or in Pisces

Molly has **Uranus in House 12,** and like her, children with this placement may be imaginative, creative and have flashes of intuition, even psychic ability. Here the need for freedom and individuality is in the inner, most secret self. There, she may have a private world of romance and perfection into which she can escape whenever she's bored, or the expectations of others are more than she wants to meet. If she "escapes" too much, you may need to pay attention to what she may be trying to shut out. Feed her creativity and quest for beauty and the ideal with opportunities for expression— music, dance, art are possibilities.

Uranus in Pisces includes the grandparent or great-grandparent generation of 1919-1927, and the kids who will be born in 2003-2011. The older group were still little kids during the crash that led to the Great Depression. Many of them had little understanding of all the problems the adults were having. Perhaps they escaped into dreams and fantasy play. By the time they grew up, World War II was beginning, and many were caught up in an idealistic fervor to march off and save the world, and many found reality to be all too harsh. Hopefully, the group to come will be able to seek its freedom and effect its changes primarily through artistic and spiritual paths.

Neptune in the Houses and Relevant Signs

Neptune in House 1

No matter what sign is rising, with Neptune in the first house, your child is, at least to some extent, a dreamer. The imagination is vivid. The expression could range from aimless fantasy or wonderful creativity; from illusion about self or others to marked intuitive senstivity. "Vibes" and feelings intuitively picked up from others may affect this little one's vulnerablility to minor illnesses. Soft music would be soothing if the mood seems sad or tense. This child may have a magnetic charisma or grace in movement that is quite attractive.

Neptune in House 2

Molly has this placement of Neptune, and she, of course, fits one of the typical adult interpretations in having developed her artistic skills into a tangible income-producing reality. Encouraging art or music in such a child is good, because it gives her the opportunity to make her imagination and dreams real—**my** painting, **my** poem, **my** song. ("My little [imaginary] friend" could possibly also be a manifestation; with Molly it was spirits.) She wants and needs to make beauty real, and make what's comfortable beautiful. Being too trusting or idealistic about money is an adult problem that you could try to avert by starting her out at an early age with a small allowance and some ongoing gentle guidance on how to manage it.

Neptune in House 3

Here is one whose thinking may always retain that early quality of the "natural magician." Or perhaps he may be a poet or a writer with great imagination that can inspire others. Or he could sometimes fall into taking the easy way out, and mistakenly trust that information from the homework he needs to do might flow in from the ether without effort on his part. A challenge will be in learning to combine his imagination and dreams with logic and objective realities, and in learning to concentrate. He may idolize a sibling or other relative, or, on the other hand, he could perhaps hide unhappy feelings even from himself, denying that the relationship just isn't the way his ideals tell him it should be.

Neptune in House 4

This child will want to idealize her home and family so much that if her experience is less than perfect, she may even deny or repress what does not live up to her ideal. "Shutting down" could also be because she's very sensitive to any tense feelings expressed around her, and needs to learn how to "tune out" what's upsetting. She needs a private place in her home where she can create her own sense of inner peace. Mother (or the more nurturing parent) is an important role model in developing this child's sense of faith, trust, and knowing what dreams are worthwhile and then following them.

Neptune in House 5 or in Leo

This one may love to perform, and have a flair for it. Shannon was like this from the time she was a tot. I remember her at the age of six singing—quite well—the English version of an operatic aria for a gathering of pros (her Dad is a singer). No shyness there—the little magician casting a spell on her audience! Or, if your tot can talk you into anything, just think what a salesman he might make someday. You may find that this one tends to overdramatize problems, too—from the bump or the broken toy to the first adolescent zit. This child is a born romantic—what, or whom, he loves, he loves to the absolute heights, which can sometimes lead to disappointment when love fails to live up to the ideal. Don't expect that downer to last for long though—his charisma soon attracts a new love; his creativity, a new ideal.

Neptune in Leo grandparents and great-grandparents, born around 1916-1929, were born when the economy was booming, and extravagance was idealized, along with the taking of risks — a lovely illusion, that was heading for a big, disillusioning fall, with the 1929 stock market crash and subsequent depression. As adults, they would come to idealize the individual who could stand proudly and self-sufficiently.

Neptune in House 6 or in Virgo

Your child with **Neptune in House 6** may drift and dream when chores are to be done—unless you are clever enough to make a fantasy game of it! Then, it may be fun. Or, perhaps if you emphasize how much you **need** the help. Helping others has appeal; doing a task for the sake of doing it (clean room) may not. Also, doing what will create beauty is a good motivation. Guide this little one to develop good habits of personal hygiene, and be careful when you introduce new foods or medicines that you know what is being given. Sometimes this placement of Neptune reflects a child who is more sensitive to drugs than the average, or has allergies. It also often indicates a child who is a natural little doctor or nurse.

This grandma was born toward the end of **Neptune in Virgo** (about 1929-1943). The ideals with which my generation was brought up were quite firmly grounded in success through hard work, acceptance of responsibility and self-discipline. No wonder so many of us lament the lack of a "work ethic" in so much of what we see today. We may even feel guilty whenever we are doing something that is not "productive!" Many had those ideals become disillusioned along the way, and have come to question to whom and to what ideals we owe our service. Still, even we who have become renegades are inclined to work toward our new ideals in a more disciplined way than some of the younger generations.

Neptune in House 7 or in Libra

In your child with **Neptune in House 7,** the focus of dreams, ideals and a quest for perfect love tends to be focused on the partner. In a child, this may be a "best friend" who is extremely special, or perhaps an older friend who becomes an idol. Disappointment can result if the other person does not live up to the child's ideals. He may expect more than is reasonable from that "best friend." If the idol has "feet of clay," or perhaps a handicap or some kind of problem, the child may go to considerable effort to try to help, and express a great deal of compassion in doing so. He is learning, through his one-to-one relationships, how to balance ideals with reality.

Neptune in Libra people, born around 1943-1957, will include some of you who, as parents of young children, are reading this book. You are the "boomers," many of whom were, in your younger days, caught up in the hippie movement and various countercultures that dissolved the more disciplined, service-to-society ideals of the years before you were born. You were born into a world that idealized and romanticized "traditional" male-female relationships, but as you grew up you saw the inequities and the illusions. In your young adulthood, the dream of "happily ever after" had faded, the divorce rate had zoomed, and the feminist movement became a high ideal for many of you.

Neptune in House 8 or in Scorpio

Neptune in House 8 reflects a dreaminess or idealizing quality focused toward a significant other person. Sharing is a major issue of this house. It may be very important to share possessions and secrets. Your child very much wants a close, special relationship. Little lessons could be learned through experiences of sharing that are uneven. Your child may want to give too much, to please her special someone, and may need your guidance as to what is appropriate. The imagination about anything hidden or mysterious is vivid. If **you're** trying to hide something, remember that. It might be better to share a bit, than to let that imagination run wild.

The largest number of parents reading this book will probably have **Neptune in Scorpio** in their charts. You, born about 1957-1970, came into a time period that idealized sexuality. The dissolution in relationships/marriages, that come out of the Neptune in Libra disillusionment with the ideals into which it was born, led to the sexual revolution. You, in turn, have grown to disillusionment with that, discovering that overt and free sexuality has its price. You were also born to an idealized view of wealth and power, which is now dissolving into economic downturn and dissolution of power structures as the "American dream" of your parents threatens to leave you holding the tab. Some of you are intently probing your psyches, searching for reasons or blame. More productively, others of you are taking your places as leaders of new ideals that will intently examine what isn't working and recreate what will.

Neptune in House 9 or in Sagittarius

Your child with **Neptune in House 9** may idealize beliefs—religion, perhaps—from an early age. I have it; and I did, from special experiences in early Sunday school and onward. But as I grew, I questioned, demanding that what I saw in church live up to the ideals preached, or I was off looking for a new ideal. (I told you this before, in Chapter 3 on adolescence.) Yet always there's a sense of wonder in life, a faith in the best in people, and that dreams can come true. It's a Sagittarian thing, no matter what Neptune's sign (reread the Sag Sun Sign poem). Education is very important for this child. He wants to know! Encourage creative expression, perhaps especially in writing and poetry.

Some of my younger parent-readers will have **Neptune in Sagittarius** (born around 1970-1984), but some of the kids of the older readers will have it, too. Sagittarius is the sign most associated with religion, and this time period has idealized a seeking after religious truths, both in the traditional religions and in a multiplicity of alternatives to tradition— eastern, metaphysical, shamanistic philosophies, and a reemergence of Goddess worship. The search is for meaning, and for values and ethics that had become lost or confused during the two previous periods. Many of you have become disillusioned with the traditions of your parents, but are finding a primarily secular culture to be somehow empty. You are searching for a new path.

Neptune in House 10 or in Capricorn

Your child with **Neptune in House 10** can display a special charisma— another kid with a magic smile that can sell you anything. This may also be a good, little actor. Ideals may be focused on the parent who is the authority, or perhaps one who has a career or identity that seems glamorous to the child. If that is you, you'd better stay on your pedestal, or at least bring the child gently to the realization that you are human. On the other hand, this placement sometimes reflects a child whose parent is expecting too much of her. Either alternative can result in disillusioning experiences. This is a child who needs to turn her dreams into accomplishment in the world. Just take care they are **her** dreams, not yours.

Most of the children about whom this book is being read are, or will be, born with **Neptune in Capricorn**, sign of conservatism and tradition. The approximate time period of their births, 1984-1998, began during the Reagan presidency, a time that glorified "traditional" values. The religious revival (of the previous period) in a more fundamentalist form of Christianity was dominant and vocal — most of the alternative religions were autonomous minorities with no organized voice. The conservatives held the power and authority was respected. As the time period moved on, disillusionment set in. TV religious leaders fell to scandal. Doubts about the Reagan administration set in. The big business of illegal drugs allowed all too many to escape the reality of an established order that was dissolving with no viable dream to replace it. Now we have a mammoth, incredible deficit, a new president who would like to "rebuild government from the ground up," but who must work within a context of too many people whose illusions are still stuck on recreating an idealized past that is gone, rather than creating a new ideal out of what is. Hopefully, your kids will be able to see "what is," and help find that new ideal that can manifest into a new and workable reality.

Neptune in House 11 or in Aquarius

With **Neptune in House 11**, the friends, including groups in clubs, or working together for some goal, are idealized and provide inspiration for the child's own goals. This can be very good in some cases, from an early, creative play group through such experiences as Brownies and Cub Scouts or the like. It may reflect a problem if the attraction is to groups that do not share your values, or to those who are up to mischief. Part of what the child is seeking through these experiences is a personal sense of individuality. This may have to do with why a bunch of kids conforming to each other think they are being different, individual, and even a bit shocking. They are defining themselves and their own aspirations. Provide the resource of affiliations with desirable groups early.

I'll speculate a bit on the illusions and disillusionments of a **Neptune in Aquarius** generation, for the first births will come in 1998, which may include some of your children-yet-to-be-born. Coming after a period in which the ideal of top-down authority is dissolving into self-directed work teams and networking in business, term limit movements and general disillusionment with government, and rapid growth of alternative religious movements that seek God/Goddess within rather than on a throne on high, these kids will probably be born in a world that idealizes individuality. Too much individual freedom (anarchy) could dissolve into a search for a new ideal of social structure.

Neptune in House 12

Your child with **Neptune in House 12** has a very rich and vivid imagination that can be a great strength in life, or an avenue of escape from whatever does not measure up to the dream. If one wants too much, it can be a temptation to give up. It's important to give this child plenty of opportunities for creative outlets—and that does not mean letting her sit in front of the TV too much, letting it create all her fantasies. Encourage her with dancing, with music, with arts and crafts, with making up little rhymes, with playing make-believe games. Art will help her ground her dreams into something tangible, and it might even lead to a career someday. Also, this placement often reflects one who cares for others with compassion—a budding nurse or doctor, perhaps.

Pluto in the Houses and Relevant Signs

Pluto in House 1

Here you have a kid who is very intense about being in control, and is likely to react emotionally when his control is threatened. He's much more deeply emotional than he may appear on the surface. Expect him to test you, competitively or with manipulation, just to see how far he can go. Once he has a goal, he's very determined and compromise won't be easy. You'll have to help him learn to give in gracefully when he must. An appeal in regard to others' feelings might work better than logic. Remember his emotions are at stake, too.

Pluto in House 2

Control urges are directed toward comfort and material things. You can try to change the way your child wants her room, her space, her idea of comfort, what she cares about—but I wish you luck. Liz is my personal experience with this placement. I've found it much more conducive to my own sense of emotional control to close the door to her room, accept that maybe she really can read effectively with that slouching position in bad light, and that if allowed to choose things for herself, will generally make good choices.

Pluto in House 3

This is a child who may seek a sense of control through words, or alternatively, through silence. You could have the "wheedler" who will talk it to death until you finally give in, or one who will withdraw in a profound silence until someone comes to find out what is wrong, and…gives in. Just realize what's going on, while maintaining consistency about what can and cannot be, and give him plenty of chances to learn and develop mentally. After all, words, knowledge and the power to persuade are very good, too. Maybe he'll become a marketing genius!

Pluto in House 4 or in Cancer

Mom (or the more nurturing parent) is an especially important role model for the **Pluto in House 4** child's attitudes toward power and self-control. A close, nurturing bond—but NOT smothering—is highly important in the child's development of the ability to share with others and feel secure. Feelings about home and family, and the security or lack of it within, are very emotionally intense and may be unconscious.

Grandparents or great-grandparents may have been born with **Pluto in Cancer**, 1913-1938. Strong feelings of patriotism (my homeland) all over the world led to World War I and the beginnings of World War II. Agriculture underwent a revolution in order to increase food production — chemicals, insecticides, irrigation, power equipment. The wars and increased industrialization both led to a breakdown of extended families and much upheaval in previous patterns of family life. Women gained the vote in the United States.

Pluto in House 5 or in Leo

Your **Pluto in House 5** tyke may test you by raising the hairs on the back of your neck wondering if he—and you—will survive. He's testing his own sense of power and control by taking chances, perhaps by exaggerating and dramatizing. He needs challenges for his competitiveness and passion. Encourage sports, games and performing arts.

This nearly 20-year period of **Pluto in Leo** (1938-57) spans my generation to perhaps even include some of you. This period of leadership, power and drama began during World War II, climaxing with the explosion of the first atomic bomb. It continued through the build up of the cold war between the powerful forces of capitalism and communism, as the world considered the potentials of mass destruction or mass explosions of technology through the forces unleashed. Its children, inclined to probe deeply into individual creative expression, grew up to form countercultures that searched for their individuality, some even dropping out of mass society in reaction to its power abuses.

Pluto in House 6 or in Virgo

Your **Pluto in House 6** child needs a sense of personal control in her tasks and routines, and over the functions of her body. Give her that opportunity with resources and basic instruction, but with plenty of room for her to set her own details of how she accomplishes the task. Too much structure from outside could cause frustration to be internalized into illnesses. Mind this well in not overdirecting what and when she eats, or when and how she is potty trained. She is likely to be quite organized and thorough in what she does all on her own, and emotionally invested in doing it well.

Many of you who are now parents (born 1957-1971) have **Pluto in Virgo**, sign of work and health, and related techniques/technologies. Transformations in work were heralded by the beginning of the computer revolution. Increased automation streamlined production, but replaced many workers. Medical technology made great advances. The birth control pill, which separated sex from conception, contributed to the Neptunian dissolutions of Libra and Scorpio, noted previously, and also to the increase of working women. The revolutionary 60s were encompassed by this period, further influencing the children born of it to closely and intently examine the results of the technological explosion in work and health to see if it may have gone too far. Pollution and chemicals in food, for example, are a major concern.

Pluto in House 7 or in Libra

Control and self-mastery are being tested and learned through close one-to-one relationships by your child with **Pluto in House 7**. He may be one who always has a very "best friend" about whom he is very intense and absolutely loyal. Major emotional ups and downs reflect how the relationship is going at the moment. He is learning to share and to compromise, and this is his way—but steering him (and a friend) into team sports or group activities so they interact with other children, too, would be a good idea.

Pluto in Libra, 1971-1983, saw great upheaval in the areas of minority and women's rights, which had "traditionally" been decidedly out-of-balance. Even now we can look back on this period as a mammoth breakdown in traditional marriage. That theme was further emphasized during the Uranus movement through Libra, previously noted. People living together without marriage became commonplace, and children living with both parents, married happily, became the exception rather than the rule. The children, growing up in unstable homes, probe deeply to discover new ways to relate, often reluctant to make long-term commitments, but demanding fair play and equal power.

Pluto in House 8 or in Scorpio

Self-control in anything is a very strong drive for your child with **Pluto in House 8**, and the limits are tested through intensely pushing and probing the issue until the "wall breaks down" or the head that's butting into it hurts enough. A challenge is when to keep pushing, and when to just let go. I'm intimately familiar with this placement of Pluto, since I have it. Expect strong will and persistence, but if the kid finally gives up on a goal or a person, that's it. It's dead and forgotten—no use crying over spilt milk. She'll pick up the pieces and focus on a new goal with all the same intensity.

Pluto in Scorpio includes most births from the last part of 1983 until nearly the end of 1995. Ever since the period began, stories on these issues of shared resources, sexuality, life, death and power have dominated the news — abortion, right-to-life, right-to-die, gay and lesbian rights, abuse, sexual harassment, misuse of power, and of course, the national debt. It's too soon to tell for sure how all of the things will be eventually transformed, but it is clear that society is probing deeply into all of them. The children of this generation may intensely carry transformative activities in some of these areas into the next millennium. Already many of their elders are deeply concerned about the upset in ecology that has come from lack of concern for shared resources of the earth on which we all must live. Perhaps this abuse will be turned around when the children born of this era come into the prime of their adulthood. Pluto will be in Capricorn, then, suggesting an upheaval in government now in fermentation stages during Uranus and Neptune in Capricorn.

Pluto in House 9 or in Sagittarius

Intensity and a sense of control are sought through issues of faith, religion, philosophy, education. In your child with **Pluto in House 9,** you may see a stronger than usual early interest in issues of right and wrong, what's fair and what isn't, why the sky is blue, and what and where God is. Helping him find answers to questions, and providing some kind of religious instruction, will give the background for his later continued questioning and probing of beliefs and understanding, as he seeks his own truth.

Many of you are likely to have children born in the period of **Pluto in Sagittarius**, which will include some births in 1995 and continue into the 21st century. Sagittarius deals with the search for meaning in religion, philosophy, education, and law. Already we can see seeds of potential upheaval in all established institutions, which includes traditional religions that no longer address the realities of modern life or satisfy the needs of many for a spiritual center. We see mass dissatisfaction with public education, and a dissatisfaction with law that makes lawyers the butt of more mean jokes than any group has probably ever endured. I would expect this era to mark great transformations in all of these, and the children born of this era to be quite unorthodox and independent as they search for their own truths.

Pluto in House 10

This child may test her own sense of power against authority figures, or she may not. She will feel intensely toward an authority-type role model. The parent who makes the rules, who is the "authority," is very likely to be that person. Through this parent the child will unconsciously pick up important lessons in healthy self-control (or lack of it), and the ability (or inability) to share with others. Remember, your example speaks louder than any words you can say.

Pluto in House 11

A way of testing personal control for this one is likely to be through issues of freedom versus closeness, and in a child, this is likely to be played out through friends. He needs to be free and individual, but he also needs to love and be loved. He may come on too strong with others, or be intimidated by them, in the process of learning to balance his needs. While he may be inspired and influenced by his peer group, this young reformer is also capable of setting an original style.

Pluto in House 12

This child may be intensely involved in dreams and fantasies. She tests herself and her world against her dreams. Her vivid imagination may well manifest her castle in the air into a one day reality, but she may also have some fears of dragons in the dungeon that you'll have to help her transform into friendly ones. Show her that even though the world may not be perfect, she has the power to make it beautiful—at least most of the time.

Chapter Eight
Planets in Aspect

There's a strange sounding language of jargon spoken by astrologers among themselves. It draws weird looks from innocent bystanders who happen to be sharing the same hotel elevator as any two or more astrologers on their way to a typical conference lecture. One astrologer might say something like this to another: "What a year I'm having! Saturn's square my Sun-Uranus and Pluto's conjunct and opposite." To which the other might respond, "Oh, my, I do empathize. They're hitting my Moon. And what's more, the Uranus-Neptune conjunction's opposing my Mercury." This baffling conversation between two people who apparently understand each other, is about **aspects**, which is the topic of this chapter. They are speaking in a language that I call "Astrospeak." Like most occupational jargons, it is a convenient shorthand for the initiated, but it also has a tendency to discourage laypeople from trying to learn more about astrology unless they are very, very interested.

It's not going to be **that** confusing — promise! But I do think you deserve a little warning that at least a little bit of Astrospeak will have to be used to introduce this section of "cookbook" interpretations.

For those of you who have your Magical Child chart, using this chapter and the next chapter will be easy, for the aspects you should read about are listed below the chart wheel.

If you are working with the "do it yourself" tables in the appendix of this book, I must tell you up front that without a fully calculated chart you will not be able to use the interpretive paragraphs in either this chapter or in Chapter Nine. In order to know which paragraphs to read, you will need not just the signs, but the exact degrees of the planets, the Ascendant and the Midheaven. The simplified look-up tables provided in this book are just not adequate to give you this information. Send for that chart!

It would be easier, of course, not to deal with the aspects in a book intended not only for astrology students, but also for those who don't really have the time or inclination to seriously study astrology, yet are open to the idea that it might offer them some worthwhile insights. But it's important for you to realize that if we take the easy way out, and just use planets in signs, you might miss some of the most important information about your child that astrology has to offer. Also, you might make assumptions about a planet based on sign alone that would be substantially modified if you knew the nature of that planet's aspects.

The fact that various planets are closely connected with each other — in aspect to each other — is a considerably more important part of horoscope interpretation than what signs the planets are in. When planets are in close aspect, the basic function of each of them is closely blended with the other. The distinct functions are still there, but one must consider them as being more closely related than planets that are not in aspect. Aspects tell us how the planets work together. Understanding these interrelationships of the planets is the single most significant part of horoscope interpretation.

Close aspects in your child's chart may help you sort out some of the apparent contradictions you may have found in the various signs of the planets. The themes of some aspects may be considerably more noticeable in the personality than even the Sun sign.

The list of aspects below the chart wheel on the Magical Child chart names the type of aspect, for example: Sun **square** Uranus, Mercury **trine** Neptune, or Mars **conjunct** Jupiter. When you begin to look up the interpretations in this book, however, you will find that except for a few that are designated "conjunct," the paragraph headings will **not** name aspects but instead say merely Sun–Uranus, Mercury–Neptune or Mars–Jupiter, etc. Please don't be confused by this. If, for example, the list on your chart says Mercury trine Neptune, you read the interpretation headed Mercury-Neptune. If your chart list says Mercury square Neptune, you still read the Mercury-Neptune interpretation. The basic theme is the same in either case. Knowing which specific type of aspect Mercury and Neptune make to each other is worthwhile for two reasons:

1. Knowing the type of aspect helps you evaluate how strong it is, relative to other aspects in the horoscope.

2. Your Magical Child chart will be useful to you when you read other books which have different paragraphs for the various types of aspect. One of them is *Planets in Youth* by Robert Hand, which speaks to older kids, teenagers. Also, you might want to study astrology at some point and want to know which aspect is which.

The primary reason that I have **not** written separate interpretations for each different type of aspect between the same two planets is because, quite frankly, I don't see the validity of doing so, especially for the novice. The basic **theme** of two planets working together is the same, no matter what type of aspect they are making to each other. When a "cookbook" gives a different paragraph for each type of aspect, you are just getting a slightly different nuance of the same theme. The tendencey, in such books, is to assign the "good" manifestations of a two-planet theme to one type of aspect, and the "bad" ones to another type. You read only the aspect that applies, and miss understanding the full meaning of the theme. I always suggest that students, in using such books, read **all** of the aspect paragraphs applying to a given two planets, rather than just the one specific aspect they are looking for, to make sure they understand the wider range of potentials.

No aspect is all good, or all bad, and every combination in astrology has many potential manifestations, within a core theme. "Good" or "bad" is largely a matter of opinion and choice, arising out of environment and development. The type of aspect tells us something about the relative strength of the aspect and whether it is more likely to represent an active or a passive characteristic.

The Magical Child chart has two lists of aspects under two headings: **hard** and **soft**. Among the **hard** aspects, you should take special note of the **conjunctions**, *e.g.* Sun **conjunct** Venus, or Moon **conjunct** Saturn. Conjunctions are likely to be the most dominant aspects.

Understand "hard" as **strong**, rather than difficult. Because these aspects are strong, they also may reflect more challenge in learning to express the themes most appropiately. However, they also represent themes that have stronger (greater) potential for productive action than the soft aspects. Most of the challenge and the activity will be in the aspects that are listed as the hard ones.

The basic combinations of themes in each paragraph will still apply in the case of soft aspects, but the expression will be (like the name implies) much softer. "Soft" is to be understood as a milder, more passive theme.

All of the aspects symbolize the ways in which the nature of the two planets combined may be reflected in your child's personality. Whether the more or the less desirable traits predominate in the personality is not a given—**not** "fated." Growth, guidance, environmental circumstances and personal choice will be significant determining factors. Be sensitive about guiding your child with this information. Aniticipating potentials enables you to provide resources for the child to guide him/herself, and thereby guide you as to the details of his/ her needs and abilities.

The hard aspects are most likely to represent noticeable talents and successes, when challenges are met, while the soft types are more likely to represent ease. People who know a little bit about astrology may read a soft aspect interpretation and think, "Oh good," tending to then expect too much of these so-called harmonious traits. All too often, though, too much ease just goes unnoticed, or indeed may even represent a problem (challenge), if there's no incentive to do anything with the energies symbolized by the soft aspect. You see, it takes a little sand to make an oyster grow a pearl. We don't learn and grow nearly as much from ease as we do from that which takes a little effort. Read all of your child's aspect paragraphs, hard or soft, but trust me, you are most likely to notice the hard aspects at work in your child's life and growth. That's where the action is!

A good way to use information about a close soft aspect would be for hints on areas of potential ease or talent into which you might try to redirect the energy that your child is releasing through the expression of hard aspect themes — especially if those themes are trying your patience! For example, if an undesirable expression of a hard aspect is being experienced, and an activity associated with a desirable expression of a close soft aspect is available, you might have some success in giving the child a nudge in that direction. Molly has Mars square Neptune, which reflects her dreaminess and romanticism, but also an inclination to lethargy or low energy. Her Mars also is trine Jupiter, with Jupiter in House 1. She had an abundance of energy, enthusiasm and ambition when her romantic dreams were directed into expressing herself in dance. Now she can be tirelessly caught up for hours when she's transforming a personal vision into a painting.

If one potential expression of a hard aspect does not seem to you to be appropriate, you might succeed in redirecting the child's energy toward one of the more acceptable options of that same aspect. Just understand that it is not in your child's best interests for you to expect the complete repression of the theme of these active aspects. The child's energy, as symbolized by that aspect, needs to be expressed in one way or another. So please redirect — do not suppress.

Blend the aspect interpretations with the information you have already read about sign placements. Look for repeated themes as being the most important ones for you to consider in understanding and guiding your child.

The Planetary Aspect "Cookbook"

The following paragraphs interpret each combination of two planets in your child's horoscope. In order to eliminate unwieldy "he and she" stuff, I will alternate gender pronouns in each paragraph, and also at the beginning of each new planetary sequence, if it is necessary to associate specific planets with one sex in one series, and the other in the next. Just substitute the pronouns, if your child is the opposite sex of that used in a paragraph.

In just a few cases, I think the conjunction "works" differently enough from other types of aspects that I have provided a separate paragraph for the conjunction. In most cases I have not, because as I said before, the mix of symbolism for those two planets working together simply does not change that much from one type of aspect to another. It's sufficient to consider whether the aspect is hard or soft in order to evaluate strength and potential for the more challenging parts of the interpretive text.

The general symbolism of the planetary combinations for either sex is very similar. I said that before, too — just in case you jumped ahead to this part and missed it... (Grandma knows how inclined you are to skip past the explanations and get right to the personal stuff!) I'll repeat it now, because it's important.

If your little girl takes a softer approach in reflecting her Mars aspects, for example, or your little boy, a noisier approach to a Venus aspect, it's not the planets that are "doing" it. More likely, it's environmental programming. Even with all the progress in eliminating male/female stereotypes in recent history, most people still tend to treat girl and boy babies somewhat differently right from the start. If you don't agree, just quietly observe and listen to the different manner in which people behave with little boys and little girls — even step back and observe yourself — and you'll see what I mean. Regardless, your girl may be a very active, extroverted type by nature, or your boy may be a sensitive, artistic introvert. They'll be much more successful — and happier in life — if allowed to be themselves, and even encouraged in their natural directions. And, trust me, so will you!

Sun conjunct Moon

Your child, born near the New Moon, has an instinctive flair, no matter what the Sun/Moon sign placements. Consider whatever you read about Sun and Moon signs to be more than doubly strong — in both desirable and not so desirable manifestation. There's a basic harmony between the basic personality expression and the inner emotional needs. In whatever talents and skills your child develops, he is likely to take the lead — so long as he has a basic emotional comfort. Emotional reactions are pronounced — read again, most carefully, the emotional needs of the Moon sign, and consider how best to nurture this child's sense of security.

Sun-Moon

Your child's basic personality expression and her fulfillment of purpose in life are very closely tied to her inner emotional needs. Especially with the hard aspects, some inner conflict exists between her underlying motivations — how she feels — vs. the mode of her self expression, *e.g.*: how she best can "shine" in the world. In early childhood this might manifest as uncertainty about when, and under what circumstances, to put oneself forward assertively and when to hold back and be receptive rather than active. Inappropriate choices may be made until inner balance is achieved. Balance in role models (active/passive, masculine/feminine) and harmonious interactions between parents (ability to both give and take when appropriate) is of enormous help for her development in this area.

Sun and Moon related in passive aspects are not likely to be associated with challenge, but they are different. Read again the Sun and Moon sign combinations for hints as to how your child's style of "shining" may be enhanced or hindered by her emotional needs.

Sun conjunct Mercury

Your child's vital expression (Sun) and his "messenger" (Mercury) are working together closely. The result is additional clarity of mind and ability to understand and organize the life according to the best qualities suggested by the Sun sign. His thinking and style of communication supports his conscious objectives in life. This aspect increases the ability to articulate, and quite probably will also mean that this child may talk early and a lot!

(Mercury is not far enough from the Sun for any aspect other than conjunction to form between them.)

Sun conjunct Venus

Your child is blessed with the gift of charm. She will seem to have a natural, instinctive gift for making people like her. She will probably be perceived as attractive by others, no matter what her actual physical features, for she will be sociable, friendly and "easy" to be with. This aspect will most likely be a real asset — unless it is overdone. Possible misuses would be being too compromising — too inclined to do what is agreeable to others when she really ought to be sticking up for her own point of view — or placing too much emphasis on surface appearances. Any talent in or inclination toward the arts will be emphasized and supported by this aspect.

(Venus can never be more than 46° from the Sun, so the only other aspects possible are the 30° semi-sextile, which is very soft and may not be particularly significant, and the 45° semi-square. The latter is a hard aspect, which means it is significant, but not as strong as the conjunction.)

Sun conjunct Mars

Your child is likely to be quite strong willed and assertive. He has an extra amount of energy, determination, courage and ability to go after what he wants in life. He is inclined to be competitive, and is unafraid of most any challenge. This kid may not pick a fight, but he won't back off from one, either. A possible downside could take the form of "bull-headedness" in insisting on his own way no matter what. Giving in could seem like a too personal defeat. This child will need physical activity to help burn off his excess energy. Encourage sports.

You may also have to suggest techniques to burn off anger. If you send him to his room to simmer alone, his bottled up anger is likely to explode later, and even more inappropriately. The energy and the feelings need to be released, but in a way that does not hurt others. Your willingness to listen a bit and acknowledge the anger, without necessarily agreeing, might help. Or send him to his room, but with the possibility of release through a punching pillow or the private drawing of angry pictures, and then coming back to talk about it after calming down.

This aspect, if you as caregiver are too "programmed" by old-fashioned ideas of how boys and girls "should" be, is likely to be a much harder one to handle for your little girl. "Traditional" girls would more likely be "programmed" to suppress this type of Mars energy. Suppression can create more problems than healthy release. Passive aggression can be just as destructive. Whether boy or girl, the child with this aspect needs physical activity and guidance toward acceptable, safe and constructive means of releasing anger.

Sun-Mars

Your child is inclined to be very assertive and competitive, especially with the active aspects, although even the passive ones will indicate extra emphasis to her basic Sun expression. She could be very obstinate about "my own way or else." There's an overabundance of energy that needs an outlet. Sports should be encouraged. No matter what the Sun sign, this aspect suggests an element of rashness in the personality. With the ability to accept a challenge and fight, in the positive sense, there is also the tendency to perceive a challenge even when one has not been given. In this case, she may be too quickly defensive, and/or the temper could flare.

Another possible manifestation of this aspect could be a tendency to overdo, to take on too much, which could result in "burn-out." Or, particularly if other planets of the chart suggest a nonassertive or suppressed personality, your child may attract overly aggressive friends. She could be very subtly provocative in a way that triggers others to pick a fight with her. You could help by being alert to these possibilities, and able to acknowledge your child's feelings (listen), and then suggest ways of redirecting her energy.

Sun-Jupiter

This aspect combination is usually quite favorable. It suggests a warm, healthy, optimistic and happy ("jovial") personality, who is capable of much success in the world. Your child could be described as expansive and self-confident. He can usually be counted upon to take the optimistic point-of-view toward any challenge. The potential downside can be a tendency toward over-expansiveness, which could take the form of extravagance or perhaps carelessness, or arrogance. Too much emphasis on the material aspects of life are more likely to lead to the problems, while examples (role models) with integrity and spiritual ideals are supportive of the most favorable qualities.

Sun-Saturn

No matter what the Sun sign, this aspect will add an overtone of seriousness and reserve to the personality. Your child could seem old for her age. She may seem somewhat shy and/or inhibited, or tend to be too self-critical. An over-perception of limitation from outside the self could result in problems with authority figures, or feelings of being blocked or frustrated. In a positive sense, however, this planetary combination often describes a person of great perseverance, who has a strong ability to focus and concentrate, and to be quite self-disciplined at whatever work she undertakes. She may need more encouragement from you, at least at earlier ages. Genuine respect shown for this child's accomplishments will build self-esteem that will help to bring out the best in her.

Sun-Uranus

No matter what the Sun sign, this planetary combination indicates an extra need to be free and to express individuality. This kid is in some way a bit of a rebel, who wants to find a new way of doing things. He is inventive and original in his expression of whatever characteristics are suggested by the Sun sign. Because he likes to do things his own way, or just in a different way, it follows that this could sometimes place him in conflict with others, perhaps including you, or other authority figures, who might then describe him as self-willed, obstinate or even as a "'trouble-maker." Or such traits as "excitable" or "tense" might also apply. Balance? In what area do you REALLY need to insist on your way? Everything? Doubtful. Allow original expression in every way that you comfortably can — encourage it, to bring out his innovative best. Try to choose a progressive, creative school environment rather than a highly structured one. Encourage creativity. This kid has a lot of it!

Sun-Neptune

One could say that Neptune wears a mask. No matter what the Sun sign, a close aspect with Neptune may cast an aura of mystery or fogginess over the overt expression of the Sun sign characteristics. There are multiple possibilities for the Neptune "mask" and your child may express one or more of them. She may be extremely sensitive, with strong empathy for feelings around her, even when they are not expressed openly. This could result in a tendency to withdraw or seem inhibited. With understanding, she could grow to be a person with great helping and healing skills. She may be extra sensitive on a physical level. If colic or fussiness, later hyperactivity or other health problems, should manifest, be sure you look into the possibility of allergies. Realize — it's not "bad behavior." It's probably only "sensitivity" that can quite possibly be modified if you can find out what's causing it. She could be romantic and dreamy, with a private world of her own and maybe even imaginary friends. Such creative fantasy, encouraged and trained, could lead to the creation of great beauty in the arts.

Sun-Pluto

Pluto adds an overtone of power to whatever Sun sign characteristics you've already read about your child. He'll be a very strong willed kid, who may be likely to carry almost anything to extremes. He is an intense personality who is not inclined to do anything halfway. Whether this is "good" or "bad," of course depends upon what he is being intense about! Conflicts with authority figures are possible, so you could be in for some power struggles. On some things you will need to be firm. Be clear on what they are. But it would be best to encourage self-discipline and mutual trust. The positive potential of this aspect is very strong. This one is ambitious, persistent, and he is a survivor. Nothing will keep him down for long. He will keep trying no matter what. And he will probably achieve considerable success in whatever he tries.

Moon-Mercury

It is difficult for this child to separate his FEELINGS from what he THINKS. He tends to approach every issue subjectively, personalizing things that would be better handled with reason and objectivity. On the other hand, he might rationalize away his feelings. Habits of thinking or "programming" that he picks up in very early childhood, often subconsciously, will be of utmost importance in the future. What he "thinks" about anything is likely to fall back on that programming. Your child will need to learn to differentiate between objective reality and his feelings, lest the emotions take over at the wrong time. Yet suppressing the emotions is not the answer, for without feeling, life can be pretty drab. The trick will be awareness of which is which.

Moon-Venus

This aspect generally belongs to a person who is gracefully and cordially kind and affectionate. It will greatly support any artistic talents or inclinations that your child may have. She is likely to be quite socially adept, cheerful and charming. One thing to note: this child NEEDS affection (Moon) and comfort (Venus). As a tot, she'll especially like touchy, feely toys. Any downside of this aspect would come from overdoing what it takes to satisfy those needs. Building a secure foundation for her, as a baby and tot, will mean seeing that she feels loved for her inner qualities, rather than for surface appearances.

Moon-Mars

With this aspect there is a strong NEED (Moon) to assert oneself (Mars). Feelings tend to be pretty near the surface, and can easily flare up if the sensitivities are provoked. This child is not likely to take teasing well at all, and he needs to be in a fairly calm environment. His relationship with Mother, or the primary nurturing caregiver, is very significant. He needs tranquillity, but at the same time, needs to be taught to express angry or moody, upset feelings in a manner that gets them out without hurting others. The strength of this aspect is that this kid will fight for what he wants and/or believes in. His strong will and honest directness, coupled with a powerful sense of purpose, can be a considerable asset toward his success in life.

Moon-Jupiter

This is generally a very positive aspect that belongs to a cheerful, upbeat person who feels good about herself and is fun to be with. She probably has lots of energy and uses it very generously. The potential problem, of course, for any energetic "doer" is overdoing! This kid can "go" until she drops, so you may have to be the one to rein her in at times, and try to instill some examples of the value of self-control. This issue of self-control could also arise in regard to spending money or food indulgences.

Moon-Saturn

No matter how jovial the planets in signs may suggest your child might be, with this aspect he will be considerably more serious and reserved. He NEEDS emotional security (Moon), but that which he needs seems limited (Saturn). Thus he may feel somehow unsupported and alone, even unloved. It is possible that this aspect may reflect some conflict or imbalance in the mother/father role models, or tension between the parents. There may be issues here that you, as parent, cannot control. What you can do is provide as emotionally supportive an environment as possible, including lots of hugs and other expressions of affection. Nurture your child with love, while at the same time encouraging his self-sufficiency. With inner balance he can develop security within himself, and conservatively and productively achieve. This child may seem grown-up when young, and can be a good manager of his work. He is likely to be quite conscientious and responsible.

Moon-Uranus

With this aspect the emotions (Moon) are tense (Uranus). Your child NEEDS (Moon) to express her independence as an individual (Uranus). Some constructive expressions of this energy are determined striving for goals, strong will and ambition, sometimes aided by sudden flashes (Uranus) of intuition (Moon). Some destructive expressions are a tendency to magnify feelings out of proportion, over-stressed nervousness or being extremely self-willed. This child may seem somewhat emotionally detached, preferring not to get too closely involved with anyone, even though he may have many casual friends. It is best to encourage her uniqueness, and as much as acceptably possible, to encourage her need for freedom. Possessiveness and "smother-love" are NOT supportive. Appreciation, with a quick and sincere hug, for her creativity and specialness, is.

Moon-Neptune

This is a child who is very intuitive and may well have some form of psychic ability. If he tells you of impressions or experiences of that nature, don't discount them. This may be quite real, and in any case, it's real to him. You don't have to "swallow" everything as fact, but do not make fun of him and do not brush him off with disbelief. Listen with interest. At the same time, you don't want him lost in fantasy. Give your child opportunities to channel his fantasies and dreams and visions into constructive expressions, such as art, music or poetry. Be aware that he is likely to pick up negative feelings from those around him, and may not be able to evaluate whether or not they are really directed at him. You may need to help him understand that he is not responsible for other's feelings, and that often they have nothing to do with him. He will have to learn how to separate reality from imagination, and perhaps also how to shut out impressions from others when he needs to.

Moon-Pluto

Your child has such intense, deep feelings, it is often difficult for her to understand them at all, much less articulate them to anyone else. Because her emotions are so strong, they can sometimes get in her way, causing erroneous perceptions of what is really going on. Moods can swing from the heights to the depths. For these reasons, her problems in life may take the form of feeling misunderstood (silently), or perhaps being overly possessive of a loved one, or suspicious and/or manipulative, when there is really no threat of loss. The relationship with the Mother is probably emotionally complex, and will be of great significance in how this child learns to use her emotional power. Strive to teach, and set examples of, self-control and inner mastery. Your child can grow to be one who will transfer her emotional insights into the ability to lead others toward positive transformative experience.

Mercury-Venus

Any talents or inclinations that your child has in the arts are supported and enhanced by this aspect. He is likely to have an excellent sense of form and design, and you should encourage his interests in art. This aspect also suggests an intellect that is strongly influenced by his desires for comfort and pleasure. This could mean a rather light-hearted approach to life, but if encouraged, it could also mean a love (Venus) of learning (Mercury).

Mercury-Mars

This aspect combines the thinking and assertive functions. Put quite simply, that means that this child is probably going to let you know what she thinks, in no uncertain terms! This kid should probably be steered toward the debate team when she is older, and perhaps that will lead to a career that involves public speaking or persuasion. For now, you may note a tendency to speak out first and think later, a love of talking and arguing, and also perhaps a love of spinning a tale with no small amount of exaggeration. You'd better be on your toes. This kid won't give ground easily!

Mercury-Jupiter

Mercury symbolizes the thinking process, and Jupiter symbolizes higher thought processes, like philosophy. The two in close aspect can indicate the potential for considerable wisdom, and plain old common sense — assuming other aspects do not offer too much conflict, and that the talent potentials of this child are constructively channeled. The potential downsides of this combination are of the "overdone" variety: arrogance, exaggeration, tactlessness. Your child needs a good education — that is primary. He will have good ideas and a gift for speech, and probably will be quite optimistic most of the time.

Mercury-Saturn

This aspect combines the thinking process with the capacity for discipline, responsibility and the building of structures. Obviously, then, a constructive application suggests that your child has the ability to concentrate on her studies, to organize material systematically, and to work quite industriously. The aspect may also indicate a shyness or reserve in her personality. It could also mean a tendency to take a rather narrow view, to be skeptical or to be quite stubborn in her thinking. These traits, too, could serve her well in pursuits that involve research and investigation.

Mercury-Uranus

Here we could imagine that the thinking process is permanently plugged into an electric current that's frequently hit by a lightening bolt. The intuition is strong, punctuated with flashes of inventiveness. The mind is innovative and shrewd. This child might do well in technical fields, in science. He is likely to be good at grasping abstract concepts such as in math. In any case, this is an independent thinker with a revolutionary spirit. Ideas come so fast that sometimes he may be scattered, with too much going on at once. Words may come out in a flash, too, all too frankly to the point of tactlessness (others may think). Excitement could become nervousness. Independence could "read" as eccentricity. The tyke may actually enjoy shocking you. If you don't like it, don't be shocked. Ignoring him will probably be a better strategy to "tone him down." Save your reactions for positive appreciation of his little innovative flashes of genius!

Mercury-Neptune

Your child's thinking process is hitched to her dreams, imagination and fantasies. On the downside, this conjures up the possibility that facts may get confused with fiction, anywhere from little, white lies to great, big fibs. On the other hand, such possibilities, properly channeled, can become talents and careers for those whose work demands that they "play a role": actors, lawyers, diplomats, etc. Just be aware that you may have to check things out, and perhaps help your child sort out fantasy from reality on occasion. She may show psychic abilities, including the ability to "see" some things in advance. Her imagination will be vivid, and her capacity for empathy may come out in a great capacity for compassion toward others. This aspect is also good for creative writing, art and super sales ability.

Mercury-Pluto

The thinking process in this child is supported by his capacity to be in control. This implies a person who can speak or write very persuasively, who can exert a strong influence over others. He has a deep, penetrating mind, with a strong ability to concentrate — to probe and dig until he gets to the bottom of what he is trying to figure out. If he feels a need to understand something, nothing will stop him and nothing will frighten him, either — not the dark, the hidden or even the forbidden. He will learn to see power in knowledge and in words, and how to use them to advantage. All this can be strongly beneficial toward a number of career areas, or possibly manipulative and obsessive, depending upon his direction and ethical sense. A good education is very important. Even more important is an ethic of personal responsibility for himself (including not blaming anything outside himself) and respect for the free will of others.

Venus-Mars

The principle of this combination is the ACTION (Mars) of LOVE (Venus). The most obvious connotation of this is sexual, and with this aspect your child has "it" — a magnetic, charismatic type of attractiveness. He may be one who becomes quickly attracted — but also one who swings between the Venus tendency to compromise and defer, and the Mars tendency to exert his own independence and want his own way. Venus is also art interest, and the action of that can mean both talent and drive. Relax about "it" for now, parent! While he is so young, begin by encouraging him in the arts. Try him out on everything from drawing to dance and see what "takes."

Venus-Jupiter

In this child , the capacity for love and pleasure is very expansive, and infused with the desire for growth and a quest for higher ideals. Potential challenges in this combination could involve difficulty in grounding romantic ideas with everyday reality. The idea that "there's something more" could mean inability to take pleasure in what she has now. On the definitely plus side, she will likely be one who is known for her warm-hearted generosity and charm. She is likely to be very popular, to get along well with others. She is just naturally friendly — but may be inclined toward overindulgence and extravagance.

Venus-Saturn

For this child, the capacity for love and pleasure is shadowed by an overtone of reserve, self-control and even inhibition. Somehow he seems to feel that his desires for love and comfort must be disciplined, kept within bounds. His sense of duty exceeds his wish for pleasure. Something very early in life may have given a subconscious feeling of deprivation that has created a very cautious attitude toward love. It must be earned, perhaps. Or "I must be very careful, or I'll be hurt." In any case, the result of this aspect is likely to be a very practical personality, inclined to be thrifty, reliable and sensible. Be very generous with affection and hugs for this little one. He may not show it, but he needs love, perhaps even more so than more demonstrative types. To the Venusian appreciation of the arts, Saturn adds an element of structure that can translate into profit. Encourage your child in the arts. If he develops a love for an art form, he will also have the business sense to make it pay. It could mean a future career.

Venus-Uranus

For your child, the capacity for love and pleasure is attached to a lightning rod. Impulsive "strikes" could mean falling in love at first sight, but also a "flash in the pan." This one could be interesting to watch as a teenager — if YOUR nerves can stay relatively calm! Don't expect her to settle down too fast. If the new love is possessive of her, she is likely to move on as fast as she "fell." In earlier childhood, this could take the form of instant likings for new friends or something new, but it's hot one day, cold the next. The tastes will run toward the unusual and the innovative. This combination is also associated with rhythm, and this child may be quite attracted to dance and/or rhythmic music.

Venus-Neptune

For this child, the capacity for love and pleasure is tied to his dreams and illusions. In his imagination is a lovely world of his own, where everything is beautiful and where princes and princesses dwell, and where all dragons are easily conquered. So idealistic is he, that disappointment is almost inevitable at some time or another. Who could possibly live up to his fantasies? Or, he could project what is in his dreams on someone who is unworthy, and then be just sure that his love will surely help that person become the love of his dreams. This is an aspect of being "in love with love." His idealism and empathy could be redirected into the wider world, toward helping or healing. Also, he is likely to have considerable flair for beauty and the arts. Give him opportunities to explore these areas.

Venus-Pluto

For your child, the capacity for love and pleasure is wedded to her power urges. Love can take on an intense, all-or-nothing quality, and can have a transformative effect on her. Whether her love is directed at people, pets, pleasures or possessions, you are not likely to see much resembling moderation in this kid's attitude. If she cares about someone, she is deeply loyal, and would go to the ends of the earth for that person. Naturally, it follows that possessiveness may be likely and jealousy may be a problem, too. She will need to learn that self-control is an asset, and trying to control others is a liability. Her capacity to probe to the depths can be an asset in the development of art forms, or perhaps as a catalyst for transformation in others (if she learns to relate to people in a non-manipulative way). This is a person who is likely to be quite magnetic and sensual in her attractiveness.

Mars-Jupiter

The capacity to act is expansive, exuberant and enthusiastic. Excitement attracts. Ideals inspire actions and choices for work. Your child will most likely be a confident and optimistic little character who will derive a lot of joy from life. He could be somewhat daring or impulsive, or inclined to overdo, and may need to learn some lessons of moderation. He may be most inclined to leap into the fray if his sense of morals, ethics or ideals are offended. On the whole, though, this aspect is strongly supportive of success in all of his undertakings. He'll have lots of energy, ambition to go with it, and probably a sense of humor and delight.

Mars-Saturn

For this child, the capacity to act is tethered to a structure of reality that may sometimes be perceived as limitation. "I want to do it, but I just can't." It's against the rules, Dad (or some authority figure) won't let me, the wall is too high, I don't know how... Or it may be perceived as "I HAVE to do this, no matter what, no matter how long it takes, according to the rules..." Overdoing either feeling blocked or feeling overburdened can be a problem for your child. It may not be easy for her to find a good balance between the conflicting themes of Mars and Saturn. Yet at their best, with self-discipline and the inner security of good self-esteem, she can accomplish much in life. Her endurance is endless, and her sense of timing may be quite good. She is practical and she has very good potential organizational abilities.

Mars-Uranus

Like a bolt out of the blue, this kid is zapped into action and takes off like a jet, leaving lesser mortals in the dust. He is free as the breeze, daring, independent and very much his own person. Don't try to change him. Such energy won't go away. If repressed, it is likely to come out in a much less desirable form. Accidents happen — usually when people aren't looking for them. Not when they are running a race by choice. Instead of restricting, direct this kid's excess energy into some areas where his adrenaline and innovative spirit can excel. This could be a wide variety of things: sports, science, computers, art. It isn't so much the activity, but the freedom within it to innovate, invent, problem-solve — to find a new way, a way that uniquely expresses him!

Mars-Neptune

For your child, the capacity for action is woven into a web of mystical, magical fantasy and dreams of perfect beauty. Sometimes it is so much easier to dream than to do, and lethargy sets in. The dreamer finds it difficult to cope with the demands of reality. Yet the urge to act can also be inspired by imagination, intuition or a compassionate sense of helping, healing or spiritual mission. It may be very important for her to have a sense of service beyond her personal needs in order to have the impetus to work and translate dreams into action. Or the form of action must have a connection with the realms of beauty and fantasy. Fantasy in action might be dance, figure skating, water ballet, gymnastics. Transcendent service might be work for a cause or a spiritual ideal. Do not try to suppress this child's sensitivities, intuition and love of fantasy — just try to channel them into productive expressions. Sometimes extreme sensitivity is internalized physically, so you might be extra cautious with her in regard to any hint of allergies or susceptibility to adverse reactions to medications.

Mars-Pluto

The capacity to act, for this child, has a permanent, pulsating power surge. There is an overtone of intensity, passion and do-or-die cast over everything he does. He is a strong competitor in games or sports, but may be a poor loser. He has tremendous stamina, but may not know when to quit or how to relax. He absolutely thrives on challenge. Self-control is very important to him, and this may spill over into the urge to control everything and everyone else around him. It will be important for your child to learn self-mastery, and to learn NOT to infringe on the rights of others to have that same privilege and responsibility.

Yet at the same time, do not attempt to suppress this child's power drives. It is important for him to find constructive outlets to claim and express his personal power. If he fails to claim his own power, he may constantly attract others who will pick on him. Angers and resentments could then build up and explode at the wrong time in a destructive manner. Your child has a very strong survival instinct, and can cope with most anything when necessary.

Age Group Aspects

The remainder of the aspects in this chapter are shared with your child's age group. They will be more individually significant if one of the planets is also in aspect to a personal planet or point.

Jupiter-Saturn

Since Jupiter represents expansion and growth, while Saturn represents limitation, there are some obvious potential conflicts of energy here. This child could swing from one focus to another. Or get stuck in the middle. There can be tension in balancing ideals and faith with the realities with which one must deal. With proper balance, the combination can be a real asset in which he blends the will to grow and the belief in a goal with the practical steps and stability to achieve it.

Jupiter-Uranus

For your child and others her age, the capacity for growth and the personal belief system is charged with the spirit of revolution, which may be exuberant and could be tense. Mental stimulation is important. All things new, innovative, inventive, eccentric, and exciting are appealing. These kids are bound to want to change things. Your world views, traditions, rules, standards, religion and other ideas are all up for question. "Because I say so" or "that's the way it always has been" just won't wash. Especially if there's an aspect to Mercury, you'd better be prepared to talk about it! This aspect increases any tendency toward optimism, independence and a sense of adventure.

Jupiter-Neptune

With this aspect optimism can be lifted to the realms of fantasy, or idealism to the outer boundaries of mystical vision. Kids with this combination have the ability to visualize a better, more humane way of doing things. Whether vision becomes reality probably depends on links to other aspects. For individuals, this planetary theme can take a number of forms. Speculation and risk taking is one — optimism leading to faith in Lady Luck. Your child could be overly impressionable, be consequently taken advantage of, and feel misunderstood. Or his rich imagination and humanitarian impulses could lead to altruism, spirituality or pursuit of beauty through art.

Jupiter-Pluto

Here the capacity for growth and the belief system are linked to the power to transform. If this combination is also linked with an aspect to a personal planet or point, your child could be quite a leader. She could have a real gift for organization, and be capable of influencing groups of people. She could develop into a good teacher, spiritual leader or politician, with the power to persuade. Potential problems could be power struggles, if her goals are at odds with others. This aspect supports any other success indicators in the horoscope.

Saturn-Uranus

The principle of structure and stability clashes with the principle of change and innovation. The result is tension, and the kids that have this combination are likely to be a generation that breaks down some worn out structure and replaces it with a new one. Your child, depending upon how closely this aspect may be linked with more personal ones, will have some challenge in balancing the old with the new, or perhaps freedom with restriction. If the balance is found he may accomplish much through his ability to bring discipline and structure to his creative and innovative ideas.

Saturn-Neptune

A major theme of this aspect is reality vs. fantasy. It can be associated with the suffering, anxiety and depression of a longing for impossible dreams, or it can be associated with the ability to turn dreams into reality. Which way it goes for an individual has a lot to do with environment and role-models, and may be indicated by the strength of this aspect's contacts with more personal planets. It may be important for you, through your own example, to strike a balance for her between faith in dreams and fear about trying for what may, at the moment, seem out-of-reach. Be open to her dreams, and try to find realistic opportunities for her to work toward them.

Saturn-Pluto

Mixing the principles of structure/reality with that of power/control can be quite a strong combination. To the degree that this aspect may be linked with personal planets, your child may be involved with power issues as a major theme in his life. He will learn much by his experiences in handling or denying power. You can help him strike a constructive balance by not being controlling, but by teaching and setting an example of self-discipline and responsibility. If your child learns to claim his own power without feeling the need to exert power over others, he will acquire the positive qualities of this aspect — endurance, discipline, patience, and a general toughness that will enable him to take on the most difficult of tasks and bring them to success.

Uranus-Neptune

This could be the combination of an individualistic idealist, a revolutionary artist, a psychic visionary. Most kids born during 1991-96 have the conjunction of this planet in their charts, and they could be a generation that makes major changes in areas of growing concerns such as equal opportunity, ethics in government, protection of the environment, etc. If personal planets are involved in aspects to this combination, your child may be uniquely involved in social/humanitarian concerns. Or she could be uniquely creative, innovative in expressing her fantasies, dreams and ideals.

Uranus-Pluto

This is a combination of intensity and power brought to bear on issues of humanitarian principle, social change, and freedom. Personal planets involved with this combination could indicate that this child is one who will be extremely committed to some social change in which he believes. He could be quite a reformer — determined, hard-working, unwilling to compromise or ever give up. He may have personal issues of balancing control with freedom, which could blow hot and cold on personal relationships as he tries to balance intense involvement with a need for space.

Neptune-Pluto

Idealism, fantasy and intuition is linked with intensity, passion and power. A generation of this combination could bring about transformations in social ideals. Individually, much depends on how this combination may be aspected by other more personal planets. This is a soft aspect, if anything, for kids of the ages covered by this book, so it probably isn't significant unless one or both of the planets are also closely aspected to a personal planet or point. Your child could have considerable psychic ability. Or she could be one who could become a healer. Or an artist of great expressive power. She could have both the sense of awareness of the invisible or elusive, and the stamina and will to probe to the depths to discover the meaning of it.

Chapter Nine

Aspects of Planets to Midheaven and Ascendant

As with Chapter 8, you will not be able to use the interpretive information in this chapter without a fully calculated birth chart. For those of you who have obtained your Magical Child chart, using this chapter will be easy, for the aspects you should read are listed below the chart wheel, right along with the planetary aspects that were covered in the last chapter.

The degrees of Ascendant and Midheaven, are of course, not planets. They are mathematical points. I've found that planets in close aspect to these two points often point to the most dominant themes in the personality. I consider them so important that I didn't feel right about leaving them out of this book. This, in fact, was a primary reason for my decision to include that free chart coupon! So, if you haven't already taken advantage of it, please do!

Midheaven and Ascendant. What they are; why they are especially significant.

Mathematically, the Midheaven is the point (degree) in the horoscope which is derived from the exact time and the longitude of birth. It marks the cusp (cusp means the beginning degree) of the 10th House of a horoscope. Its opposition point is the cusp of the 4th House. The Ascendant degree is mathematically derived from the Midheaven plus the latitude of birth. It is the cusp of the 1st House.

Midheaven and Ascendant are the most personal points in any horoscope because they change one full degree for every four minutes of birth time. Even identical twins born five minutes apart will have different degrees on their Ascendants and Midheavens. Children born at very close to the same time in the same place are likely to share the same signs for these points, although even this could have changed. Only a small change in degrees for these points can mean that different planets are in aspect to them.

This difference in degrees based on exact time and place is why astrologers will always say that if you don't know your time of birth, the information that can be derived about you can only be general in nature. Everyone born on the same day — anywhere in the world — will have their planets in the same signs, and the general characteristics associated with sign interpretations do "ring a bell" for most people when they are told about them. But when the **date of birth** is combined with the **time** and the exact **location** (longitude and latitude) the astrologer can calculate a chart that is nearly as unique to you as your fingerprint. The main reason it is so unique is because of the Midheaven and Ascendant and where the planets are in relationship (aspect) to those two points.

The Midheaven

You were given personality characteristics associated with the sign of the Ascendant, or Rising Sign, earlier in this book. You were not given personality characteristics for the sign of the Midheaven. Not much is generally written in any book about the sign of the Midheaven. Because signs are the main symbols used in "pop" astrology, not many nonastrologers are even aware that the Midheaven exists.

I did not write individual sign look-ups for the Midheaven, either, because it has not been my experience that its sign, in itself, contributes that much to the understanding of basic personality, particularly for a young child. Sometimes I have seen the sign of the Midheaven prominently reflected in the chart of an older person whose life purpose had become well defined. For ideas of what the sign on your child's Midheaven might possibly mean in terms of his or her longer range potential choices, you might read the description for that sign given under the Sun sign look-ups. The Sun sign may be more overtly expressed in the personality, but the basic zodiac archetype for the sign of the Midheaven might tell you something about the areas in which your child will strive to gain recognition.

The primary reason for including the Midheaven in the book at this point is because planetary aspects to it are so important. I'm trying to get you into a more accurate level of astrology than you can get through signs alone, and that is why we have been dealing with aspects. Aspects of one planet to another are important, but aspects of planets to Midheaven and Ascendant are even more significant because of their more individualized nature. And, even though you may have never heard of a Midheaven before, it is just as important as the more popularized Ascendant. Indeed, some astrologers (including this one) consider Midheaven even **more important than Ascendant.**

The Midheaven is a primary personal point in the methods of astrology (Uranian/Cosmobiology) in which I specialize. According to them, and to my own experience, the Midheaven is much more than a focal point of career and reputation, with its opposition degree a point of foundation, roots and home, as some texts will say. Midheaven tells us something of the soul — where a person seeks beyond, for the highest in Self, and its opposition degree, the cusp of the 4th House, shows what deep roots of soul memory may influence that seeking.

Midheaven aspects may show in career choice, for it is through striving in the world that a person often seeks his or her highest potential. To think about what careers might be associated with each Midheaven sign, though, is a little too simplistic. It would be perhaps more accurate to say that the Midheaven shows how a person identifies Self — where one might say "I am ..." (and consequently, what achievements in life bring "me" the greatest satisfaction). So, if the career is just a job to make a living, but a hobby or skill (avocation) is the area that the individual most savors in life, the Midheaven is more likely to suggest the avocation. The potentials for careers or avocations are too vast to contemplate, and those associated with various signs are often overlapping. The Midheaven, through aspects to the degree and to the opposition degree, might also suggest what gives fulfillment to the inner sense of being, and what elements in the foundation of that being contribute to or hinder that fulfillment.

Though you may not "see" the Midheaven in your child's chart as a career indicator, while he or she is so young, I think you'll see evidence that the theme of a planet very close to the Midheaven has much to do with the child's concept of who "I am."

The Four Angles

As I've hinted, but not yet specifically said, the Midheaven and Ascendant are axes, meaning that the degrees that are exactly opposite each of them are equally important. Together, these four degree points are called the **angles**.

As said earlier, preceding the Rising Sign interpretations, the **Ascendant** is associated with outer personality. Its opposite point is called the **Descendant,** and it is associated with one-to-one relationships.

The **Midheaven** (also often called MC for *medium coeli*, point of culmination), is most often symbolically associated with career choice and the individual's reputation or status in the world. Its opposite point is called the **IC** (stands for *imum coeli*, or undersky), and it is most often associated with one's roots, inner foundation of being or home life.

Any planet, either personal or outer, that is "on" any of the four angles will most likely be a dominating factor in a personality. To say the same thing another way, any planet that is either conjunct or opposite Midheaven or Ascendant is especially emphasized in the horoscope.

Planets Aspecting Ascendant

For the Rising Sign interpretations in this book, I wrote of outer personality and relationships. A planet "on" (conjunct) the Ascendant degree is even more important. If the theme of the planet is contradictory to the sign characteristics (such as serious Saturn right on a normally outgoing and optimistic Sagittarius Ascendant, for example), it will nearly always be the planet theme that will predominate. Our Sag Rising, with Saturn conjunct the Ascendant, might more likely be a subdued, philosophical type.

If, however, a planet is on the Descendant (or, in other words that mean the same thing, opposite the Ascendant), that planet's theme might describe close one-to-one relationships, or it might still modify the Ascendant (outer personality) itself. Some people "own" all of their own chart, while others tend to "project" some of it, attracting or choosing other people with whom to relate, who will "be" some part of their inner self that they need to express, but are not comfortable expressing. To carry out the same example, our Sagittarius Rising, if Saturn should be on the Descendant, might still be a more serious philosophical-type Sag rather than a happy-go-lucky one. It is also very likely that he or she might instead choose a very serious, practical partner who will keep Sag in check (and possibly be resisted or even resented until Sag matures enough to use his or her own Saturn themes).

As for the aspects other than conjunction/opposition, it is my experience that a planet aspecting either Ascendant or Descendant could just as easily relate to ourselves or to how we handle our relationships—either one or the other or both. Expressions of outer personality, in any case, are more about how others perceive us — and relate to us — rather than how we perceive ourselves.

Planets Aspecting Midheaven

Planets conjunct the Midheaven are more likely to describe career/avocation, how one handles responsibility, authority, achievement and recognition, and how one relates to the more authoritive parent.

Planets opposite the Midheaven (conjunct the IC) are more likely to be just the reverse. Here the emphasis is more likely to be on the home or on nurturing issues. But this may not always be the case. Issues of what we strive for in life and of what foundations we are coming from are very closely related to each other. As for other kinds of aspects to Midheaven and IC, I feel that they could as easily relate to the matters of one end of the axis as the other.

If the Midheaven and Ascendant axes are in or very close to 90° angles to each other, which will happen in many locations, it gets even more confusing, because then the same planets will aspect all four angles.

Organization of the Interpretations

For the purposes of the look-up interpretations in this book, I have treated the Midheaven and Ascendant as axes, rather than as separate points.

Inner foundations affect career choice and aspirations, and that, in turn, affects home life. How we behave affects our relationships, and who we are relating to affects how we behave.

For Sun and Moon, I've given you one look-up paragraph for conjunction/opposition and one for all other aspects. For the other planets, I have only given you one look-up for each planet in aspect to Midheaven and one for each planet in aspect to Ascendant. This is because the basic themes are essentially the same for all aspects, and I see little point in inventing methods to say the same things in several slightly different ways.

On the Magical Child chart you should take special note of any planet that is listed as conjunct/opposite either Midheaven or Ascendant, because these are especially important. Within each look-up for planets other than Sun and Moon, I have pointed out some of the possible variations from the basic theme, depending on whether the planet is "on" Midheaven or IC, or "on" Ascendant or Descendant, but you should keep in mind that the symbolism of one end of each axis is very closely related to the symbolism of the other end.

In some cases I've included notes about how hard aspects may work as contrasted with soft ones. As before, consider that if an aspect is "hard" the theme of the planet will be stronger and more noticeable. "Soft" aspects will have a softer theme, and will be less noticeable, but may suggest a harmonious and interesting avenue to which you might redirect parental-insanity-producing energy that your child may be expressing through other more challenging aspects.

Sun conjunct/opposite Midheaven

Your child has an unusually strong desire to achieve personal recognition in the world. Also, he needs to feel that he is in charge. Because of this concern, and the willingness to work to achieve, he is more than likely to gain considerable success in the world. This is a person who may be inclined to choose a field in which he can be his own boss (or strive to be the boss), because he prefers to do things independently. In childhood, this could manifest as resistance to authority. In this case it may be well to point out that others can help or hurt him in the quest to get ahead, and that diplomacy is a valuable art. The influence and guidance of a parent (or parent-figure) as a self-disciplined, professional role model is very important to this child's perception of what success means. Such a figure can greatly add to the child's self-confidence, or decrease it. Be aware.

With Sun on the Midheaven he is more likely to be concerned about status and reputation in the world (what do others think), while with Sun on the IC, he is more inclined to suit himself. Or, Sun on the IC might suggest a work focus in or out of the home, or a strong emphasis on home and family interests.

Sun conjunct/opposite Ascendant

No matter what the sign characteristics, this aspect doubles them, and gives your child the aura of one in the spotlight. This kid shines. When she walks into a room, everyone notices. And if they don't, she is likely to do something to make SURE they do! She craves attention, and she wants to be in the leading role. The reaction of others to this, of course, depends upon the appropriateness of her behavior to the time, place and audience. This may take some diplomacy and some firmness when she is young. But don't squelch too hard. You'll need to be a willing and approving audience frequently in order to nurture the best in this child. You will also need to teach her how to judge when the considerate thing to do is to yield the stage to others—and why yielding is not only considerate, but also in her own best interests in the long run.

If Sun is on the Descendant, it is possible that your child may tend to shy away from the limelight herself, and instead pick a best friend to "shine" for her. Don't push her — pushing kids often has a way of getting just the opposite behavior from what you want. But be aware that she may be attracted to "stars" because she'd secretly like to be one. Praise and appreciation will be very encouraging to her.

With a Rising Sign such as Virgo or Capricorn which tends to be self-critical it is possible that Sun conjunct either Ascendant or Descendent could be associated with a high degree of self-consciousness. Again, don't push.

Sun-Midheaven

The child's Self is infused with the desire to do something vital, to be recognized for it, to "make a difference" in doing things that are worthwhile. The sign of the Sun and other planets in aspect to it offer ideas about the areas in which the vitality might be expressed, and in which she might be especially wanting to be noticed and appreciated. Whatever the area, however, success is very important to this child. The hard aspects indicate a more energetic thrust, but they may also indicate a larger possibility for conflict with parental or other authority. The "Sun child" has a strong sense of Self, remember. There are, of course, some things upon which parents must insist, but if you are getting a large amount of resistance, it would also be well to consider whether there are other ways in which you can comfortably allow your child's own individuality to "shine."

Sun-Ascendant

This child will tend to be very concerned about interactions with others. It is very important to him to be recognized and to win approval. A "sunny" demeanor will win friends and popularity, and the soft aspects may show ease in this. Hard aspects, particularly, may indicate that there are frequent issues to resolve in regard to balancing personal needs and wants with those of others. Your child may be too inclined to put his own interests first, or he may compromise too much in order to please friends. He may have some difficulty deciding whether someone is friend or foe, for he both needs others and competes with them. Yet it is through relationships that he learns, and others will always be important to him. Just understand!

Moon conjunct/opposite Midheaven

Powerful emotions, and empathic understanding of others' emotions, desires and needs, often give a person with Moon on the Midheaven a winning charisma with the public. She is able to "touch a chord" to which other people respond. For this reason, this combination has been linked with careers that involve politics, sales, advertising and public relations.

The above could also be said of Moon opposite Midheaven, on the IC, but here, the attachment to home and family may be an especially significant factor. A strong psychological link with Mother (a Mother-image, or the most nurturing parent) could be very significant in the career this child eventually chooses.

The thing to be most aware of in dealing with children who have this very strong lunar emphasis is that inner security, as it is developed in the home, is of utmost importance. Warmth and caring from parents will help this deeply emotional child grow into a secure, generous and sympathetic person who will want to help others. With that foundation, in whatever career she chooses, she will remember, appreciate and respect the values of family and its traditions.

Moon conjunct/opposite Ascendant

Nobody has to guess how this kid feels about anything. It's right out there, where it can be read on his face, or on the heart he wears on his sleeve. For the most part, this can be positive, for most people respond well to honesty and directness — as long as he learns to also be direct, with grace and some diplomacy. Moon on Ascendant is also a good aspect for a politician, salesperson, or anyone else who deals with the public. Whether he is feeling deeply inside or not, your child has a way of expressing sympathy for others, and this usually results in positive feedback.

With Moon opposite — on the Descendant — the lunar themes may be projected onto his closest relationships. He may be constantly attracted to people who are especially sympathetic and emotional. He may depend too much on having a "best friend" for his own emotional support, or to "mother" him. When he grows up, he is likely to seek a very motherly type partner.

A good relationship with Mother (or a nurturing mother-figure) is important in developing the child's inner security.

Moon-Midheaven

Any Moon aspect to Midheaven may indicate a person who will forge a career in the public, because there is an empathic understanding of others' needs. Your child may be instinctively good at dealing with groups of people, at showing sympathy for them and eliciting sympathy in return — sort of "Mother to many," one might say. Deep and powerful emotions and sensitivity to the feelings and desires of others can someday translate into a strong message of service, and you could see evidence of this even in a small child's play or desires to help persons or animals who hurt. A strong, supportive relationship with Mother will be important in bringing out the best of this combination. The flow will be easier, but softer with the soft aspects. With hard aspects he may experience considerable tension in learning to make good choices because his emotional needs and desires may sometimes seem in conflict with what others expect, or even what the child's own reason tells him.

Moon-Ascendant

Especially with the hard aspects, there could be a conflict between how your child is perceived by others (her image or outward personality) and how she really feels inside. Read the Moon and Ascendant in signs again for ideas of what forms this might take. There could be a tendency to be too dependent upon relationships, hiding her feelings for fear of loss. Or she might withdraw from relating. The conflict could be "Will others like me if I show how I really feel?" or perhaps "If I'm too close to you, can I still be free to be me?" or maybe "How and when must I be the one to give, and what do I have the right to expect from you?" With the softer aspects, the child might be quite open about expressing her feelings, but in either case, the child does tend to relate to others emotionally, rather than intellectually, and moodiness may be an issue. A close, secure and supportive relationship with Mother (or nurturing mother-figure) is important in providing a foundation for your child in her future relationships.

Mercury-Midheaven

This child sees herself as a thinking person, a communicator. Her mental processes are closely tied to her perception of who she is and what she has to bring to the world. Because of this, it is very likely that her career choices will have to do with some Mercury-associated vocation, such as teaching, writing, speaking, sales, communications media, etc. This is an especially strong possibility with Mercury conjunct the Midheaven, although any close Mercury aspect may be expressed through career.

A good education is an essential foundation for this child in order to assist her in making the most of any Mercury-Midheaven aspect. She is thinking every minute, is likely to be intellectually sharp, possibly advanced for her age. She is likely to develop quite decided opinions about things, and to be articulate in expressing them. Restlessness may be an issue, and a need to develop the discipline to stay with a topic long enough to really get something out of it. With the hard aspects, there may be more tension between the child's own views and those which she is taught. Mercury on the IC suggests deeper thinking, perhaps more influenced by feelings, the past, and the beliefs and opinions of parents than on the child's own objective observations.

Mercury-Ascendant

A strong aspect of this child's identity, as seen by others in his environment, is dominated by his way of thinking and communicating. He is likely to be thought of as a communicator―one who talks a lot, or perhaps is "an intellectual," is "logical," a good speaker, a "gossip," is critical, writes well, is a practical joker, etc. Not all of these descriptions will apply, of course. The point is: he is most likely to be defined by others by some theme which has to do with Mercury. His mind works overtime, but he is not at his best when alone. He bounces his thoughts off other people — he is stimulating and he receives stimulation, in return. Whether this helps him or causes him trouble in school (or home) probably depends a lot on his personality mix with his teacher or parent. If the adult can deal well with lots of questions and having his or her ear talked off, it'll be fine. Keep this kid busy. Distractions toward books and things to do with his hands are good, when you're talked and listened out. Mercury on the Descendant might indicate more of a mentally competitive streak (though other aspects could mean this, too), and debate might be a good outlet. This position also accents the need for others. Studying with another kid is probably worthwhile to encourage.

Venus-Midheaven

For this child, the Venusian ideals of love, beauty and harmony are closely tied to his concept of who he is. He is likely to define his role in the world, and his career, according to these ideals. The most obvious possibility would be the artist, and your child may have a strong flair for the arts. Certainly you should provide him with opportunities to explore various art forms — visual arts, music, drama, dance, etc. Venus may also reflect an inclination toward the enhancement of physical beauty — his own, or for the benefit of others. Or the direction might be toward harmony and peace — diplomacy, mediation of disputes. A bit of conceit may also be possible. An affectionate disposition — a person who is kind and helpful toward others, is very likely.

The refinement and beauty of the home is also probably important to this child. This may be most emphasized with Venus conjunct the IC. Relationships with parents and other authority figures are probably harmonious. Some tension may occur with the hard aspects between what the child instinctively feels in regard to his own taste, and what he thinks he needs to do and like in order to gain the approval of others.

Venus-Ascendant

Others are likely to describe your child with words like attractive, charming, cordial, sociable, refined, tactful, has good taste, artistic. She relates to others in a sociable, friendly manner, and so that is how others see her. She will prefer surroundings that are aesthetically beautiful and peaceful, and will go out of her way to try to seek harmony and balance in her environment and in her associations. Discord and ugliness may be quite upsetting to her, and consequently she may be sometimes too compromising in order to keep the peace. But her concept of fairness is likely to be highly developed and if necessary, she will fight to reestablish balance and harmony.

Any Venus aspect indicates charm, appeal and popularity, as well as a tendency to be quite sociable. About the only possible problems (most likely with hard aspects) might be a tendency to be a little lazy (because charm gets her by) or to waver between what she really thinks and the overdone compromises she may think she has to make to have others like her. Relating (and consequently, approval of others) is important with any aspect — probably most of all with Venus conjunct Descendant.

Mars-Midheaven

For this child, the concept of who she is may be strongly linked with her ability to act decisively and energetically, with taking the lead, or with expressing courage. Her work in the world is likely to be derived from these basic characteristics. Whatever she does, she is likely to be a leader and a doer, strong willed and competitive. You will probably find her to be very determined, and possibly even headstrong. Try to stop her in what she really wants to do, and she might even get angry. With Mars on the Midheaven, especially, but also with the aspects, the future career had best allow a considerable amount of independence, where she can set her own pace. Something that uses actual physical effort may be likely. Athletics would be good to encourage when she is young, because she'll put effort into it and have a competitive spirit.

Mars on the IC places greater emphasis on the child's own inner needs and what pleases her, while Mars on the Midheaven may indicate more willingness to do what gains recognition in the world. Greater tension, anger or competitiveness may be evident with the hard aspects. Lots of energy and enthusiasm are still likely with the soft aspects, but probably less competitiveness.

Mars-Ascendant

This child is likely to be seen as an assertive person, a fighter, one who has a great deal of drive and push in any activity he undertakes. He could also be known as a quarrelsome person, and if this should be the case, a redirecting of his ample energy is in order. Argumentiveness could become an asset in debate, for example, or channeled toward persuasive speech, in selling or in leadership activities where "cheerleading" or an urge to action is involved — so long as an urge to be too dominant can be resisted. It is especially important that this child be taught to take responsibility for his own actions, and for the consequences of them. A strong sense of self-identity and self-control will enable him to make the best use of his very considerable energy.

Encourage sports, including competitive sports. He may work better on his own than with a team. Conflicts with others will probably be more of an issue with the hard aspects, though even the soft aspects indicate an independent person who will stick up for himself. Mars on the Descendant may be projected, meaning that the child will attract relationships with people who are very aggressive and challenging to him. He may not be consciously looking for a fight with anyone, but will attract them just the same. This may be a case of your child suppressing his own assertive energy too much. If you are the one who is overly "holding him down," you may need to think of acceptable things in which you might encourage him to express some of his own needs to be assertive, active and independent.

Jupiter-Midheaven

This child has a concept of self that is likely to develop in a way that is strongly linked with his ideals and the quest for higher wisdom. He is likely to be optimistic and upbeat about his possibilities of growth and influence in these areas. Because his sense of honor is very strong, this placement generally indicates a person of favorable reputation. The choice of a career may follow, and may involve teaching, persuasion, upholding the law, or spiritual ideals.

Whatever religious upbringing you give your child is likely to make a very strong impression on him, and even if you don't practice any particular faith, he may find his own and become quite active in it, when he gets in school and is exposed to religion through others. In any case, he is likely to give more thought to ethical standards and ideals than the average. He may be one who in upper grades or as a teen will be interested in class offices or student government. What he believes is important to him, and he'll stick up for those beliefs.

With Jupiter on the IC, home, family and root traditions and beliefs may have the greatest emphasis, and will stay with the child through adulthood. Home is a place of emotional security — a retreat. With the hard aspects there could be conflicts with parents or authorities, particularly over beliefs. He could have unreasonably high expectations in regard to home or family status. With the soft aspects, he'll probably get along quite easily with his elders.

Jupiter-Ascendant

Most people are going to like being around your child, for Jupiter tends to be jovial, and one who has Jupiter in close contact with the Ascendant is likely to be identified as a generally happy, generous, and harmonious person with high ideals and optimistic attitudes. She will want an environment that befits her high aspirations; she will want things to be "nice." She will tend to work and play well with other people. She is broadminded and tolerant, and may surprise you with how many things she will be interested in. One thing she is likely not to be particularly tolerant about, however, is when she perceives that someone is doing something "wrong." She has a strong sense of ethics, and she expects those she associates with to agree with them and behave accordingly. This could present some conflict (Jupiter on the Descendant or in hard aspect) because her wide ranging interests could attract her to relationships with people who are different. Then, with time, she may realize that those very differences include beliefs/ethics/morality that do not jibe with her own.

For the most part, though, any Jupiter aspect is likely to be mostly expansive and positive. Sometimes, the expansion is physical — Jupiter on the Ascendant (or perhaps the hard aspects), could reflect a child who is big for her age or grows taller than average.

Saturn-Midheaven

This child has a self-concept of conservatism and reserve. She respects and reveres tradition, and values organization and structure. She is disciplined in her work, and has patience and endurance in pursuing what she wants out of life. The choice of career is likely to emerge from these traits. Her attributes generally contribute to an excellent business sense, and she may make a good manager. She might also be a teacher, or even if in another career field, in some sense she may be involved in teaching within that field. She is basically serious and she sets a high standard for herself, and may be excessively hard on herself if she feels she's not living up to it. For this reason, you do not need to push this one, and indeed shouldn't, for if expectations are excessively high (from you), she could become discouraged and then, quite counterproductively, feel like a failure.

A sense of aloneness could be accentuated with Saturn on the IC, with even more need for support and reassurance from the parental home. Unfortunately, this placement sometimes reflects too much "conditional love," which creates that sense of aloneness. Be aware. Behavior that is mature for her age is likely with any Saturn-Midheaven combination. The soft aspects show more ease, the hard aspects may reflect a greater sense of aloneness or emotional withdrawal. The influence of Father, father-figure or the more disciplinary parent is very important. The emotional support that aids the best of this aspect requires discipline that is accompanied by love.

Saturn-Ascendant

Even if the Rising Sign is associated with an extroverted personality, a close aspect with Saturn is likely to mean that your child will be perceived as rather quiet and reserved and serious. He may be shy, and may seem to prefer the company of people who are older — a child who really enjoys being with adults, and who thrives on little chores and responsibilities. He will seem mature for his age, and the adults are therefore likely to like being with him, too. This child may also be seen as somewhat of a loner, preferring to spend a considerable amount of his time in privacy. You might find it very difficult to pry out of him what he thinks or how he feels about anything, unless he is the one who initiates the conversation, and then it may be only what he wants to talk about, not what you wanted to know.

If Saturn is on the Descendant, the seriousness might be projected in the friends he attracts, or in the close relationships he might someday choose. One whose other planets lean toward a much less serious or flighty type might be even more apt to choose someone else to be serious, practical and stable for him — and then, perhaps, resist those very qualities as being too restrictive. With any aspect a practical realist is likely, with good capacity for self-discipline. With hard aspects, emotional withdrawal may be more evident, with concerns about self-worth. Appreciation and emotional support from you are important.

Uranus-Midheaven

Your child has a self-concept of originality and individuality. He is creative, inventive, independent, and perhaps somewhat eccentric. He should, and probably will, choose a life's work that expresses those traits. Since he will be attracted to anything new and futuristic, the career field could be in high technology or science, or perhaps in an innovative art form. Or, we could say, just about anything that is decidedly different than what his early environment might have "programmed" him to think is a suitable and appropriate career — like the one who is expected to go into Dad's business, but instead became an opera singer. Who knows? He might even become an astrologer!

With Uranus on the IC, the parental home, itself, may be unusual and eccentric in some way, or it may indicate parents who are so busy with their own lives that independence in the child is not only encouraged but is necessary. In any case, home is a place for the child and later for the adult he will become, in which emotional detachment and free-spiritedness may be evident.

With all Uranus-Midheaven aspects, an air of excitement is likely, along with creativity, innovation, and an interest in technology or anything unusual. Rebellion and conflicts with authority are possible expressions of differentness with the hard aspects, which of course includes the conjunction. Tension and nervousness may also be an issue. Encourage independence and try to become comfortable with eccentricity in some areas. If you do, you may ease the tension and be more successful in winning respect for the values you consider to be very critical.

Uranus-Ascendant

Others are likely to describe your child as original, independent, innovative, creative, one who loves changes, and maybe one who is a bit eccentric. She is restless and excitable — probably nervous, if expected to suppress her natural tendencies and sit still! However her environment is arranged, this kid will probably want to change it, often. Friends had better be ready to give her lots of space and freedom, because she won't stand for being possessed or confined.

Now, if other planets in the chart are much more serious, or if she's "sat on" too hard and suppressed, she may project her Uranian freedom needs — especially with Uranus on the Descendant. She'll attract offbeat, free-spirited, eccentric or rebellious friends, which could either get her in trouble or really rattle her sense of security or stability because she'll never be able to count on them. Be aware that she needs to express her own originality and creativity.

With any Uranus-Ascendant aspect, freedom needs are a very significant part of her personality. She must express freedom and independence herself, and she must both allow and respect the freedom needs of those with whom she relates. Tension with parents or authorities, or projection, is more likely with the hard aspects. Even with the soft aspects, she'll demand the right to be herself, and will be drawn to excitement and the unusual.

Neptune-Midheaven

The self-concept of this child involves her own experience of living within her ideals and dreams of what the world should be. She may create a fantasy and believe that she can make it real, and perhaps she can. Support will be needed from other aspects to bring structure to the illusionary quality of Neptune, or insecurities and difficulty in defining goals might be a problem. In some way or other, this child is a visionary, and her career choice will likely emerge from that. She may achieve her recognition as an actor, artist, writer, poet or musician, and the art she produces may have a mystical bent. She may create illusion through acting or dance. Work in the realms of the occult, psychic phenomena, spirituality or astrology are other possibilities.

With Neptune on the IC, the more nurturing parent may be "Neptunian" in either a positive (artistic, mystical) or negative (escapist) sense. In any case, the child may be especially sensitive to the "vibes" within the home, and probably picks up feelings around her there like a sponge, which will support or hinder her aspirations depending on what kind of feelings she is picking up.

With any aspect, a great deal of idealism and empathy are likely. Also likely is the ability to create illusion, which could overdo fantasy or even deceit, particularly with the hard aspects. This, too, can also be channeled positively, though. Positive ability to create illusion (a nicer term for deceit) is necessary for acting, a skill which is also necessary for other fields such as trial law or advertising, for example. People in such careers usually have a strongly placed Neptune.

Neptune-Ascendant

Others might describe your child as dreamy, sensitive, sympathetic, romantic, imaginative, mysterious, ethereal, impressionable — or perhaps, a bit flaky or confused. His aspirations or his hobbies and interests are probably out-of-the norm, and involve his very vivid imagination. Lack of clarity could emerge as deception. He could be very compassionate and caring — one to whom others bring their problems.

Relationships with others could be over idealized. This child could expect too much of them, with consequent disappointment. Especially with tendencies to suppress his own dreaminess and sensitivity and needs for romance, Neptune may be projected (most likely with Neptune conjunct Descendant). He could attract friends (and later significant relationships) who deceive, or disappoint, because he sees in them what he wants to see (idealizes) rather that seeing them for who they really are.

With any Neptune-Ascendant aspect, he may be inclined to bring home waifs or hurt animals or whomever he feels a need to help or save. He is very sensitive to others' feelings, and is probably quite intuitive. Don't chide him for his insights, his dreams, or even perhaps for his imaginary friends. He may know more than you think. Encourage his creativity and imagination, while also being alert to what may be an outright fib from time to time. Try to gently help him understand his own feelings and perceptions — don't put them down. Intuition can be very valuable in many areas of life.

Pluto-Midheaven

Your child has a self-image of power and strength. He expects to be in the lead, to be in control and to be an authority — and so he is likely to strive to be, in whatever life's work he chooses. Because he sees his possibilities as wide-ranging and limitless, the sky is the limit, and considerable recognition is possible. He will likely have the determination, the intensity of will, and the passion to excel in whatever he sets his mind to accomplish. Pluto suggests leadership in career possibilities. It also suggests a psychological understanding, and an interest in research, investigation, and problem-solving. The kid thrives on probing a mystery.

Because he is so intense about making an impact on his world, some conflict with authority is, of course, possible. In some cases Pluto-Midheaven is associated with a parental relationship in which the parent is very domineering or too controlling. This may be more likely with Pluto conjunct IC, but it could be any hard aspect. Such a situation could result in psychological distortion for the child, which could foster compulsive behaviors that hinder development. And/or it is likely to symbolize power struggles. With all children, but especially children with strong Pluto aspects such as this, any tendency to indirectly overcontrol through guilt is counterproductive to say the least, and can be quite destructive to his psychological well-being. He needs positive, direct and honest parental relationships that encourage his own self-mastery and personal integrity.

Pluto-Ascendant

Your child is likely to impress others as a powerful personality. She may be described as strong willed, ambitious, authoritative, tough, magnetic, persuasive or influential. That is, if she is claiming her own power — which you should encourage. The alternative is attracting other people to her (more likely with Pluto on the Descendant, although it can happen with other aspects, too) who will be powerful, perhaps overly so, and could bully her in some way. Better that she is the strong one. Cultivate personal responsibility and self-control.

Whatever the aspects, she is very emotionally intense, and is intense about her relationships with others, as well. She may even be compulsive about them. Her interactions with others are very important, and will be a strong factor in major transformative changes in her life. She may have to learn to concentrate on herself and her own self-control, and learn not to attempt to manipulate others. Though she might be effective at the latter, others usually resent such maneuvers.

What you need to encourage is her responsible, honest and forthright use of her own power — not power over others, but the power to accomplish what she sets out to do, and the inner power to pick herself up after a problem or a fall, and forge ahead again. She may become very interested in psychological issues, and she may direct her capacity for reform toward some cause larger than herself.

Chapter Ten
The Magical Alchemy of Relating

For the last five chapters you've been looking up and reading material that is primarily aimed at describing your child in terms of his or her own unique magical potential — needs, style, abilities, strengths, challenges, etc. No matter how much you try to understand another person, though, it is even more essential to understand yourself in order to relate to that other person successfully. If your first reaction is "I **know** myself already," I can only say: remain open, and think about that, just a little more deeply.

Of course you know a lot about yourself, but everything? Does anyone? Most us spend the bulk of our day doing all the things we feel we have to do to live, and comparatively little time gets spent in contemplation of why. Each of us is constantly in interaction with other people, and we respond to them in various ways. It's not uncommon to explain our reactions to others in terms of what "they did," but is this really the case? Think about it. You know as well as I do that the very same incident is likely to elicit as many different reactions as there are people involved.

Astrology offers a great deal of insight into the special alchemy — chemistry — that seems to exist between people. In a similar manner to which it can provide insight into individual potential, it also offers a language of symbolism through which we can look at the magical alchemy of relating to others. Have you thought about why it is that you are attracted to some people but "turned off" by others? Why do you find it so easy to talk with some people and so difficult to communicate with others? Why are some people so easy to work with, but others seem to be constantly at odds with you? Is it the "other guy" or you, or the combination?

Of one thing I feel sure, no matter what the other person does, or doesn't do, says or doesn't say, you and only you are responsible for your reaction. Nobody else "makes" you do or feel anything. Your response is a part of you — your style, your "programming," your personality — you. This is why it is so important for you to understand you — even more important than it is for you to understand your child!

Perhaps you already have an astrological chart for yourself. If you don't, I suggest that you get one. You can even get a Magical Child chart for yourself, if you like—there's no age limit!

Of course there are plenty of "cookbooks" with interpretations written for adults. I've already mentioned an excellent one, *Easy Astrology Guide* by Maritha Pottenger. But in addition to that, I suggest you look up the interpretations of your own planets and aspects in **this** book. Even though my interpretations are written about children, the basic themes are the same for adults, too. Adults are just expected to behave …well, more adult. But do they, all the time? You might find it quite interesting to consider yourself within these child-sized interpretations. Inside you, the child you were still lives — and may come out to play, or cry out for understanding, at times when you least expect it. We'll talk more about that "inner child" later, but first, I want to tell you about one of astrology's most basic ways to look at the dynamics of relationship between two people. It involves an "elementary" method of synthesizing all of the separate parts of a chart into dominant themes and then seeing how they "mix" with others.

The following pages on elements, modes, polarities, and dominant sign assume you have the Magical Child chart, which has your child's dominant factors figured out for you and printed in a box below the wheel. If you don't have the chart yet, you can still make some use of this section by looking up your child's sign positions in the appendix tables. It's simply a matter of counting up how many planets are in each sign type to see which type has the most. This is not difficult at all. Examples based on Tessa's chart, as we go, will show you how easy it is. (To fully use this chapter, though, you'll need to have your birth chart, too.)

The Magical Child chart is based on a weighted system that gives two points each to Sun, Moon, Ascendant and Midheaven, but only one point each to the other planets. If you are using the book tables, you won't have a Midheaven, but you can use the Rising Sign for Ascendant. Not including the Midheaven will change the dominant factors only in cases where it's close between two, so in any case, you'll still have useful information about which sign types are more significant.

The Four Elements

Each person's basic type can be more or less defined according to a system that is so much a part of our idiom that most everyone just takes it for granted. We hear all kinds of statements of evidence:

What an air-head!
You're all wet!
She's so deep and fluid.
He certainly has a fiery temperament.
She's as down-to-earth as they come.
What a stick-in-the-mud.
He's so breezy.
She just flows through life, right around any obstacle.
He's a hot-blooded one.
She is a clinging vine.

The list could go on and on. Everyone has a fairly similar image of what these statements mean. The ancients saw the material world as being composed of four basic elements: fire, earth, air and water. The idea of personality types that correspond to the four elements is very old, and as the idiomatic statements above suggest, the idea has validity still. Here are short interpretations of each element type:

Fire

The fiery personality is, in many ways, an incurable romantic, with boundless enthusiasm for the latest love, be it person, thing, place or grand plan for the future. There's a great deal of energy and vitality involved in whatever inspires fire, and the fiery passion can inspire others, too. Fire people love adventure and need a great deal of freedom. Without these things, life is boring.

In any group, committee, family, or somewhere within yourself, you need fire to lift your spirits, spark your imagination, get you off your duff to forge ahead, cheer you on. Too much fire can leap ahead rashly, failing to take into account the realities of the situation — the earthy necessities that could be threatened. Too much fire could also cause the watery emotional sensitivities to rise up in steamy clouds of upset or fears. The logic of air can give fiery enthusiasm a sense of direction, or too much fire can overwhelm air, choking off the breath of reason.

Earth

The down-to-earth person is rooted to the practical matters of everyday life. Earth is strong — solid as a rock, dependable and stable, but may be somewhat stodgy, or dense to the needs of the other elements. Security is important, and uncertainty is unsettling. Earth is also very physical and sensual, aware of touching and feeling, and of what is comfortable.

In any group, committee, family, or somewhere within yourself, you need earth to keep you grounded, to see that you have adequate resources, to see the pragmatic side of issues. Too much earth could get you stuck in a rut, smothering fiery enthusiasm and new ideas before they have a chance to be explored, or refusing to budge despite air's reasonable arguments of why change is necessary. Earth tends to perceive freedom urges as a threat to security. While watery feelings are quite necessary to earth's well-being, too much earth dumped in water can also make mud, which again, can cause inertia.

Air

The airy person lives in the head, dealing with life in a manner that he or she perceives as quite rational and logical. Air thinks, rather than feels, and may be baffled by emotional responses, and deducing that which is not logically understood as irrational. Whatever the issue, the airy approach is rational — or rationalizing. Air is the intellect of the conscious mind, and can be primarily associated, in modern day jargon, with the "left brain." Air is outgoing, circulating, communicative and sociable.

In any group, committee, family, or somewhere within yourself, you need air to reason things through, weigh the pros and cons, and facilitate communication. Too much air could fail to be sensitive to watery feelings, or get carried away with rationalizations that ignore earthly practical realities. Airy rationalizations could fan fiery impulses out of control, or more gently guide its path. Too much airy logic can blow out the flames of new inspiration.

Water

The watery person feels, rather than thinks, or we could say, thinks in a manner that is very influenced by feelings and emotion. Water **knows**, in a manner that can often be as "right," and sometimes more right, as the knowing that comes from air's logical deductions. But water may not be able to easily articulate how or why this knowing came about. Water is the intuition of the subconscious mind, and can be primarily associated, in modern day jargon, with the "right brain."

In any group, committee, family, or somewhere within yourself, you need water to be sensitive to the personal issues, to how people will feel, to intuit hidden meanings, to probe beneath the surface of a matter. Too much water could fail to see the airy logic of a situation, or could over-emotionalize, perhaps dowsing fiery inspiration or enthusiasm with need-less fears. Earth is necessary to contain water, giving it security, or too much watery emotion can carve away even solid rock, breaking down the very stability which contains it.

Your Magical Child Chart has a box at the bottom that ranks which elements are strongest and weakest for that chart. This is determined from counting up all the planets in each element to see which has the most. Generally, as I've said before, one gives an extra point to the four most important factors: Sun, Moon, Ascendant, Midheaven.

Here are the elements to which each sign belongs:

Fire Signs:	Aries	Leo	Sagittarius
Earth Signs:	Taurus	Virgo	Capricorn
Air Signs:	Gemini	Libra	Aquarius
Water Signs:	Cancer	Scorpio	Pisces

Tessa's dominant element is earth. If you look back at her chart in Chapter 4, for reference, you can see that she has Sun, Rising Sign, Jupiter, Uranus and Neptune in earth signs. With Sun and Rising Sign weighted at two points, we get a total of 7 points. Including Midheaven makes it 9. Either way, earth is dominant: Mercury and Mars are fire (2), Moon and Saturn are air (3), Venus and Pluto are water (2).

The Elements in Getting Along with Others

If you are strongly one element type, you probably, for the most part, see eye to eye with other people in the same element type, and are likely to have problems with people who are strongly of an element that is most unlike you. Generally, earthy types get along well with watery ones, but not so easily with fire and air. Fiery and airy types get along well with each other, but not so easily with earth and water.

> *Water dowses fire, and fire turns water to steam.*
> *Air feeds fire and fans its flames higher, while fire*
> > *warms the air.*
> *Fire rips through the earth, while earth dumped on fire,*
> > *puts it out.*
> *Earth can stifle air, while air can blow earth to shreds.*
> *Water feeds earth, while earth contains and holds water.*

The elemental correspondences are the reason why, when in the context of the too-simple Sun sign astrology, a question such as "I'm an Aries. In a relationship, what signs are best for me?" is likely to be answered something like this:

> *"You're an Aries? OK, you'll do well with Leos and Sagittarians. Gemini, Libra and Aquarius are good, too. But the others could be difficult — unless of course you have several planets other than the Sun in compatible signs."*

To make a judgment based on Sun signs only is never a good idea, but if, in considering how people interact, you consider the dominant element of **all** the planets in each person's chart, I think that you will find some validity in this idea of basic elemental types.

It is fascinating to me to observe how people are so often attracted to the elements that are most opposite their own dominant one. This is probably because the element that attracts us is the one we most need for inner balance. We instinctively find people to help teach us balance, even as we may also often chafe with discomfort over our incompatibilities with their basic natures. Any two elemental types can work well together, or any two can work against each other. Generally, though, it is true that fire and air harmonize with each other more easily than with earth or water, and earth and water harmonize more easily with each other than with fire or air.

Some people (as is reflected in their charts) have a good balance within themselves. As an all-over personality, the elemental types will be most notable in those people who have a clearly dominant element. Once in a while, a person may seem to over- express an element that is "missing" in their chart. Perhaps this is an instinctive overcompensation for a trait that is not naturally comfortable, such as in the strongly airy type who "loses it" when confronted with an emotional situation.

The best use of any astrological knowledge in getting along well with another person, is awareness. If you find that you are in a relationship with another person who is of a personality type that is decidedly different from yours, and that makes you uncomfortable — or drives you nuts — you'd best start out by trying to understand just why that is, and if it could mean that you could learn something from them that would bring more balance into your own life.

You cannot change another person's basic, elementary way of being unless that person really wants to change. It's a waste of time to try, even with children, and potentially destructive. Instead, you should try to understand and accept other people for what they are, and encourage the best of that.

The Importance of Elemental Balance

Do you ever find yourself stuck in inertia, when your mind tells you that you should change? Or jumping into situations before you've thought them through? Or sabotaging your own enthusiasm with fears of what will happen? Or getting a great, new idea that comes to nothing because you rationalize why it won't work, or just can't seem to get started? All of these may be examples of elements out of balance within you. You might help yourself achieve a better balance by first realizing what is going on, and then meditating on the elemental imagery. The first step toward any change is awareness of the need for it.

If, on the other hand, you are playing one elemental role and your child is playing another, do not automatically assume that you are "right" and the child is "wrong." It may be that the child needs to be "reined in" or nudged forward a bit, but you wouldn't want to stifle or unnecessarily discourage that child through your own lack of understanding of a difference between your basic elementary types. One reason that this child (whose style is so different from yours) may be in your life is to help you learn what is out-of-balance in you. Again, reflect on the elemental imagery. Are you perhaps too quick or pushy, too insensitive to feelings, too stodgy, too fearful? Think about it.

If a chart shows a clearly dominant element you will probably be able to easily "see" that person as one of the following four elemental types. Sometimes a person will be equally strong in two elements, and a major challenge for growth will be found through achieving a blance between those two themes. As said before, if the chart lacks an element (zero), overcompensation may be the case. The important thing here, is for you to be aware if you and your child are "playing" elemental roles that are in conflict with each other. Awareness and understanding are always helpful in achieving a more productive relationship. If you, as the "adept", understand what is going on, you are empowered to modify your own approach to bring out the best in the child's natural magical style.

The Three Modes or Qualities of Action

A further refinement of how people might behave can be determined through another typing of the signs into three modes or qualities of action. The three modes are **cardinal, fixed** and **mutable**.

The Magical Child Chart lists the dominant mode next to the element. For those of you using the tables in the back of the book, refer to Tessa's chart again and then the table just below. Note that her dominant mode is cardinal: Sun, Moon, Midheaven, Uranus and Neptune, for a total of 8. Even without Midheaven, she'd have 6, still dominant over 5 for fixed signs and 3 for mutuable.

Again, an apparent conflict in relating between you and your child might be improved by understanding the mode of action that is natural for each of you. You can encourage the child in the way that works best for the child, and avoid being impatient because he or she doesn't operate as you do. The signs that belong to each mode are:

Cardinal:	Aries	Cancer	Libra	Capricorn
Fixed:	Taurus	Leo	Scorpio	Aquarius
Mutable:	Gemini	Virgo	Sagittarius	Pisces

Cardinal

Cardinal signs, of whatever element, are most inclined to take the initiative and get things moving. They are better at starting than they are at following through. Aries is the most obvious charge-ahead, let's go type, but each of the others initiates in its own way. Cancer is emotionally "out front," a veritable tigress or tiger if perceiving a threat to family. (Some tout the cat as a more proper symbol for Cancer than the crab.) Libra initiates socially, seeking contacts and relationships. Capricorn takes the lead in striving to reach the top of whatever mountain (goal) is ahead.

Fixed

Fixed signs, of whatever element, are just what the name implies, stubbornly fixed. They don't like change, and may dig in their heels hard, to avoid it. They may not take the initiative, but they are very good at follow-through. Taurus, of all things most wants to be comfortable and materially secure, with all matters dependable. Leo likes its place on that pedestal or throne, and is not about to relinquish it. Scorpio will dig and probe forever until it accomplishes what it feels must be done. Aquarius may be eccentric, but once having adopted an idea, stubbornly resists any attempt to change its mind.

Mutable

This word also suggests flexibility, and that is a keyword for this type. Mutable signs are very adaptable, and make changes rather easily, but may be difficult to hold down to anything for long. They live in their heads and might be said to sort of dance around life. Gemini flits from one bright new thought to another with quicksilver speed. Virgo has so many, many details to sift through in order to find what works. Sagittarius searches far and wide for the ideal, for the ultimate, that may be ever over the next rainbow. Pisces conjures visions and dreams and endless fantasies.

All Modes are Essential!

In any group, committee, family, or somewhere within yourself, you need the impulse and the courage to begin, the persistence to follow through, and the flexibility to cope with and adapt to situations as they develop.

Too much cardinality could mean lots of energy and initiative, but perhaps clashes over who is to lead, or get there first, or who is to clean up after.

Too much fixity may be stable and focused, but stuck, stubbornly refusing to budge.

Too much mutability rides through all kinds of changes, but may be scattered all over the place, moving from one thing to another, never settling down long enough for concrete decisions or accomplishments.

The Polarities

Astrological signs are traditionally divided into two polar opposite groups. All of the earth and water signs are in one group, and all the fire and air signs in the other. The Magical Child Chart ranks the two polarities next to the modes and elements.

I really don't care for some of the traditional keywords for these two groups, because they have uncomfortable connotations. I'll deal with them, but want to be sure you understand them for what they are, particularly if you have a little girl who is predominant in the so-called "masculine" group, or a little boy who is predominant in the so-called "feminine" group. This happens with probably about 50% of births.

The masculine signs are also called positive and the feminine signs negative, which are equally uncomfortable words, because in our language, we tend to associate "negative" with bad and positive as "good." In the past this has also been true of feminine and masculine, in many connotations, but fortunately that manner of thinking is well on its way out. Some astrologers have chosen to duck the issue of the uncomfortable keywords by substituting the Chinese words "yin" for feminine/negative and "yang" for masculine/positive. It means pretty much the same thing, but without the "bad/good" implications — and if you don't understand Chinese, at least it obscures the issue. Other keywords for "yin" are passive, and for "yang," active. The two polarities are also often notated with + or − symbols. Ouch! Another bad/good implication (plus = more, minus = less). The + polarity is frequently said to be associated with extroversion, and the − polarity with introversion.

We are all a mixture of both polarities. Jungian psychologists have told us that each of us is both masculine and feminine, in that whatever we are physically, we have the other within, in our psyche. The masculine within a woman is called the *animus* and the feminine within the man is called the *anima*. If we suppress that other half too much, "he" or "she" can give us a great deal of trouble.

I prefer to think of positive and negative as a **battery charge** — both are equally necessary to make the thing work.

Active and passive work fairly well in my understanding of the polarities within, and I also like two words that you won't find in many astrology books, since I thought of them as possible polarity keywords myself. That would be "magnetic" for feminine/negative/passive and "kinetic" for masculine/positive/active. The first — OK, just for fun, let's say the little girl within — is the part of us that desires, wants, needs. The little boy within is the part that, attracted by that need (magnetism), goes charging out in the world (kinetic, active motion) to get it, and then brings it right back to that magnetic, responsive part who receives it saying, "Thanks, now I think I might like…" The question here could be just who is **really** getting things accomplished!

Kidding about the sexes aside, the important thing to realize here, is that everybody, no matter whether occupying a male or female physical body, has both of these polarities within their personality, but may have one very predominantly over the other. Some people, of course, are nicely balanced.

The problem with "traditional" sex roles, is that if you happen to be a very outgoing, assertive, active little girl, you tend to get clamped down on and admonished to be ladylike, instead of being encouraged to make the most of it like you would if you were a boy.

On the other hand, if you happen to be a very sensitive, introverted, passive little boy, you tend to get pushed to be "more of a man" or even called "sissy," instead of being valued and encouraged to do your best in what you are, as you would if you were a girl. Many children of both sexes have been damaged by these stereotypes. Stereotyping is changing, but only gradually.

With that background, I will, for brevity, label the columns of the two polarities with + and − signs, but mind you, think of these symbols as battery charges and NOT "more" and "less"!

For those using the tables, and referring to Tessa's chart as example, your count, including Midheaven, should be 11 in negative (-) signs and 5 in positive (+) signs. Without Midheaven, she's still negative-dominant.

+	-
Aries	Taurus
Gemini	Cancer
Leo	Virgo
Libra	Scorpio
Sagittarius	Capricorn
Aquarius	Pisces

Two people who are both very dominantly + will have a lot of energy in their relationship, but may clash over who is in charge.

Two people who are both very dominantly – will probably get along quite harmoniously, but may get stuck in a rut because neither one prefers to take the lead.

A relationship between one person who is very + and another who is very – may work fine if the – person is really content to let the + person dominate, and enjoys going along. (This would best characterize the old "traditional" ideal of male/female roles, or the ideal of "children should be seen and not heard" role, resulting sometimes in a very + female taking a "power behind the throne" role, or a very + child learning to dominate by subversive manipulation, rather than by speaking up directly.)

The trouble with a strongly +/– opposition relationship could come if the – person feels suppressed, uncomfortably pushed or disregarded, or if the + person perceives that the – person is constantly holding back, being a drag, pulling guilt strings, or the like.

Working with the Three Sign Types

As example of how you might work with the basic element, mode and polarity types, let's return to the chart of my granddaughter Tessa, whose chart form lists Earth, Cardinal and – as her dominant types. Her mother Shannon's chart would list Fire, Mutable and +. How might Shannon consider this information in terms of understanding and guiding Tessa? Perhaps she could think:

"My main element is Fire, and Tessa's is Earth. Tessa may not always react as enthusiastically about my new ideas for her as I do. She will take her time, and need to see the practical value of whatever it is, before she's willing to try it. I may need to learn to be patient with her. I might be successful in getting her to do what I'd like her to do by pointing out something concrete she would have to gain through doing it.

"Tessa is Cardinal, and I am Mutable. When she decides she wants to do something, she'll do it. With that, and her down-to-earth characteristics, she'll probably be good at achieving what she sets out to do. I have a lot of ideas, hopes and aspirations for her — maybe too much. But I am flexible. I'll watch to see what she expresses interest in, and as long as its reasonably appropriate, I'll help provide the resources for her to pursue it.

"Tessa is a strongly – type, and I am slightly more on the + side. I may be more naturally out-going than she will be. I'll try to remain aware of that, and not be pushy if she goes through shy stages. I'll just do what I can to help see that she feels safe in the situation."

I remember when the first edition of this book was published, and Tessa was just a toddler (she's now 6), Shannon and I discussed the fact that in spite of all this earth/- emphasis, Tessa is still cardinal-dominant, and has her Mars in fiery, spunky Sagittarius. She's a good illustration of the fact that the sign-styles of personal planets other than the Sun are more easily seen in a small child. Mars, you remember, shows action. Tessa's parents provide her with the structure and security that her earthiness needs, and at the same time, encourage activity and fun. Tessa has her shy moments, but she's spunky, too, and she shows the athletic ability that is often a Sagittarian expression. This capacity for fiery action will serve her well when she discovers which Capricornian mountain she wants to climb!

This little digression offers you an small example of how everything in a chart influences everything else. Nothing can be taken out of context. Putting all the separate pieces of a chart together to discover the most significant themes is called synthesis.

Synthesis of the Three Sign Types into One

It is possible to use the three methods of typing I've just told you about to come up with one dominant sign. Let's review again the list of signs, this time listing each one with all three types: element, mode and polarity:

Aries	Fire	Cardinal	+
Taurus	Earth	Fixed	–
Gemini	Air	Mutable	+
Cancer	Water	Cardinal	–
Leo	Fire	Fixed	+
Virgo	Earth	Mutable	–
Libra	Air	Cardinal	+
Scorpio	Water	Fixed	–
Sagittarius	Fire	Mutable	+
Capricorn	Earth	Cardinal	–
Aquarius	Air	Fixed	+
Pisces	Water	Mutable	–

As you can see, no two signs have all three types in common. Tessa is dominant in Earth, Cardinal and – , and the only sign that fits all three is Capricorn. Shannon is Fire, Mutable and +, and the only sign that fits all three of those is Sagittarius. By this system of synthesis, then, Tessa's single dominant sign is Capricorn and Shannon's single dominant sign is

Sagittarius. In this case, it coincindentally happens that each one has the Sun sign as her dominant sign. For many of you, this will **not** be the case.

For example, I am a Sun in Scorpio, but according to this system of finding primary sign emphasis in my chart, I am by a slim margin, more Earth than Water, definitely Fixed and –. The only sign that fits all three of those categories is Taurus.

Sometimes you will be unable to get an absolutely clear single sign. This is true with both of my other daughters. Molly, who has Sun in Sagittarius, has absolutely equal emphasis on Fire and Earth, a clear emphasis on Fixed, and equal points in + and –. Fire, Fixed and + is Leo, and Earth, Fixed – is Taurus. While balance is desireable, sometimes an equal balance between two naturally opposing elements, represents an inner conflict. A challenge for Molly is to find her own inner balance between her desire to shine brightly with her own individual creative expression (Leo), and her need to be safe, secure and comfortable (Taurus). Since she is Fixed, the dilemma is accentuated by a reluctance to initiate change.

Elizabeth, who has Sun in Libra, also has equal points in + and -signs. She has a very clear cut emphasis on the mutable mode, and emphasis in Air signs by a slight edge of only one point more than water. The sign with Air, mutable and + is Gemini. Even though Liz has not one single planet in Gemini, a Gemini flavor can easily be seen in her personality, which can quick-change in a flash from being so quiet and serious I can't pry a word out of her, to very bright, talkative, even funny.

At this point, it can be enlightening to go back into the look-up section and read all the interpretations that apply to planets in your dominant sign—those for **every** planet in that sign. This will give you a more complete overview of the sign style.

Having said that, however, I must remind you that no matter what the dominant sign, a planet right on an angle (Midheaven or Ascendant) will probably still be the most dominant factor in the chart. To repeat my earlier analogy, the nature and function of the planet is the "light." The sign is only the colored pane of glass that light shines through. The planet predominates over the sign, and the degrees of the angles are the most personally individual factors in a birth chart. For example, I have Neptune closely conjunct my Midheaven. The decidedly "unearthly" and idealistic Neptune, in spite of being in earthy Virgo, still points to the art and the metaphysical studies that have been so important in my life.

Liz, with her Pisces Moon conjunct Descendant, as the most closely angular planet, also has extra emphasis on Water. Water is very close in emphasis to Air in her chart, making Water, mutable and –, or Pisces very nearly as much a candidate for "dominant sign" as Gemini. Her very deep feelings come out in the sculpture, poetry and prose she creates. Following my own advice for this book, for Liz I'd read all the planets in both Gemini and Pisces for extra insight into her personal style.

Molly has two closely angular planets—Jupiter on the Ascendant and Saturn on the Descendant. This is another indicator of a potential inner conflict similar to that of her two equally dominant signs. Expansive Jupiter is open, independent and idealistic; limit-conscious Saturn is concerned with security and approval in relationships.

Shannon, with Saturn right on her Midheaven, even though in Aries, has a very Saturnine seriousness that will make it much easier for her to understand and blend with Tessa's Capricorn nature than a "pure" Sagittarian type might.

Saturn is the planetary "ruler" of Capricorn. We say "ruler" not because the planet person "rules" the sign person (even if it IS the Mom who has the planet here!) but because there is one planet that astrologers generally consider to be closely aligned in basic symbolism with each sign. The "rulers" of the signs are:

Sun	Leo
Moon	Cancer
Mercury	Gemini and Virgo
Venus	Taurus and Libra
Mars	Aries
Jupiter	Sagittarius
Saturn	Capricorn
Uranus	Aquarius
Neptune	Pisces
Pluto	Scorpio

Synastry: The Relationship of Your Child's Aspects to Yours

Astrologers call the art of comparing one birth chart with another synastry. This book is not specifically designed for synastry, yet there is a way that you could use it fairly effectively for that purpose. You could use the aspect interpretations for some more detailed ideas as to how you and your child (or children) get along (or how any pair of individuals get along with each other, or in what areas they might conflict).

You will need to have your fully calculated chart, as well as that of your child (or any other person's chart) to do this aspect comparison. Look at the number right next to each planetary glyph on the wheel chart. That is the number of the degree of the zodiac the planet is in. (Next to the degree number you'll see the sign glyph, and then another number that represents the minutes, or portion of a whole degree.) You need to know the degrees in order to tell whether two planets are in aspect.

Although what I am suggesting here is a simplified method of looking at aspects, and won't give you the type of aspect, it will tell you which planetary themes in your chart have significant impact on your child's chart, and vice versa.

There are 30 degrees in each sign of the zodiac. Customarily they are numbered zero through 29. (30 is the same as zero of the next sign.) If you mark each planet, according to its degree number, on a 30 degree grid, you will be easily able to see which ones are close in degree to each other. Knowing which ones are close together will not tell you which type of aspect they are in (square, trine, or whatever), but it does tell you that they are in some kind of aspect.

For this grid analysis, I recommend you pay special attention to planets on the same degree number or those that are no more than two degrees away from each other. Major aspects will be valid at a greater distance (called "orb" in Astrospeak), but you can't tell from a 30° grid which ones are major and which minor. For that reason, let's stick with small orbs.

You could compare the charts of everyone in your family by this method. Choose a different color marker for each person and enter their planets on the same grid. By studying how the themes of planets in the same places interact, you should learn some interesting things about how the people to whom those planets belong interact with each other!

The basic combinations of planets remain quite similar, even if one planet belongs to one chart, and the planet it aspects belongs to another. Mars in one chart in close aspect to Sun in another chart, for example, means that the Mars person is very stimulating to the Sun, and sometimes challenging. It's a very energetic relationship. Saturn in one chart can mean that the person represents some kind of limitation or seriousness in communicating with another person whose Mercury that Saturn aspects. The two might collaborate well on a research project, but probably wouldn't easily engage in chatter. I think you'll get the idea, but I'll give you an example — a potentially tough one. Here is a grid that shows my planets on the left and my daughter Shannon's planets on the right

Shannon has Mars at 10° Aquarius. I have Mercury at 12° Scorpio, Jupiter at 8° Taurus and Saturn at 10° Taurus. These are all fixed signs, which if you remember from earlier in this chapter, means that whatever these planetary combinations signify in our relationship, we are likely to be somewhat stubborn about it. Planets in the same mode or quality, that are also in aspect, are in "hard" aspect. That means

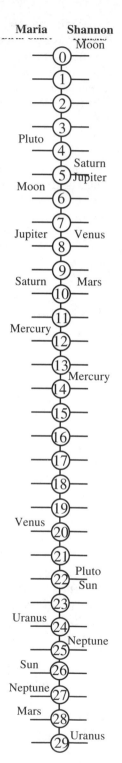

Maria		Shannon
		Moon
	0	
	1	
	2	
	3	
Pluto	4	
		Saturn
	5	Jupiter
Moon	6	
	7	
Jupiter	8	Venus
	9	
Saturn	10	Mars
	11	
Mercury	12	
	13	
		Mercury
	14	
	15	
	16	
	17	
	18	
	19	
Venus	20	
	21	
		Pluto
	22	Sun
	23	
Uranus	24	
		Neptune
	25	
Sun	26	
Neptune	27	
Mars	28	
	29	Uranus

Shannon's Mars is in "hard" aspect to my Mercury, my Jupiter and my Saturn.

Now, the interpretations in this book are written to interpret one child's chart, not a comparison between parent and child. Still, as I've said, the general theme of a planetary pair is the same, no matter what the aspect. Take another look at the interpretation for Mercury-Mars, in Chapter 8. You can see that lots of assertive, persuasive talking is an issue. It's **her** Mars — remember what I said earlier about S.A.S.? She rattled my nerves on more than one occasion when she was little. Well, we still talk a lot — always have. Usually it's a very stimulating dialogue, each respecting the other's opinions, but not easily giving ground. At least I always heard what was going on in this one's head — it's easier to deal with than silence, and wondering what the kid is thinking and doing.

My Saturn, I am sure, was often perceived as limits on what she could do and when (read again the interpretation labeled Mercury-Saturn). It is not unusual for a parent to have Saturn in some key aspect to the child's chart, symbolizing the limitations placed on the child, or the responsibility the parent expects. On the other hand, for the child's Saturn to aspect a parent's planet symbolizes the responsibility that child represents to the parent. A parent would do well to be especially aware of how his or her Saturn aspects a planet in a child's chart. There can sometimes be a very fine line between the discipline or structure that builds security and skill, and the discipline or structure that harshly squelches the magic of creative individuality.

Review the basic function of each planet, as they are explained at the beginnings of chapters 5, 6 and 7. This will help you decide who's doing what, in thinking about the aspect combinations as having one planet from one person's chart and the other planet from another person's chart.

I think my Jupiter, to Shannon's Mars-action function, has symbolized both the optimistic encouragement for her to try whatever she was trying — and, on other occasions, has represented an impulse or an overdoing on my part that she wasn't quite ready for. Certainly she has always been very stimulating (Mars) to my sense of joy (Jupiter) and to my sense of responsibility (Saturn).

All in all, I think I've been most aware of the Mercury-Mars contact between us, and it has helped me calm down sometimes and regain my sense of "who is the parent, here, anyway" to remember that it is my choice, ultimately, whether to be irritated or stimulated.

For insights into same planet to same planet (parent's Sun in aspect to child's Sun, etc.), just read the sign interpretations for each one, and think of how the two different styles of personality might understand, or fail to understand, each other.

This is far from complete, of course, and if you want to pursue it further, there are books specifically on synastry available, some listed in the bibliography. Also, Astro offers a number of computerized comparison reports. One of them, the Compatibility Profile for Mother/Child, or for Father/Child, is described on one of the back pages.

Finding Yourself in Your Child's Horoscope

There's an astrological tradition for interpreting how an individual perceives his or her parents. In this day and age, I can't promise it will always work, since traditional parental roles are changing. Still, it's worth thinking about, for additional insight into how you can be a positive role model for your child—and how your own perception of your parents influences you.

In it's simplest form, the tradition has it that the Moon in a horoscope describes the individual's perception of Mother, and Saturn describes the father. Moon is the planet most associated with nurturing qualities, and Saturn with discipline and conditions. A full interpretation of parents in the chart would also take into account aspects to Moon or Saturn, and also the planetary rulers (and their aspects) of House 10 and House 4. House 10 and its ruler traditionally tells us something about the father, or in a more contemporary interpretation, the parent who "sets rules and makes me follow them." House 4 and its ruler traditionally tells us something about Mother, but in a more contemporary interpretation, the parent who is caring and understanding. (The traditional theory, here, could break down if it turns out that Mom is the primary authority figure, and Dad is the more nurturing parent.)

The planetary ruler of a house is the planet most closely associated with the sign on the house cusp. The planets most closely associated with the signs are listed on page 48, e.g. Mars "rules" Aries, Venus "rules" Taurus, etc.

What I will offer you here is food for thought—another facet of astrology to observe as your child grows. If you become aware of how your child sees you (which may be quite different than how you see yourself) you'll gain insight into how you, as a role model, might play to the child's perception in a positive sense, and avoid the negative. You'll also better understand how each one of your children may perceive you in a different way, each according to his or her own horoscope. I know, it hardly seems fair to say you play a different role for each child, after everything else I've told you to think about. But, that's the way it is, and it is worth considering.

So, look at the Moon in your child's horoscope if you're the Mom; Saturn if you're the Dad, as well as the rulers of Houses 10 and 4, and read the paragraphs in this book about those planets in sign, house and aspect. Reflect on the ways in which you embody both the constructive and destructive qualities of those interpretations. This may help you understand how you may "come off" to your child, and show you how you can become a better role model.

This level of interpretation introduces more advanced astrological technique than the rest of this book. If you are interested in taking the next step toward understanding how to blend all the separate facets of a horoscope into major themes (such as how does this individual perceive his/her parents), I suggest *The Next Step: Complete Horoscope Interpretation*, by Maritha Pottenger, and *The Only Way to Learn Astrology, Vol. III: Horoscope Analysis*, by Marion D. March and Joan McEvers.

Your Inner Child

Throughout this book we've been sharing the special attributes of your child as a naturally magical little person, whom we hope to guide in becoming skillfully adept at achieving his or her highest potential. Now we have also considered the special alchemy of relating that is likely to exist between you. In conclusion, I want to talk about just you, because in one way or another (as I've said repeatedly), **what you do** and **who you are** will mean more than anything you can ever say, in terms of what your child learns from you. Let's consider who **you** are.

Are **you** a magical person? We know you were — just as your child is now, and so is every little baby who comes into the world. You were born with tremendous power — infinite potential and possibilities — the center of your personal Universe, carrying the essence of God/Goddess within. Food, attention and comfort appeared at your cry-command. You believed that you could create and do what you wanted, and in one magical year you achieved marvelous feats of growth and development. Your magic was spontaneous, instinctive and wonderful — at first — but eventually, doubts in the omnipotence of your power began to creep in. Your reality, your perception of "what works," all too often came into conflict with the realities of others who inhabited your Universe. You learned that what you commanded didn't always manifest the way you wanted it to, and you had to learn to adapt. Your "natural magic" of "if I do this, it will bring ..." was no longer quite adequate. It became increasingly necessary for you to develop skills and strategies. Instinct had to be combined with intellect, and impulse with planning.

When you were behaving in accordance with the realities, the expectations, of the powerful bigger people who provided many things you needed, you were "good." You had considerable motivation to adopt their reality as your own. But there are many realities. For the most part you grew steadily in your ability to cope, to conform and to create your world. You pushed ever more deeply inside you that little child who cried and caused the world to be magically changed for the better. The little child was still there, though, and still is, even now.

That child within you is still quite capable of being "bad," which I will define as acting very much in conflict with the preferences of your adult self. Without that child's cooperation, though, you just can't be a magical person. Effective, mature magic depends upon all aspects of you behaving in concert. No matter what you consciously think you believe or want, if that child within is in opposition, or even in doubt, you are in trouble. Why? Because your inner child takes priority in much the same way that any baby's cry tends to prevail over whatever else the parent was doing, and redirects the parent's attention. You think, consciously, that you've definitely made up your mind about what you want and what you will do.

Then that little cry from inside surfaces in contrary doubts, assumptions and beliefs that have been previously adopted by the inner child, often even before the time of conscious memory.

The child within has been called by many names, most frequently the subconscious or the unconscious mind. Both "sub" and "un" imply something inferior, and in my opinion, that is really unfair and unrealistic — perhaps just stemming from the fact that a lot of people are a little bit afraid of the uncontrolled instincts and emotions that can come from that inner child. The truth is, that "sub"-conscious part of you is extremely powerful — capable of overwhelming all of your conscious intentions and "better judgment."

Think about it. Who are you, deep inside? Look down through all the layers of adult thinking and behavior, down to the little child you were, and still are ...sometimes, when you're not expecting it. Aren't there times when you're under some kind of emotional stress — upset, anger, fear, excitement, joy — and all your adult composure and best intentions are overcome by that little kid who creeps out and screams or cries or acts on impulse or says something that you regret later? That little child within influences you with hidden memories and responses long forgotten. It's experiencing all kinds of new things with you, too, and storing them away within its own framework of perceptions and beliefs that were established long before your logical, conscious mind was trained in a more "realistic" framework.

If you were fortunate as a young child, the adults within your environment appreciated and supported your uniqueness and your magic. They gently guided you to adapt to your world and to acquire logical and objective skills. They corrected your behavior when necessary, but still made it clear that they loved and valued you. They accomplished these things without squelching your instinctive style, and most of all without squelching your belief in yourself and your own power. You grew up with an all-important feeling of self-worth, and therefore, creating magic in your life seems "natural." You are one of those people who, even in the face of crisis, can not only cope, but "turn lemons into lemonade."

Unfortunately, for a great many people, this is not the case. The child within is fearful and full of doubts. To some extent, all of us lose some of our "natural magic." The "shoulds" and "shouldn'ts" take over, and the child-magician within can become so diminished and suppressed that it can be expressed only in the uncontrolled outburst that hurts self or someone else. If this fits you in any way, then it is well worthwhile for you to become reacquainted with your inner child, and what it needs to feel secure, confident and loving.

New-age or self-help type seminars on "healing the inner child" are fairly common these days, and they can be helpful — so long as they do **not** encourage participants to become "victims." If you feel your childhood is not all that it should have been, blaming your parents or your environment can be a nicely convenient excuse for today's problems. Sorry, this grandma is not impressed.

Magic, if forgotten or long suppressed, can be relearned. The natural magic of childhood can be transmuted into the creatively skilled focus of the adept, and the joy and wonder of life can be renewed in even greater measure. It may take work, but it can be done. And the power to change is not in the planets, or in any outside authority. The power is in YOU! (And the only person who can sabotage that power is YOU.)

If you feel that your life is not as magical as it could be, and your inner child might be neglected, you might begin to get back in touch with that child by reading my child-oriented astrological delineations about your chart. In reflecting on what you were like as a child from your now adult perspective, and noting how the interpretations I've written fit or don't fit with who that child was, I think you might still see your adult self, too, in certain ways. Think about that child as profiled in the interpretive text. Think about yourself now, and try to remember how you were as a child. Ask yourself:

"What do/did I need to be able to "shine? What made/makes me feel secure? How do/did I think and communicate? When do/did I feel most loving? What did I need to "get going" as a child? What incites me into action now? What are my core beliefs, and when did I first adopt them?"

Thinking about these things should give you fresh insight into how you instinctively react when you are stressed, or when your emotional buttons are pushed, or why you may be carrying around some long-past hurt. On the other hand, you might see the areas of life that give you the most joy and satisfaction, and be led to consider whether or not you are letting yourself "play" enough in those areas. Thinking about these things may show you ways in which you can restore or increase the magic in your life — the sparkle and the sense of personal worth and satisfaction that makes life worth living.

Who's the Parent, Anyway?

Toward the beginning of this chapter, I used the phrase above that heads this final section. In conclusion, let's return to a contemplation of your inner child and the parent you've become.

Face it. Any child worth its salt will learn how to "get around" — manipulate — parents (and often, teachers, too) in short order. Kids learn how to "push your buttons." They learn to play one adult against another, how to get what they want even when your first answer is "no," when you mean what you say and when you don't. It's endless. Why? Maybe because they instinctively recognize your inner child, even if you don't.

Adults have their own lives, too, of course. They tend to get caught up in their own issues — projects, goals, stresses, worries. When the child intrudes, the adult may often take the easy route. "Easy" tends to mean instinctive — and there we are, back with the inner child — reacting, rather than thinking things through. If you are just starting out as a parent, you may think that my next statement sounds pretty terrible, but I'm going to say it anyway. Any "normal," well-intentioned parent (or teacher) who is really honest with herself or himself, can understand why child abuse **can** happen. Even if you **never** give in to your impulses and **always** transmute those impulses into constructive behavior (you saint!), **there are times** you **feel** like...#!@?#!.

Raising a child may well be the most complex and the most challenging single project you undertake in your life. Certainly there is none more important, for the future lies with our children. There is nothing you'll ever undertake that has a greater potential for joy — or for frustration and even despair. No one should embark on this path lightly — and yet few really think about the commitment they are making before the child is conceived.

This grandma believes that one thing is for certain. Whether you planned your child's coming carefully, or whether your little inner child decided for you, "un"–consciously, in the impulse of a moment, **this** path of parenting you have **chosen**. I know that you want to do the very best you can.

Just be aware that when your child exasperates you, your own inner impulse to flee or to strike back is like the natural, uncontrolled darkly magical world of the littlest child. It can be very powerful, can sometimes be very effective at that moment — and can also boomerang back at you in unpleasant ways that you never intended. Remember, **you are the parent,** and therefore it is you who must behave with the maturity that the child lacks. If you are to guide your magical child to learn skill while retaining an all-important belief in self, you must strive to be the "adept." You must strive to be an example of the serenity, courage, and wisdom, and the self-mastery and belief-in-self that enables anyone to focus and direct desired change. This is mature magic!

Love and respect your child's uniqueness, spend quality time with the child, provide as best you can the resources he or she needs to learn, foster security through consistency — all the things we've been considering throughout this book. But love and respect your own uniqueness, too, and don't neglect to find some quality time for yourself — and for yourselves as a couple, if you are raising this child as partners.

The more adept you are at creating your own magical life, the easier it will be for you to convey your skill to your child. Always remember, no matter what your child is like as an individual, the most important lessons of life that child will learn from you are simply what you do and who you are. The Earth and the Cosmos of your personal Universe can be no more or no less than you create them. Create magic!

Appendix
Look Up Your Child's Planets

**Planetary Ingresses into Signs 1985-2005
plus Rising Sign Table**

How to Look Up Your Child's Planets

With the planetary tables that follow you'll be able to look up the sign placements for all the planets for any child born from 1985 through 2005. They are provided so you can at least read the sign interpretations for your child, while you are waiting for your free Magical Child computer chart to arrive in the mail.

Do send for that chart, though, or obtain a fully calculated chart by another means. Computer charts are best, and chart orders called in to Astro Communications Services, Inc., are sent out within a day of when the order is received, or can be faxed back if you're really in a hurry. If you have a home computer, you could purchase ***Electronic Astrologer*** software for Windows. It's by far the easiest and lowest-cost really accurate astrological software on the market. Not only does it calculate charts, but it provides an excellent and comprehensive interpretation.

Let's Get Started

Step One —

Convert Birth Time to Eastern Standard

As you all know, time varies across the country. The Planet Tables in this book are calculated for Eastern Standard Time. (You lucky readers whose children were born in Eastern **Standard** Time can skip this part and jump ahead to Step Three!) For Eastern **Daylight** Time, or **any Daylight Time birth**, read on:

A. Subtract one hour for daylight time births.

Examples: 9:15 AM Daylight Time
-1:00
8:15 AM Standard Time

12:30 PM Daylight Time
-1:00
11:30 AM Standard Time

An example where the **day changes**:

12:45 AM Daylight Time on June 9
-1:00
11:45 PM Standard Time on June 8

B. Now that everyone has the birth time in Standard Time, those with **births in any time zone other than Eastern must convert to Eastern Time (ET).** Following are conversions for the USA:

For **Central** Time, **add one** hour to get ET
For **Mountain** Time, **add two** hours to get ET
For **Pacific** Time, **add three** hours to get ET

For **YST** (Alaska) **add four hours** to get ET
For **AHST** (Hawaii), **add five hours** to get ET

If your child was **born outside the continental USA**, and you do not know how many hours your time zone is from Eastern Standard, you should easily be able to find out from your local library . Since most time zone references use hours from Greenwich, it may help you in your conversion to know that Eastern Standard Time is Greenwich Mean Time minus 5 hours.

STEP THREE —

Looking up the Signs of Planets

The planets appear in the tables in the same order that they are covered in the book's text, Sun first, followed by Moon, Mercury, Venus, Mars, Jupiter, Saturn, Uranus, Neptune and Pluto. The dates and times shown are exactly when the planet changed from one sign to the next, in Eastern Standard Time. This way there can be no concern about being "on the cusp" (born on a day when the planet changed signs). For example, if your child was born on September 28, 1997, at 5:21 pm EST, Mars is in Scorpio. If the birth was at 5:22 pm EST, Mars is in Sagittarius—no "almosts," no approximations. Just fit your child's birthday in between any two dates and times, and you'll have the right sign. To follow through on the example already given, a child born any time from 3:42 am EST on August 14, 1997 until 5:21 pm EST September 28, 1997, has Mars in Scorpio. Any child born from 5:22 pm EST September 28 through 12:33 am EST November 9, 1997 has Mars in Sagittarius.

STEP FOUR —

Finding the RISING SIGN

It is not within the scope of this book's limited tables to assure you the exact accuracy on the Rising Sign as was possible for the planet's signs. This is because Rising Sign requires knowing the city of birth, in addition to the time and date. What we are providing is an approximate Rising Sign table for each USA time zone, based on the median latitude in three bands across the map illustration. This method will give the correct Rising Sign in most cases. If, however, your child was born close to a given time change, don't count on the Rising Sign being accurate. Even a few degrees difference in latitude could change it. Get that computer chart to be sure!

SUN POSITIONS 1985-2005

1985

Jan 19	9:58 pm	Aquarius
Feb 18	12:08 pm	Pisces
Mar 20	11:15 am	Aries
Apr 19	10:27 pm	Taurus
May 20	9:44 am	Gemini
Jun 21	5:45 am	Cancer
Jul 22	4:37 am	Leo
Aug 22	11:37 am	Virgo
Sep 22	9:08 pm	Libra
Oct 23	6:23 am	Scorpio
Nov 22	3:52 am	Sagittarius
Dec 21	5:09 pm	Capricorn

1986

Jan 20	3:47 am	Aquarius
Feb 18	5:58 pm	Pisces
Mar 20	5:04 pm	Aries
Apr 20	4:13 am	Taurus
May 21	3:29 am	Gemini
Jun 21	11:31 am	Cancer
Jul 22	10:25 pm	Leo
Aug 23	5:27 am	Virgo
Sep 23	2:60 am	Libra
Oct 23	12:15 pm	Scorpio
Nov 22	9:45 am	Sagittarius
Dec 21	11:03 pm	Capricorn

1987

Jan 20	9:41 am	Aquarius
Feb 18	11:51 pm	Pisces
Mar 20	10:53 pm	Aries
Apr 20	9:58 am	Taurus
May 21	9:11 am	Gemini
Jun 21	5:12 pm	Cancer
Jul 23	4:07 am	Leo
Aug 23	11:11 am	Virgo
Sep 23	8:46 am	Libra
Oct 23	6:02 pm	Scorpio
Nov 22	3:30 pm	Sagittarius
Dec 22	4:47 am	Capricorn

1988

Jan 20	3:25 pm	Aquarius
Feb 19	5:36 am	Pisces
Mar 20	4:40 am	Aries
Apr 19	3:46 pm	Taurus
May 20	2:58 pm	Gemini
Jun 20	10:57 pm	Cancer
Jul 22	9:52 am	Leo
Aug 22	4:55 pm	Virgo
Sep 22	2:30 pm	Libra
Oct 22	11:45 pm	Scorpio
Nov 21	9:13 pm	Sagittarius
Dec 21	10:29 am	Capricorn

1989

Jan 19	9:08 pm	Aquarius
Feb 18	11:21 am	Pisces
Mar 20	10:29 am	Aries
Apr 19	9:40 pm	Taurus
May 20	8:54 pm	Gemini
Jun 21	4:54 am	Cancer
Jul 22	3:46 pm	Leo
Aug 22	10:47 pm	Virgo
Sep 22	8:21 pm	Libra
Oct 23	5:36 am	Scorpio
Nov 22	3:06 am	Sagittarius
Dec 21	4:23 pm	Capricorn

1990

Jan 20	3:03 am	Aquarius
Feb 18	5:15 pm	Pisces
Mar 20	4:20 pm	Aries
Apr 20	3:28 am	Taurus
May 21	2:38 am	Gemini
Jun 21	10:34 am	Cancer
Jul 22	9:22 pm	Leo
Aug 23	4:22 am	Virgo
Sep 23	1:56 am	Libra
Oct 23	11:15 am	Scorpio
Nov 22	8:48 am	Sagittarius
Dec 21	10:08 pm	Capricorn

1991

Jan 20	8:48 am	Aquarius
Feb 18	10:59 pm	Pisces
Mar 20	10:03 pm	Aries
Apr 20	9:09 am	Taurus
May 21	8:21 am	Gemini
Jun 21	4:20 pm	Cancer
Jul 23	3:12 am	Leo
Aug 23	10:14 am	Virgo
Sep 23	7:49 am	Libra
Oct 23	5:06 pm	Scorpio
Nov 22	2:37 pm	Sagittarius
Dec 22	3:55 am	Capricorn

1992

Jan 20	2:33 pm	Aquarius
Feb 19	4:44 am	Pisces
Mar 20	3:49 am	Aries
Apr 19	2:58 pm	Taurus
May 20	2:13 pm	Gemini
Jun 20	10:15 pm	Cancer
Jul 22	9:10 am	Leo
Aug 22	4:11 pm	Virgo
Sep 22	1:44 pm	Libra
Oct 22	10:58 pm	Scorpio
Nov 21	8:27 pm	Sagittarius
Dec 21	9:44 am	Capricorn

1993

Jan 19	8:24 pm	Aquarius
Feb 18	10:36 am	Pisces
Mar 20	9:42 am	Aries
Apr 19	8:50 pm	Taurus
May 20	8:03 pm	Gemini
Jun 21	4:01 am	Cancer
Jul 22	2:52 pm	Leo
Aug 22	9:51 pm	Virgo
Sep 22	7:23 pm	Libra
Oct 23	4:38 am	Scorpio
Nov 22	2:08 am	Sagittarius
Dec 21	3:27 pm	Capricorn

1994

Jan 20	2:08 am	Aquarius
Feb 18	4:23 pm	Pisces
Mar 20	3:29 pm	Aries
Apr 20	2:37 am	Taurus
May 21	1:49 am	Gemini
Jun 21	9:49 am	Cancer
Jul 22	8:42 pm	Leo
Aug 23	3:45 am	Virgo
Sep 23	1:20 am	Libra
Oct 23	10:37 am	Scorpio
Nov 22	8:07 am	Sagittarius
Dec 21	9:24 pm	Capricorn

1995

Jan 20	8:01 am	Aquarius
Feb 18	10:12 pm	Pisces
Mar 20	9:15 pm	Aries
Apr 20	8:22 am	Taurus
May 21	7:35 am	Gemini
Jun 21	3:35 pm	Cancer
Jul 23	2:31 am	Leo
Aug 23	9:36 am	Virgo
Sep 23	7:14 am	Libra
Oct 23	4:33 pm	Scorpio
Nov 22	2:02 pm	Sagittarius
Dec 22	3:18 am	Capricorn

1996

Jan 20	1:54 pm	Aquarius
Feb 19	4:02 am	Pisces
Mar 20	3:04 am	Aries
Apr 19	2:11 pm	Taurus
May 20	1:24 pm	Gemini
Jun 20	9:25 pm	Cancer
Jul 22	8:20 am	Leo
Aug 22	3:24 pm	Virgo
Sep 22	1:01 pm	Libra
Oct 22	10:20 pm	Scorpio
Nov 21	7:50 pm	Sagittarius
Dec 21	9:07 am	Capricorn

SUN POSITIONS 1985-2005

1997		
Jan 19	7:44 pm	Aquarius
Feb 18	9:53 am	Pisces
Mar 20	8:56 am	Aries
Apr 19	8:04 pm	Taurus
May 20	7:19 pm	Gemini
Jun 21	3:21 am	Cancer
Jul 22	2:16 pm	Leo
Aug 22	9:20 pm	Virgo
Sep 22	6:57 pm	Libra
Oct 23	4:16 am	Scorpio
Nov 22	1:49 am	Sagittarius
Dec 21	3:08 pm	Capricorn

1998		
Jan 20	1:47 am	Aquarius
Feb 18	3:56 pm	Pisces
Mar 20	2:56 pm	Aries
Apr 20	1:58 am	Taurus
May 21	1:06 am	Gemini
Jun 21	9:04 am	Cancer
Jul 22	7:56 pm	Leo
Aug 23	2:60 am	Virgo
Sep 23	12:38 am	Libra
Oct 23	9:60 am	Scorpio
Nov 22	7:35 am	Sagittarius
Dec 21	8:58 pm	Capricorn

1999		
Jan 20	7:38 am	Aquarius
Feb 18	9:48 pm	Pisces
Mar 20	8:47 pm	Aries
Apr 20	7:47 am	Taurus
May 21	6:53 am	Gemini
Jun 21	2:50 pm	Cancer
Jul 23	1:45 am	Leo
Aug 23	8:52 am	Virgo
Sep 23	6:33 am	Libra
Oct 23	3:53 pm	Scorpio
Nov 22	1:26 pm	Sagittarius
Dec 22	2:45 am	Capricorn

2000		
Jan 20	1:24 pm	Aquarius
Feb 19	3:34 am	Pisces
Mar 20	2:36 am	Aries
Apr 19	1:41 pm	Taurus
May 20	12:50 pm	Gemini
Jun 20	8:49 pm	Cancer
Jul 22	7:44 am	Leo
Aug 22	2:50 pm	Virgo
Sep 22	12:29 pm	Libra
Oct 22	9:49 pm	Scorpio
Nov 21	7:20 pm	Sagittarius
Dec 21	8:38 am	Capricorn

2001		
Jan 19	7:17 pm	Aquarius
Feb 18	9:28 am	Pisces
Mar 20	8:32 am	Aries
Apr 19	7:37 pm	Taurus
May 20	6:45 pm	Gemini
Jun 21	2:39 am	Cancer
Jul 22	1:27 pm	Leo
Aug 22	8:28 pm	Virgo
Sep 22	6:06 pm	Libra
Oct 23	3:27 am	Scorpio
Nov 22	1:02 am	Sagittarius
Dec 21	2:23 pm	Capricorn

2002		
Jan 20	1:03 am	Aquarius
Feb 18	3:14 pm	Pisces
Mar 20	2:17 pm	Aries
Apr 20	1:22 am	Taurus
May 21	12:30 am	Gemini
Jun 21	8:25 am	Cancer
Jul 22	7:16 pm	Leo
Aug 23	2:18 am	Virgo
Sep 22	11:56 pm	Libra
Oct 23	9:19 am	Scorpio
Nov 22	6:55 am	Sagittarius
Dec 21	8:15 pm	Capricorn

2003		
Jan 20	6:54 am	Aquarius
Feb 18	9:01 pm	Pisces
Mar 20	8:01 pm	Aries
Apr 20	7:04 am	Taurus
May 21	6:13 am	Gemini
Jun 21	2:12 pm	Cancer
Jul 23	1:05 am	Leo
Aug 23	8:09 am	Virgo
Sep 23	5:48 am	Libra
Oct 23	3:10 pm	Scorpio
Nov 22	12:44 pm	Sagittarius
Dec 22	2:05 am	Capricorn

2004		
Jan 20	12:43 pm	Aquarius
Feb 19	2:51 am	Pisces
Mar 20	1:50 am	Aries
Apr 19	12:51 pm	Taurus
May 20	12:00 pm	Gemini
Jun 20	7:58 pm	Cancer
Jul 22	6:51 am	Leo
Aug 22	1:54 pm	Virgo
Sep 22	11:31 am	Libra
Oct 22	8:50 pm	Scorpio
Nov 21	6:23 pm	Sagittarius
Dec 21	7:43 am	Capricorn

2005		
Jan 19	6:23 pm	Aquarius
Feb 18	8:33 am	Pisces
Mar 20	7:34 am	Aries
Apr 19	6:38 pm	Taurus
May 20	5:48 pm	Gemini
Jun 21	1:47 am	Cancer
Jul 22	12:42 pm	Leo
Aug 22	7:47 pm	Virgo
Sep 22	5:24 pm	Libra
Oct 23	2:43 am	Scorpio
Nov 22	12:16 am	Sagittarius
Dec 21	1:36 pm	Capricorn

MOONPOSITIONS 1985

January

1	Taurus		
2	Taurus		
3	Taurus	7:00 am	Gemini
4	Gemini		
5	Gemini	3:18 pm	Cancer
6	Cancer		
7	Cancer	8:28 pm	Leo
8	Leo		
9	Leo	11:40 pm	Virgo
10	Virgo		
11	Virgo		
12	Virgo	2:13 am	Libra
13	Libra		
14	Libra	5:07 am	Scorpio
15	Scorpio		
16	Scorpio	8:48 am	Sagittarius
17	Sagittarius		
18	Sagittarius	1:29 pm	Capricorn
19	Capricorn		
20	Capricorn	7:38 pm	Aquarius
21	Aquarius		
22	Aquarius		
23	Aquarius	4:02 pm	Pisces
24	Pisces		
25	Pisces	3:05 pm	Aries
26	Aries		
27	Aries		
28	Aries	3:53 am	Taurus
29	Taurus		
30	Taurus	4:01 pm	Gemini
31	Gemini		

February

1	Gemini		
2	Gemini	12:59 am	Cancer
3	Cancer		
4	Cancer	6:02 am	Leo
5	Leo		
6	Leo	8:09 am	Virgo
7	Virgo		
8	Virgo	9:10 am	Libra
9	Libra		
10	Libra	10:49 am	Scorpio
11	Scorpio		
12	Scorpio	2:09 pm	Sagittarius
13	Sagittarius		
14	Sagittarius	7:27 pm	Capricorn
15	Capricorn		
16	Capricorn		
17	Capricorn	2:36 am	Aquarius
18	Aquarius		
19	Aquarius	11:38 am	Pisces
20	Pisces		
21	Pisces	10:43 pm	Aries
22	Aries		
23	Aries		
24	Aries	11:27 am	Taurus
25	Taurus		
26	Taurus		
27	Taurus	12:11 am	Gemini
28	Gemini		

March

1	Gemini	10:23 am	Cancer
2	Cancer		
3	Cancer	4:28 pm	Leo
4	Leo		
5	Leo	6:43 pm	Virgo
6	Virgo		
7	Virgo	6:47 pm	Libra
8	Libra		
9	Libra	6:47 pm	Scorpio
10	Scorpio		
11	Scorpio	8:29 pm	Sagittarius
12	Sagittarius		
13	Sagittarius		
14	Sagittarius	12:55 am	Capricorn
15	Capricorn		
16	Capricorn	8:11 am	Aquarius
17	Aquarius		
18	Aquarius	5:50 pm	Pisces
19	Pisces		
20	Pisces		
21	Pisces	5:20 am	Aries
22	Aries		
23	Aries	6:06 pm	Taurus
24	Taurus		
25	Taurus		
26	Taurus	7:02 am	Gemini
27	Gemini		
28	Gemini	6:13 pm	Cancer
29	Cancer		
30	Cancer		
31	Cancer	1:51 am	Leo

April

1	Leo		
2	Leo	5:25 am	Virgo
3	Virgo		
4	Virgo	5:54 am	Libra
5	Libra		
6	Libra	5:10 am	Scorpio
7	Scorpio		
8	Scorpio	5:18 am	Sagittarius
9	Sagittarius		
10	Sagittarius	7:57 am	Capricorn
11	Capricorn		
12	Capricorn	2:04 pm	Aquarius
13	Aquarius		
14	Aquarius	11:30 pm	Pisces
15	Pisces		
16	Pisces		
17	Pisces	11:18 am	Aries
18	Aries		
19	Aries		
20	Aries	12:12 am	Taurus
21	Taurus		
22	Taurus	1:01 pm	Gemini
23	Gemini		
24	Gemini		
25	Gemini	12:26 am	Cancer
26	Cancer		
27	Cancer	9:10 am	Leo
28	Leo		
29	Leo	2:24 pm	Virgo
30	Virgo		

May

1	Virgo	4:22 pm	Libra
2	Libra		
3	Libra	4:17 pm	Scorpio
4	Scorpio		
5	Scorpio	3:56 pm	Sagittarius
6	Sagittarius		
7	Sagittarius	5:11 pm	Capricorn
8	Capricorn		
9	Capricorn	9:38 pm	Aquarius
10	Aquarius		
11	Aquarius		
12	Aquarius	5:56 am	Pisces
13	Pisces		
14	Pisces	5:25 pm	Aries
15	Aries		
16	Aries		
17	Aries	6:23 am	Taurus
18	Taurus		
19	Taurus	7:01 pm	Gemini
20	Gemini		
21	Gemini		
22	Gemini	6:05 am	Cancer
23	Cancer		
24	Cancer	2:54 pm	Leo
25	Leo		
26	Leo	9:06 pm	Virgo
27	Virgo		
28	Virgo		
29	Virgo	12:41 am	Libra
30	Libra		
31	Libra	2:07 am	Scorpio

June

1	Scorpio		
2	Scorpio	2:33 am	Sagittarius
3	Sagittarius		
4	Sagittarius	3:34 am	Capricorn
5	Capricorn		
6	Capricorn	6:52 am	Aquarius
7	Aquarius		
8	Aquarius	1:46 pm	Pisces
9	Pisces		
10	Pisces		
11	Pisces	12:24 am	Aries
12	Aries		
13	Aries	1:11 pm	Taurus
14	Taurus		
15	Taurus		
16	Taurus	1:45 am	Gemini
17	Gemini		
18	Gemini	12:22 pm	Cancer
19	Cancer		
20	Cancer	8:32 pm	Leo
21	Leo		
22	Leo		
23	Leo	2:32 am	Virgo
24	Virgo		
25	Virgo	6:48 am	Libra
26	Libra		
27	Libra	9:37 am	Scorpio
28	Scorpio		
29	Scorpio	11:30 am	Sagittarius
30	Sagittarius		

MOONPOSITIONS1985

	July		
1	Sagittarius	1:22 pm	Capricorn
2	Capricorn		
3	Capricorn	4:36 pm	Aquarius
4	Aquarius		
5	Aquarius	10:40 pm	Pisces
6	Pisces		
7	Pisces		
8	Pisces	8:20 am	Aries
9	Aries		
10	Aries	8:44 pm	Taurus
11	Taurus		
12	Taurus		
13	Taurus	9:23 am	Gemini
14	Gemini		
15	Gemini	7:54 pm	Cancer
16	Cancer		
17	Cancer		
18	Cancer	3:25 am	Leo
19	Leo		
20	Leo	8:29 am	Virgo
21	Virgo		
22	Virgo	12:10 pm	Libra
23	Libra		
24	Libra	3:16 pm	Scorpio
25	Scorpio		
26	Scorpio	6:12 pm	Sagittarius
27	Sagittarius		
28	Sagittarius	9:21 pm	Capricorn
29	Capricorn		
30	Capricorn		
31	Capricorn	1:25 am	Aquarius

	August		
1	Aquarius		
2	Aquarius	7:33 am	Pisces
3	Pisces		
4	Pisces	4:43 pm	Aries
5	Aries		
6	Aries		
7	Aries	4:41 am	Taurus
8	Taurus		
9	Taurus	5:31 pm	Gemini
10	Gemini		
11	Gemini		
12	Gemini	4:28 am	Cancer
13	Cancer		
14	Cancer	11:57 am	Leo
15	Leo		
16	Leo	4:15 pm	Virgo
17	Virgo		
18	Virgo	6:44 pm	Libra
19	Libra		
20	Libra	8:51 pm	Scorpio
21	Scorpio		
22	Scorpio	11:36 pm	Sagittarius
23	Sagittarius		
24	Sagittarius		
25	Sagittarius	3:24 am	Capricorn
26	Capricorn		
27	Capricorn	8:31 am	Aquarius
28	Aquarius		
29	Aquarius	3:25 pm	Pisces
30	Pisces		
31	Pisces		

	September		
1	Pisces	12:42 am	Aries
2	Aries		
3	Aries	12:28 pm	Taurus
4	Taurus		
5	Taurus		
6	Taurus	1:27 am	Gemini
7	Gemini		
8	Gemini	1:10 pm	Cancer
9	Cancer		
10	Cancer	9:27 pm	Leo
11	Leo		
12	Leo		
13	Leo	1:52 am	Virgo
14	Virgo		
15	Virgo	3:34 am	Libra
16	Libra		
17	Libra	4:17 am	Scorpio
18	Scorpio		
19	Scorpio	5:40 am	Sagittarius
20	Sagittarius		
21	Sagittarius	8:49 am	Capricorn
22	Capricorn		
23	Capricorn	2:11 pm	Aquarius
24	Aquarius		
25	Aquarius	9:50 pm	Pisces
26	Pisces		
27	Pisces		
28	Pisces	7:43 am	Aries
29	Aries		
30	Aries	7:35 pm	Taurus

	October		
1	Taurus		
2	Taurus		
3	Taurus	8:36 am	Gemini
4	Gemini		
5	Gemini	8:59 pm	Cancer
6	Cancer		
7	Cancer		
8	Cancer	6:33 am	Leo
9	Leo		
10	Leo	12:09 pm	Virgo
11	Virgo		
12	Virgo	2:12 pm	Libra
13	Libra		
14	Libra	2:13 pm	Scorpio
15	Scorpio		
16	Scorpio	2:06 pm	Sagittarius
17	Sagittarius		
18	Sagittarius	3:35 pm	Capricorn
19	Capricorn		
20	Capricorn	7:54 pm	Aquarius
21	Aquarius		
22	Aquarius		
23	Aquarius	3:27 am	Pisces
24	Pisces		
25	Pisces	1:47 pm	Aries
26	Aries		
27	Aries		
28	Aries	1:59 am	Taurus
29	Taurus		
30	Taurus	2:59 pm	Gemini
31	Gemini		

	November		
1	Gemini		
2	Gemini	3:31 am	Cancer
3	Cancer		
4	Cancer	2:04 pm	Leo
5	Leo		
6	Leo	9:18 pm	Virgo
7	Virgo		
8	Virgo		
9	Virgo	12:52 am	Libra
10	Libra		
11	Libra	1:31 am	Scorpio
12	Scorpio		
13	Scorpio	12:52 am	Sagittarius
14	Sagittarius		
15	Sagittarius	12:53 am	Capricorn
16	Capricorn		
17	Capricorn	3:25 am	Aquarius
18	Aquarius		
19	Aquarius	9:42 am	Pisces
20	Pisces		
21	Pisces	7:42 pm	Aries
22	Aries		
23	Aries		
24	Aries	8:07 am	Taurus
25	Taurus		
26	Taurus	9:08 pm	Gemini
27	Gemini		
28	Gemini		
29	Gemini	9:23 am	Cancer
30	Cancer		

	December		
1	Cancer	7:59 pm	Leo
2	Leo		
3	Leo		
4	Leo	4:14 am	Virgo
5	Virgo		
6	Virgo	9:33 am	Libra
7	Libra		
8	Libra	11:56 am	Scorpio
9	Scorpio		
10	Scorpio	12:13 pm	Sagittarius
11	Sagittarius		
12	Sagittarius	11:59 am	Capricorn
13	Capricorn		
14	Capricorn	1:15 pm	Aquarius
15	Aquarius		
16	Aquarius	5:50 pm	Pisces
17	Pisces		
18	Pisces		
19	Pisces	2:37 am	Aries
20	Aries		
21	Aries	2:41 pm	Taurus
22	Taurus		
23	Taurus		
24	Taurus	3:45 am	Gemini
25	Gemini		
26	Gemini	3:44 pm	Cancer
27	Cancer		
28	Cancer		
29	Cancer	1:44 am	Leo
30	Leo		
31	Leo	9:43 am	Virgo

MOON POSITIONS 1986

January

1	Virgo		
2	Virgo	3:45 pm	Libra
3	Libra		
4	Libra	7:44 pm	Scorpio
5	Scorpio		
6	Scorpio	9:47 pm	Sagittarius
7	Sagittarius		
8	Sagittarius	10:42 pm	Capricorn
9	Capricorn		
10	Capricorn		
11	Capricorn	12:01 am	Aquarius
12	Aquarius		
13	Aquarius	3:39 am	Pisces
14	Pisces		
15	Pisces	11:03 am	Aries
16	Aries		
17	Aries	10:14 pm	Taurus
18	Taurus		
19	Taurus		
20	Taurus	11:12 am	Gemini
21	Gemini		
22	Gemini	11:15 pm	Cancer
23	Cancer		
24	Cancer		
25	Cancer	8:47 am	Leo
26	Leo		
27	Leo	3:51 pm	Virgo
28	Virgo		
29	Virgo	9:10 pm	Libra
30	Libra		
31	Libra		

February

1	Libra	1:19 am	Scorpio
2	Scorpio		
3	Scorpio	4:31 am	Sagittarius
4	Sagittarius		
5	Sagittarius	7:02 am	Capricorn
6	Capricorn		
7	Capricorn	9:35 am	Aquarius
8	Aquarius		
9	Aquarius	1:32 pm	Pisces
10	Pisces		
11	Pisces	8:21 pm	Aries
12	Aries		
13	Aries		
14	Aries	6:38 am	Taurus
15	Taurus		
16	Taurus	7:17 pm	Gemini
17	Gemini		
18	Gemini		
19	Gemini	7:39 am	Cancer
20	Cancer		
21	Cancer	5:25 pm	Leo
22	Leo		
23	Leo	11:58 pm	Virgo
24	Virgo		
25	Virgo		
26	Virgo	4:07 am	Libra
27	Libra		
28	Libra	7:06 am	Scorpio

March

1	Scorpio		
2	Scorpio	9:51 am	Sagittarius
3	Sagittarius		
4	Sagittarius	12:56 pm	Capricorn
5	Capricorn		
6	Capricorn	4:42 pm	Aquarius
7	Aquarius		
8	Aquarius	9:48 pm	Pisces
9	Pisces		
10	Pisces		
11	Pisces	5:03 am	Aries
12	Aries		
13	Aries	3:04 pm	Taurus
14	Taurus		
15	Taurus		
16	Taurus	3:23 am	Gemini
17	Gemini		
18	Gemini	4:04 pm	Cancer
19	Cancer		
20	Cancer		
21	Cancer	2:38 am	Leo
22	Leo		
23	Leo	9:39 am	Virgo
24	Virgo		
25	Virgo	1:22 pm	Libra
26	Libra		
27	Libra	3:05 pm	Scorpio
28	Scorpio		
29	Scorpio	4:20 pm	Sagittarius
30	Sagittarius		
31	Sagittarius	6:25 pm	Capricorn

April

1	Capricorn		
2	Capricorn	10:11 pm	Aquarius
3	Aquarius		
4	Aquarius		
5	Aquarius	4:03 am	Pisces
6	Pisces		
7	Pisces	12:12 pm	Aries
8	Aries		
9	Aries	10:36 pm	Taurus
10	Taurus		
11	Taurus		
12	Taurus	10:51 am	Gemini
13	Gemini		
14	Gemini	11:42 pm	Cancer
15	Cancer		
16	Cancer		
17	Cancer	11:10 am	Leo
18	Leo		
19	Leo	7:24 pm	Virgo
20	Virgo		
21	Virgo	11:50 pm	Libra
22	Libra		
23	Libra		
24	Libra	1:15 am	Scorpio
25	Scorpio		
26	Scorpio	1:16 am	Sagittarius
27	Sagittarius		
28	Sagittarius	1:41 am	Capricorn
29	Capricorn		
30	Capricorn	4:06 am	Aquarius

May

1	Aquarius		
2	Aquarius	9:30 am	Pisces
3	Pisces		
4	Pisces	6:01 pm	Aries
5	Aries		
6	Aries		
7	Aries	4:59 am	Taurus
8	Taurus		
9	Taurus	5:26 pm	Gemini
10	Gemini		
11	Gemini		
12	Gemini	6:18 am	Cancer
13	Cancer		
14	Cancer	6:15 pm	Leo
15	Leo		
16	Leo		
17	Leo	3:45 am	Virgo
18	Virgo		
19	Virgo	9:41 am	Libra
20	Libra		
21	Libra	12:02 pm	Scorpio
22	Scorpio		
23	Scorpio	11:57 am	Sagittarius
24	Sagittarius		
25	Sagittarius	11:15 am	Capricorn
26	Capricorn		
27	Capricorn	12:00 pm	Aquarius
28	Aquarius		
29	Aquarius	3:54 pm	Pisces
30	Pisces		
31	Pisces	11:43 pm	Aries

June

1	Aries		
2	Aries		
3	Aries	10:45 am	Taurus
4	Taurus		
5	Taurus	11:26 pm	Gemini
6	Gemini		
7	Gemini		
8	Gemini	12:16 pm	Cancer
9	Cancer		
10	Cancer		
11	Cancer	12:11 am	Leo
12	Leo		
13	Leo	10:18 am	Virgo
14	Virgo		
15	Virgo	5:38 pm	Libra
16	Libra		
17	Libra	9:36 pm	Scorpio
18	Scorpio		
19	Scorpio	10:36 pm	Sagittarius
20	Sagittarius		
21	Sagittarius	10:00 pm	Capricorn
22	Capricorn		
23	Capricorn	9:50 pm	Aquarius
24	Aquarius		
25	Aquarius		
26	Aquarius	12:12 am	Pisces
27	Pisces		
28	Pisces	6:35 am	Aries
29	Aries		
30	Aries	4:54 pm	Taurus

MOON POSITIONS 1986

July

1	Taurus		
2	Taurus		
3	Taurus	5:32 am	Gemini
4	Gemini		
5	Gemini	6:19 pm	Cancer
6	Cancer		
7	Cancer		
8	Cancer	5:56 am	Leo
9	Leo		
10	Leo	3:50 pm	Virgo
11	Virgo		
12	Virgo	11:40 pm	Libra
13	Libra		
14	Libra		
15	Libra	4:58 am	Scorpio
16	Scorpio		
17	Scorpio	7:34 am	Sagittarius
18	Sagittarius		
19	Sagittarius	8:10 am	Capricorn
20	Capricorn		
21	Capricorn	8:17 am	Aquarius
22	Aquarius		
23	Aquarius	9:59 am	Pisces
24	Pisces		
25	Pisces	3:02 pm	Aries
26	Aries		
27	Aries		
28	Aries	12:11 am	Taurus
29	Taurus		
30	Taurus	12:19 pm	Gemini
31	Gemini		

August

1	Gemini		
2	Gemini	1:04 am	Cancer
3	Cancer		
4	Cancer	12:26 pm	Leo
5	Leo		
6	Leo	9:44 pm	Virgo
7	Virgo		
8	Virgo		
9	Virgo	5:05 am	Libra
10	Libra		
11	Libra	10:36 am	Scorpio
12	Scorpio		
13	Scorpio	2:17 pm	Sagittarius
14	Sagittarius		
15	Sagittarius	4:22 pm	Capricorn
16	Capricorn		
17	Capricorn	5:44 pm	Aquarius
18	Aquarius		
19	Aquarius	7:52 pm	Pisces
20	Pisces		
21	Pisces		
22	Pisces	12:27 am	Aries
23	Aries		
24	Aries	8:36 am	Taurus
25	Taurus		
26	Taurus	8:00 pm	Gemini
27	Gemini		
28	Gemini		
29	Gemini	8:40 am	Cancer
30	Cancer		
31	Cancer	8:08 pm	Leo

September

1	Leo		
2	Leo		
3	Leo	5:06 am	Virgo
4	Virgo		
5	Virgo	11:33 am	Libra
6	Libra		
7	Libra	4:12 pm	Scorpio
8	Scorpio		
9	Scorpio	7:40 pm	Sagittarius
10	Sagittarius		
11	Sagittarius	10:28 pm	Capricorn
12	Capricorn		
13	Capricorn		
14	Capricorn	1:07 am	Aquarius
15	Aquarius		
16	Aquarius	4:27 am	Pisces
17	Pisces		
18	Pisces	9:33 am	Aries
19	Aries		
20	Aries	5:25 pm	Taurus
21	Taurus		
22	Taurus		
23	Taurus	4:13 am	Gemini
24	Gemini		
25	Gemini	4:44 pm	Cancer
26	Cancer		
27	Cancer		
28	Cancer	4:39 am	Leo
29	Leo		
30	Leo	1:57 pm	Virgo

October

1	Virgo		
2	Virgo	8:03 pm	Libra
3	Libra		
4	Libra	11:35 pm	Scorpio
5	Scorpio		
6	Scorpio		
7	Scorpio	1:48 am	Sagittarius
8	Sagittarius		
9	Sagittarius	3:52 am	Capricorn
10	Capricorn		
11	Capricorn	6:45 am	Aquarius
12	Aquarius		
13	Aquarius	11:03 am	Pisces
14	Pisces		
15	Pisces	5:13 pm	Aries
16	Aries		
17	Aries		
18	Aries	1:35 am	Taurus
19	Taurus		
20	Taurus	12:15 pm	Gemini
21	Gemini		
22	Gemini		
23	Gemini	12:37 am	Cancer
24	Cancer		
25	Cancer	1:02 pm	Leo
26	Leo		
27	Leo	11:20 pm	Virgo
28	Virgo		
29	Virgo		
30	Virgo	6:04 am	Libra
31	Libra		

November

1	Libra	9:19 am	Scorpio
2	Scorpio		
3	Scorpio	10:19 am	Sagittarius
4	Sagittarius		
5	Sagittarius	10:49 am	Capricorn
6	Capricorn		
7	Capricorn	12:29 pm	Aquarius
8	Aquarius		
9	Aquarius	4:30 pm	Pisces
10	Pisces		
11	Pisces	11:14 pm	Aries
12	Aries		
13	Aries		
14	Aries	8:24 am	Taurus
15	Taurus		
16	Taurus	7:26 pm	Gemini
17	Gemini		
18	Gemini		
19	Gemini	7:46 am	Cancer
20	Cancer		
21	Cancer	8:25 pm	Leo
22	Leo		
23	Leo		
24	Leo	7:46 am	Virgo
25	Virgo		
26	Virgo	3:59 pm	Libra
27	Libra		
28	Libra	8:13 pm	Scorpio
29	Scorpio		
30	Scorpio	9:08 pm	Sagittarius

December

1	Sagittarius		
2	Sagittarius	8:28 pm	Capricorn
3	Capricorn		
4	Capricorn	8:23 pm	Aquarius
5	Aquarius		
6	Aquarius	10:48 pm	Pisces
7	Pisces		
8	Pisces		
9	Pisces	4:49 am	Aries
10	Aries		
11	Aries	2:10 pm	Taurus
12	Taurus		
13	Taurus		
14	Taurus	1:41 am	Gemini
15	Gemini		
16	Gemini	2:09 pm	Cancer
17	Cancer		
18	Cancer		
19	Cancer	2:44 am	Leo
20	Leo		
21	Leo	2:30 pm	Virgo
22	Virgo		
23	Virgo		
24	Virgo	12:05 am	Libra
25	Libra		
26	Libra	6:06 am	Scorpio
27	Scorpio		
28	Scorpio	8:19 am	Sagittarius
29	Sagittarius		
30	Sagittarius	7:54 am	Capricorn
31	Capricorn		

MOON POSITIONS 1987

January

1	Capricorn	6:54 am	Aquarius
2	Aquarius		
3	Aquarius	7:36 am	Pisces
4	Pisces		
5	Pisces	11:51 am	Aries
6	Aries		
7	Aries	8:13 pm	Taurus
8	Taurus		
9	Taurus		
10	Taurus	7:39 am	Gemini
11	Gemini		
12	Gemini	8:18 pm	Cancer
13	Cancer		
14	Cancer		
15	Cancer	8:45 am	Leo
16	Leo		
17	Leo	8:15 pm	Virgo
18	Virgo		
19	Virgo		
20	Virgo	6:09 am	Libra
21	Libra		
22	Libra	1:30 pm	Scorpio
23	Scorpio		
24	Scorpio	5:35 pm	Sagittarius
25	Sagittarius		
26	Sagittarius	6:42 pm	Capricorn
27	Capricorn		
28	Capricorn	6:17 pm	Aquarius
29	Aquarius		
30	Aquarius	6:24 pm	Pisces
31	Pisces		

February

1	Pisces	9:09 pm	Aries
2	Aries		
3	Aries		
4	Aries	3:53 am	Taurus
5	Taurus		
6	Taurus	2:23 pm	Gemini
7	Gemini		
8	Gemini		
9	Gemini	2:55 am	Cancer
10	Cancer		
11	Cancer	3:21 pm	Leo
12	Leo		
13	Leo		
14	Leo	2:26 am	Virgo
15	Virgo		
16	Virgo	11:44 am	Libra
17	Libra		
18	Libra	7:04 pm	Scorpio
19	Scorpio		
20	Scorpio		
21	Scorpio	12:09 am	Sagittarius
22	Sagittarius		
23	Sagittarius	2:57 am	Capricorn
24	Capricorn		
25	Capricorn	4:08 am	Aquarius
26	Aquarius		
27	Aquarius	5:07 am	Pisces
28	Pisces		

March

1	Pisces	7:37 am	Aries
2	Aries		
3	Aries	1:11 pm	Taurus
4	Taurus		
5	Taurus	10:26 pm	Gemini
6	Gemini		
7	Gemini		
8	Gemini	10:24 am	Cancer
9	Cancer		
10	Cancer	10:54 pm	Leo
11	Leo		
12	Leo		
13	Leo	9:55 am	Virgo
14	Virgo		
15	Virgo	6:34 pm	Libra
16	Libra		
17	Libra		
18	Libra	12:57 am	Scorpio
19	Scorpio		
20	Scorpio	5:32 am	Sagittarius
21	Sagittarius		
22	Sagittarius	8:48 am	Capricorn
23	Capricorn		
24	Capricorn	11:18 am	Aquarius
25	Aquarius		
26	Aquarius	1:46 pm	Pisces
27	Pisces		
28	Pisces	5:12 pm	Aries
29	Aries		
30	Aries	10:46 pm	Taurus
31	Taurus		

April

1	Taurus		
2	Taurus	7:16 am	Gemini
3	Gemini		
4	Gemini	6:33 pm	Cancer
5	Cancer		
6	Cancer		
7	Cancer	7:04 am	Leo
8	Leo		
9	Leo	6:28 pm	Virgo
10	Virgo		
11	Virgo		
12	Virgo	3:06 am	Libra
13	Libra		
14	Libra	8:41 am	Scorpio
15	Scorpio		
16	Scorpio	12:02 pm	Sagittarius
17	Sagittarius		
18	Sagittarius	2:21 pm	Capricorn
19	Capricorn		
20	Capricorn	4:45 pm	Aquarius
21	Aquarius		
22	Aquarius	8:02 pm	Pisces
23	Pisces		
24	Pisces		
25	Pisces	12:41 am	Aries
26	Aries		
27	Aries	7:06 am	Taurus
28	Taurus		
29	Taurus	3:43 pm	Gemini
30	Gemini		

May

1	Gemini		
2	Gemini	2:39 am	Cancer
3	Cancer		
4	Cancer	3:06 pm	Leo
5	Leo		
6	Leo		
7	Leo	3:07 am	Virgo
8	Virgo		
9	Virgo	12:29 pm	Libra
10	Libra		
11	Libra	6:09 pm	Scorpio
12	Scorpio		
13	Scorpio	8:41 pm	Sagittarius
14	Sagittarius		
15	Sagittarius	9:37 pm	Capricorn
16	Capricorn		
17	Capricorn	10:42 pm	Aquarius
18	Aquarius		
19	Aquarius		
20	Aquarius	1:24 am	Pisces
21	Pisces		
22	Pisces	6:23 am	Aries
23	Aries		
24	Aries	1:39 pm	Taurus
25	Taurus		
26	Taurus	10:55 pm	Gemini
27	Gemini		
28	Gemini		
29	Gemini	9:59 am	Cancer
30	Cancer		
31	Cancer	10:25 pm	Leo

June

1	Leo		
2	Leo		
3	Leo	10:56 am	Virgo
4	Virgo		
5	Virgo	9:24 pm	Libra
6	Libra		
7	Libra		
8	Libra	4:06 am	Scorpio
9	Scorpio		
10	Scorpio	6:53 am	Sagittarius
11	Sagittarius		
12	Sagittarius	7:05 am	Capricorn
13	Capricorn		
14	Capricorn	6:45 am	Aquarius
15	Aquarius		
16	Aquarius	7:54 am	Pisces
17	Pisces		
18	Pisces	11:56 am	Aries
19	Aries		
20	Aries	7:09 pm	Taurus
21	Taurus		
22	Taurus		
23	Taurus	4:54 am	Gemini
24	Gemini		
25	Gemini	4:22 pm	Cancer
26	Cancer		
27	Cancer		
28	Cancer	4:52 am	Leo
29	Leo		
30	Leo	5:34 pm	Virgo

MOON POSITIONS 1987

July

1	Virgo		
2	Virgo		
3	Virgo	4:55 am	Libra
4	Libra		
5	Libra	1:03 pm	Scorpio
6	Scorpio		
7	Scorpio	5:05 pm	Sagittarius
8	Sagittarius		
9	Sagittarius	5:43 pm	Capricorn
10	Capricorn		
11	Capricorn	4:49 pm	Aquarius
12	Aquarius		
13	Aquarius	4:36 pm	Pisces
14	Pisces		
15	Pisces	7:00 pm	Aries
16	Aries		
17	Aries		
18	Aries	1:04 am	Taurus
19	Taurus		
20	Taurus	10:33 am	Gemini
21	Gemini		
22	Gemini	10:13 pm	Cancer
23	Cancer		
24	Cancer		
25	Cancer	10:50 am	Leo
26	Leo		
27	Leo	11:26 pm	Virgo
28	Virgo		
29	Virgo		
30	Virgo	10:59 am	Libra
31	Libra		

August

1	Libra	8:09 pm	Scorpio
2	Scorpio		
3	Scorpio		
4	Scorpio	1:47 am	Sagittarius
5	Sagittarius		
6	Sagittarius	3:51 am	Capricorn
7	Capricorn		
8	Capricorn	3:37 am	Aquarius
9	Aquarius		
10	Aquarius	3:01 am	Pisces
11	Pisces		
12	Pisces	4:09 am	Aries
13	Aries		
14	Aries	8:38 am	Taurus
15	Taurus		
16	Taurus	4:59 pm	Gemini
17	Gemini		
18	Gemini		
19	Gemini	4:19 am	Cancer
20	Cancer		
21	Cancer	4:58 pm	Leo
22	Leo		
23	Leo		
24	Leo	5:23 am	Virgo
25	Virgo		
26	Virgo	4:35 pm	Libra
27	Libra		
28	Libra		
29	Libra	1:49 am	Scorpio
30	Scorpio		
31	Scorpio	8:24 am	Sagittarius

September

1	Sagittarius		
2	Sagittarius	12:04 pm	Capricorn
3	Capricorn		
4	Capricorn	1:22 pm	Aquarius
5	Aquarius		
6	Aquarius	1:37 pm	Pisces
7	Pisces		
8	Pisces	2:34 pm	Aries
9	Aries		
10	Aries	5:57 pm	Taurus
11	Taurus		
12	Taurus		
13	Taurus	12:54 am	Gemini
14	Gemini		
15	Gemini	11:22 am	Cancer
16	Cancer		
17	Cancer	11:50 pm	Leo
18	Leo		
19	Leo		
20	Leo	12:13 pm	Virgo
21	Virgo		
22	Virgo	10:58 pm	Libra
23	Libra		
24	Libra		
25	Libra	7:30 am	Scorpio
26	Scorpio		
27	Scorpio	1:49 pm	Sagittarius
28	Sagittarius		
29	Sagittarius	6:08 pm	Capricorn
30	Capricorn		

October

1	Capricorn	8:51 pm	Aquarius
2	Aquarius		
3	Aquarius	10:39 pm	Pisces
4	Pisces		
5	Pisces		
6	Pisces	12:35 am	Aries
7	Aries		
8	Aries	3:57 am	Taurus
9	Taurus		
10	Taurus	10:03 am	Gemini
11	Gemini		
12	Gemini	7:31 pm	Cancer
13	Cancer		
14	Cancer		
15	Cancer	7:34 am	Leo
16	Leo		
17	Leo	8:06 pm	Virgo
18	Virgo		
19	Virgo		
20	Virgo	6:50 am	Libra
21	Libra		
22	Libra	2:41 pm	Scorpio
23	Scorpio		
24	Scorpio	7:57 pm	Sagittarius
25	Sagittarius		
26	Sagittarius	11:33 pm	Capricorn
27	Capricorn		
28	Capricorn		
29	Capricorn	2:27 am	Aquarius
30	Aquarius		
31	Aquarius	5:19 am	Pisces

November

1	Pisces		
2	Pisces	8:40 am	Aries
3	Aries		
4	Aries	1:02 pm	Taurus
5	Taurus		
6	Taurus	7:16 pm	Gemini
7	Gemini		
8	Gemini		
9	Gemini	4:10 am	Cancer
10	Cancer		
11	Cancer	3:45 pm	Leo
12	Leo		
13	Leo		
14	Leo	4:29 am	Virgo
15	Virgo		
16	Virgo	3:48 pm	Libra
17	Libra		
18	Libra	11:47 pm	Scorpio
19	Scorpio		
20	Scorpio		
21	Scorpio	4:16 am	Sagittarius
22	Sagittarius		
23	Sagittarius	6:32 am	Capricorn
24	Capricorn		
25	Capricorn	8:13 am	Aquarius
26	Aquarius		
27	Aquarius	10:40 am	Pisces
28	Pisces		
29	Pisces	2:36 pm	Aries
30	Aries		

December

1	Aries	8:05 pm	Taurus
2	Taurus		
3	Taurus		
4	Taurus	3:13 am	Gemini
5	Gemini		
6	Gemini	12:20 pm	Cancer
7	Cancer		
8	Cancer	11:40 pm	Leo
9	Leo		
10	Leo		
11	Leo	12:30 pm	Virgo
12	Virgo		
13	Virgo		
14	Virgo	12:40 am	Libra
15	Libra		
16	Libra	9:41 am	Scorpio
17	Scorpio		
18	Scorpio	2:33 pm	Sagittarius
19	Sagittarius		
20	Sagittarius	4:07 pm	Capricorn
21	Capricorn		
22	Capricorn	4:20 pm	Aquarius
23	Aquarius		
24	Aquarius	5:10 pm	Pisces
25	Pisces		
26	Pisces	8:05 pm	Aries
27	Aries		
28	Aries		
29	Aries	1:37 pm	Taurus
30	Taurus		
31	Taurus	9:29 am	Gemini

MOON POSITIONS 1988

January

1	Gemini		
2	Gemini	7:17 pm	Cancer
3	Cancer		
4	Cancer		
5	Cancer	6:47 am	Leo
6	Leo		
7	Leo	7:35 pm	Virgo
8	Virgo		
9	Virgo		
10	Virgo	8:17 am	Libra
11	Libra		
12	Libra	6:39 pm	Scorpio
13	Scorpio		
14	Scorpio		
15	Scorpio	12:58 am	Sagittarius
16	Sagittarius		
17	Sagittarius	3:15 am	Capricorn
18	Capricorn		
19	Capricorn	3:02 am	Aquarius
20	Aquarius		
21	Aquarius	2:27 am	Pisces
22	Pisces		
23	Pisces	3:31 am	Aries
24	Aries		
25	Aries	7:36 am	Taurus
26	Taurus		
27	Taurus	3:02 pm	Gemini
28	Gemini		
29	Gemini		
30	Gemini	1:11 am	Cancer
31	Cancer		

February

1	Cancer	1:06 pm	Leo
2	Leo		
3	Leo		
4	Leo	1:54 am	Virgo
5	Virgo		
6	Virgo	2:36 pm	Libra
7	Libra		
8	Libra		
9	Libra	1:42 am	Scorpio
10	Scorpio		
11	Scorpio	9:36 am	Sagittarius
12	Sagittarius		
13	Sagittarius	1:36 pm	Capricorn
14	Capricorn		
15	Capricorn	2:25 pm	Aquarius
16	Aquarius		
17	Aquarius	1:44 pm	Pisces
18	Pisces		
19	Pisces	1:35 pm	Aries
20	Aries		
21	Aries	3:50 pm	Taurus
22	Taurus		
23	Taurus	9:42 pm	Gemini
24	Gemini		
25	Gemini		
26	Gemini	7:12 am	Cancer
27	Cancer		
28	Cancer	7:12 pm	Leo
29	Leo		

March

1	Leo		
2	Leo	8:06 am	Virgo
3	Virgo		
4	Virgo	8:32 pm	Libra
5	Libra		
6	Libra		
7	Libra	7:27 am	Scorpio
8	Scorpio		
9	Scorpio	3:59 pm	Sagittarius
10	Sagittarius		
11	Sagittarius	9:31 pm	Capricorn
12	Capricorn		
13	Capricorn		
14	Capricorn	12:08 am	Aquarius
15	Aquarius		
16	Aquarius	12:42 am	Pisces
17	Pisces		
18	Pisces	12:45 am	Aries
19	Aries		
20	Aries	2:05 am	Taurus
21	Taurus		
22	Taurus	6:21 am	Gemini
23	Gemini		
24	Gemini	2:27 pm	Cancer
25	Cancer		
26	Cancer		
27	Cancer	1:54 am	Leo
28	Leo		
29	Leo	2:49 pm	Virgo
30	Virgo		
31	Virgo		

April

1	Virgo	3:05 am	Libra
2	Libra		
3	Libra	1:26 pm	Scorpio
4	Scorpio		
5	Scorpio	9:29 pm	Sagittarius
6	Sagittarius		
7	Sagittarius		
8	Sagittarius	3:19 am	Capricorn
9	Capricorn		
10	Capricorn	7:10 am	Aquarius
11	Aquarius		
12	Aquarius	9:24 am	Pisces
13	Pisces		
14	Pisces	10:47 am	Aries
15	Aries		
16	Aries	12:31 pm	Taurus
17	Taurus		
18	Taurus	4:10 pm	Gemini
19	Gemini		
20	Gemini	11:04 pm	Cancer
21	Cancer		
22	Cancer		
23	Cancer	9:34 am	Leo
24	Leo		
25	Leo	10:16 pm	Virgo
26	Virgo		
27	Virgo		
28	Virgo	10:37 am	Libra
29	Libra		
30	Libra	8:39 pm	Scorpio

May

1	Scorpio		
2	Scorpio		
3	Scorpio	3:52 am	Sagittarius
4	Sagittarius		
5	Sagittarius	8:54 am	Capricorn
6	Capricorn		
7	Capricorn	12:37 pm	Aquarius
8	Aquarius		
9	Aquarius	3:39 pm	Pisces
10	Pisces		
11	Pisces	6:23 pm	Aries
12	Aries		
13	Aries	9:22 pm	Taurus
14	Taurus		
15	Taurus		
16	Taurus	1:31 am	Gemini
17	Gemini		
18	Gemini	8:05 am	Cancer
19	Cancer		
20	Cancer	5:51 pm	Leo
21	Leo		
22	Leo		
23	Leo	6:12 am	Virgo
24	Virgo		
25	Virgo	6:49 pm	Libra
26	Libra		
27	Libra		
28	Libra	5:06 am	Scorpio
29	Scorpio		
30	Scorpio	11:57 am	Sagittarius
31	Sagittarius		

June

1	Sagittarius	3:58 pm	Capricorn
2	Capricorn		
3	Capricorn	6:34 pm	Aquarius
4	Aquarius		
5	Aquarius	9:00 pm	Pisces
6	Pisces		
7	Pisces		
8	Pisces	12:04 am	Aries
9	Aries		
10	Aries	4:02 am	Taurus
11	Taurus		
12	Taurus	9:14 am	Gemini
13	Gemini		
14	Gemini	4:19 pm	Cancer
15	Cancer		
16	Cancer		
17	Cancer	1:57 am	Leo
18	Leo		
19	Leo	2:03 pm	Virgo
20	Virgo		
21	Virgo		
22	Virgo	2:57 am	Libra
23	Libra		
24	Libra	1:58 pm	Scorpio
25	Scorpio		
26	Scorpio	9:18 pm	Sagittarius
27	Sagittarius		
28	Sagittarius		
29	Sagittarius	1:00 am	Capricorn
30	Capricorn		

MOON POSITIONS 1988

July

1	Capricorn	2:30 am	Aquarius
2	Aquarius		
3	Aquarius	3:33 am	Pisces
4	Pisces		
5	Pisces	5:37 am	Aries
6	Aries		
7	Aries	9:27 am	Taurus
8	Taurus		
9	Taurus	3:16 am	Gemini
10	Gemini		
11	Gemini	11:08 pm	Cancer
12	Cancer		
13	Cancer		
14	Cancer	9:11 am	Leo
15	Leo		
16	Leo	9:17 pm	Virgo
17	Virgo		
18	Virgo		
19	Virgo	10:22 am	Libra
20	Libra		
21	Libra	10:13 pm	Scorpio
22	Scorpio		
23	Scorpio		
24	Scorpio	6:42 am	Sagittarius
25	Sagittarius		
26	Sagittarius	11:07 am	Capricorn
27	Capricorn		
28	Capricorn	12:25 pm	Aquarius
29	Aquarius		
30	Aquarius	12:23 pm	Pisces
31	Pisces		

August

1	Pisces	12:53 pm	Aries
2	Aries		
3	Aries	3:24 am	Taurus
4	Taurus		
5	Taurus	8:43 pm	Gemini
6	Gemini		
7	Gemini		
8	Gemini	4:52 am	Cancer
9	Cancer		
10	Cancer	3:26 pm	Leo
11	Leo		
12	Leo		
13	Leo	3:46 am	Virgo
14	Virgo		
15	Virgo	4:52 am	Libra
16	Libra		
17	Libra		
18	Libra	5:12 am	Scorpio
19	Scorpio		
20	Scorpio	2:55 pm	Sagittarius
21	Sagittarius		
22	Sagittarius	8:49 pm	Capricorn
23	Capricorn		
24	Capricorn	11:05 pm	Aquarius
25	Aquarius		
26	Aquarius	11:01 pm	Pisces
27	Pisces		
28	Pisces	10:29 am	Aries
29	Aries		
30	Aries	11:22 pm	Taurus
31	Taurus		

September

1	Taurus		
2	Taurus	3:11 am	Gemini
3	Gemini		
4	Gemini	10:37 am	Cancer
5	Cancer		
6	Cancer	9:14 pm	Leo
7	Leo		
8	Leo		
9	Leo	9:48 am	Virgo
10	Virgo		
11	Virgo	10:51 pm	Libra
12	Libra		
13	Libra		
14	Libra	11:07 am	Scorpio
15	Scorpio		
16	Scorpio	9:25 pm	Sagittarius
17	Sagittarius		
18	Sagittarius		
19	Sagittarius	4:45 am	Capricorn
20	Capricorn		
21	Capricorn	8:43 am	Aquarius
22	Aquarius		
23	Aquarius	9:51 am	Pisces
24	Pisces		
25	Pisces	9:29 am	Aries
26	Aries		
27	Aries	9:29 am	Taurus
28	Taurus		
29	Taurus	11:43 am	Gemini
30	Gemini		

October

1	Gemini	5:39 pm	Cancer
2	Cancer		
3	Cancer		
4	Cancer	3:31 am	Leo
5	Leo		
6	Leo	4:01 pm	Virgo
7	Virgo		
8	Virgo		
9	Virgo	5:03 am	Libra
10	Libra		
11	Libra	4:58 pm	Scorpio
12	Scorpio		
13	Scorpio		
14	Scorpio	2:58 am	Sagittarius
15	Sagittarius		
16	Sagittarius	10:44 am	Capricorn
17	Capricorn		
18	Capricorn	4:05 pm	Aquarius
19	Aquarius		
20	Aquarius	6:58 pm	Pisces
21	Pisces		
22	Pisces	7:59 pm	Aries
23	Aries		
24	Aries	8:22 pm	Taurus
25	Taurus		
26	Taurus	9:55 pm	Gemini
27	Gemini		
28	Gemini		
29	Gemini	2:28 am	Cancer
30	Cancer		
31	Cancer	11:03 am	Leo

November

1	Leo		
2	Leo	11:02 pm	Virgo
3	Virgo		
4	Virgo		
5	Virgo	12:04 pm	Libra
6	Libra		
7	Libra	11:46 pm	Scorpio
8	Scorpio		
9	Scorpio		
10	Scorpio	9:06 am	Sagittarius
11	Sagittarius		
12	Sagittarius	4:12 pm	Capricorn
13	Capricorn		
14	Capricorn	9:36 pm	Aquarius
15	Aquarius		
16	Aquarius		
17	Aquarius	1:34 am	Pisces
18	Pisces		
19	Pisces	4:12 am	Aries
20	Aries		
21	Aries	6:02 am	Taurus
22	Taurus		
23	Taurus	8:12 am	Gemini
24	Gemini		
25	Gemini	12:20 pm	Cancer
26	Cancer		
27	Cancer	7:52 pm	Leo
28	Leo		
29	Leo		
30	Leo	7:00 am	Virgo

December

1	Virgo		
2	Virgo	7:56 pm	Libra
3	Libra		
4	Libra		
5	Libra	7:51 am	Scorpio
6	Scorpio		
7	Scorpio	4:55 pm	Sagittarius
8	Sagittarius		
9	Sagittarius	11:07 pm	Capricorn
10	Capricorn		
11	Capricorn		
12	Capricorn	3:25 am	Aquarius
13	Aquarius		
14	Aquarius	6:53 am	Pisces
15	Pisces		
16	Pisces	10:03 am	Aries
17	Aries		
18	Aries	1:11 pm	Taurus
19	Taurus		
20	Taurus	4:43 pm	Gemini
21	Gemini		
22	Gemini	9:35 pm	Cancer
23	Cancer		
24	Cancer		
25	Cancer	4:57 am	Leo
26	Leo		
27	Leo	3:27 pm	Virgo
28	Virgo		
29	Virgo		
30	Virgo	4:09 am	Libra
31	Libra		

MOON POSITIONS 1989

January

1	Libra	4:34 pm	Scorpio
2	Scorpio		
3	Scorpio		
4	Scorpio	2:12 am	Sagittarius
5	Sagittarius		
6	Sagittarius	8:14 am	Capricorn
7	Capricorn		
8	Capricorn	11:31 am	Aquarius
9	Aquarius		
10	Aquarius	1:31 pm	Pisces
11	Pisces		
12	Pisces	3:36 pm	Aries
13	Aries		
14	Aries	6:36 pm	Taurus
15	Taurus		
16	Taurus	10:57 am	Gemini
17	Gemini		
18	Gemini		
19	Gemini	4:57 am	Cancer
20	Cancer		
21	Cancer	1:02 pm	Leo
22	Leo		
23	Leo	11:32 pm	Virgo
24	Virgo		
25	Virgo		
26	Virgo	12:01 pm	Libra
27	Libra		
28	Libra		
29	Libra	12:49 am	Scorpio
30	Scorpio		
31	Scorpio	11:30 am	Sagittarius

February

1	Sagittarius		
2	Sagittarius	6:30 pm	Capricorn
3	Capricorn		
4	Capricorn	9:51 pm	Aquarius
5	Aquarius		
6	Aquarius	10:52 pm	Pisces
7	Pisces		
8	Pisces	11:18 pm	Aries
9	Aries		
10	Aries		
11	Aries	12:45 am	Taurus
12	Taurus		
13	Taurus	4:22 am	Gemini
14	Gemini		
15	Gemini	10:40 am	Cancer
16	Cancer		
17	Cancer	7:33 pm	Leo
18	Leo		
19	Leo		
20	Leo	6:34 am	Virgo
21	Virgo		
22	Virgo	7:05 pm	Libra
23	Libra		
24	Libra		
25	Libra	7:57 pm	Scorpio
26	Scorpio		
27	Scorpio	7:29 pm	Sagittarius
28	Sagittarius		

March

1	Sagittarius		
2	Sagittarius	3:58 am	Capricorn
3	Capricorn		
4	Capricorn	8:36 am	Aquarius
5	Aquarius		
6	Aquarius	9:59 am	Pisces
7	Pisces		
8	Pisces	9:36 am	Aries
9	Aries		
10	Aries	9:25 am	Taurus
11	Taurus		
12	Taurus	11:16 am	Gemini
13	Gemini		
14	Gemini	4:27 pm	Cancer
15	Cancer		
16	Cancer		
17	Cancer	1:13 am	Leo
18	Leo		
19	Leo	12:39 pm	Virgo
20	Virgo		
21	Virgo		
22	Virgo	1:24 am	Libra
23	Libra		
24	Libra	2:10 pm	Scorpio
25	Scorpio		
26	Scorpio		
27	Scorpio	1:54 am	Sagittarius
28	Sagittarius		
29	Sagittarius	11:25 am	Capricorn
30	Capricorn		
31	Capricorn	5:45 pm	Aquarius

April

1	Aquarius		
2	Aquarius	8:37 pm	Pisces
3	Pisces		
4	Pisces	8:51 pm	Aries
5	Aries		
6	Aries	8:07 pm	Taurus
7	Taurus		
8	Taurus	8:31 pm	Gemini
9	Gemini		
10	Gemini	11:58 pm	Cancer
11	Cancer		
12	Cancer		
13	Cancer	7:31 am	Leo
14	Leo		
15	Leo	6:39 pm	Virgo
16	Virgo		
17	Virgo		
18	Virgo	7:31 am	Libra
19	Libra		
20	Libra	8:13 pm	Scorpio
21	Scorpio		
22	Scorpio		
23	Scorpio	7:38 am	Sagittarius
24	Sagittarius		
25	Sagittarius	5:15 pm	Capricorn
26	Capricorn		
27	Capricorn		
28	Capricorn	12:33 am	Aquarius
29	Aquarius		
30	Aquarius	5:03 am	Pisces

May

1	Pisces		
2	Pisces	6:50 am	Aries
3	Aries		
4	Aries	6:55 am	Taurus
5	Taurus		
6	Taurus	7:03 am	Gemini
7	Gemini		
8	Gemini	9:19 am	Cancer
9	Cancer		
10	Cancer	3:23 pm	Leo
11	Leo		
12	Leo		
13	Leo	1:30 am	Virgo
14	Virgo		
15	Virgo	2:07 pm	Libra
16	Libra		
17	Libra		
18	Libra	2:48 am	Scorpio
19	Scorpio		
20	Scorpio	1:52 pm	Sagittarius
21	Sagittarius		
22	Sagittarius	10:54 pm	Capricorn
23	Capricorn		
24	Capricorn		
25	Capricorn	6:01 am	Aquarius
26	Aquarius		
27	Aquarius	11:13 am	Pisces
28	Pisces		
29	Pisces	2:25 pm	Aries
30	Aries		
31	Aries	3:59 pm	Taurus

June

1	Taurus		
2	Taurus	5:02 pm	Gemini
3	Gemini		
4	Gemini	7:17 pm	Cancer
5	Cancer		
6	Cancer		
7	Cancer	12:28 am	Leo
8	Leo		
9	Leo	9:29 am	Virgo
10	Virgo		
11	Virgo	9:31 pm	Libra
12	Libra		
13	Libra		
14	Libra	10:11 am	Scorpio
15	Scorpio		
16	Scorpio	9:12 pm	Sagittarius
17	Sagittarius		
18	Sagittarius		
19	Sagittarius	5:41 am	Capricorn
20	Capricorn		
21	Capricorn	11:57 am	Aquarius
22	Aquarius		
23	Aquarius	4:36 pm	Pisces
24	Pisces		
25	Pisces	8:06 pm	Aries
26	Aries		
27	Aries	10:45 pm	Taurus
28	Taurus		
29	Taurus		
30	Taurus	1:08 am	Gemini

MOON POSITIONS 1989

July

1	Gemini		
2	Gemini	4:19 am	Cancer
3	Cancer		
4	Cancer	9:37 am	Leo
5	Leo		
6	Leo	6:04 pm	Virgo
7	Virgo		
8	Virgo		
9	Virgo	5:30 am	Libra
10	Libra		
11	Libra	6:09 pm	Scorpio
12	Scorpio		
13	Scorpio		
14	Scorpio	5:31 am	Sagittarius
15	Sagittarius		
16	Sagittarius	2:01 pm	Capricorn
17	Capricorn		
18	Capricorn	7:35 pm	Aquarius
19	Aquarius		
20	Aquarius	11:07 pm	Pisces
21	Pisces		
22	Pisces		
23	Pisces	1:41 am	Aries
24	Aries		
25	Aries	4:10 am	Taurus
26	Taurus		
27	Taurus	7:15 am	Gemini
28	Gemini		
29	Gemini	11:32 am	Cancer
30	Cancer		
31	Cancer	5:41 pm	Leo

August

1	Leo		
2	Leo		
3	Leo	2:19 am	Virgo
4	Virgo		
5	Virgo	1:28 pm	Libra
6	Libra		
7	Libra		
8	Libra	2:05 am	Scorpio
9	Scorpio		
10	Scorpio	2:02 pm	Sagittarius
11	Sagittarius		
12	Sagittarius	11:16 pm	Capricorn
13	Capricorn		
14	Capricorn		
15	Capricorn	4:59 am	Aquarius
16	Aquarius		
17	Aquarius	7:46 am	Pisces
18	Pisces		
19	Pisces	8:59 am	Aries
20	Aries		
21	Aries	10:10 am	Taurus
22	Taurus		
23	Taurus	12:39 pm	Gemini
24	Gemini		
25	Gemini	5:13 pm	Cancer
26	Cancer		
27	Cancer		
28	Cancer	12:12 am	Leo
29	Leo		
30	Leo	9:29 am	Virgo
31	Virgo		

September

1	Virgo	8:47 pm	Libra
2	Libra		
3	Libra		
4	Libra	9:23 am	Scorpio
5	Scorpio		
6	Scorpio	9:51 pm	Sagittarius
7	Sagittarius		
8	Sagittarius		
9	Sagittarius	8:13 am	Capricorn
10	Capricorn		
11	Capricorn	3:02 pm	Aquarius
12	Aquarius		
13	Aquarius	6:07 pm	Pisces
14	Pisces		
15	Pisces	6:38 pm	Aries
16	Aries		
17	Aries	6:22 pm	Taurus
18	Taurus		
19	Taurus	7:16 pm	Gemini
20	Gemini		
21	Gemini	10:50 pm	Cancer
22	Cancer		
23	Cancer		
24	Cancer	5:44 am	Leo
25	Leo		
26	Leo	3:32 pm	Virgo
27	Virgo		
28	Virgo		
29	Virgo	3:15 am	Libra
30	Libra		

October

1	Libra	3:53 pm	Scorpio
2	Scorpio		
3	Scorpio		
4	Scorpio	4:29 am	Sagittarius
5	Sagittarius		
6	Sagittarius	3:45 pm	Capricorn
7	Capricorn		
8	Capricorn		
9	Capricorn	12:07 am	Aquarius
10	Aquarius		
11	Aquarius	4:37 am	Pisces
12	Pisces		
13	Pisces	5:41 am	Aries
14	Aries		
15	Aries	4:52 am	Taurus
16	Taurus		
17	Taurus	4:19 am	Gemini
18	Gemini		
19	Gemini	6:09 am	Cancer
20	Cancer		
21	Cancer	11:47 am	Leo
22	Leo		
23	Leo	9:15 pm	Virgo
24	Virgo		
25	Virgo		
26	Virgo	9:11 am	Libra
27	Libra		
28	Libra	9:56 pm	Scorpio
29	Scorpio		
30	Scorpio		
31	Scorpio	10:23 am	Sagittarius

November

1	Sagittarius		
2	Sagittarius	9:46 pm	Capricorn
3	Capricorn		
4	Capricorn		
5	Capricorn	7:09 am	Aquarius
6	Aquarius		
7	Aquarius	1:25 pm	Pisces
8	Pisces		
9	Pisces	4:08 pm	Aries
10	Aries		
11	Aries	4:09 pm	Taurus
12	Taurus		
13	Taurus	3:19 pm	Gemini
14	Gemini		
15	Gemini	3:51 pm	Cancer
16	Cancer		
17	Cancer	7:46 pm	Leo
18	Leo		
19	Leo		
20	Leo	3:54 am	Virgo
21	Virgo		
22	Virgo	3:25 pm	Libra
23	Libra		
24	Libra		
25	Libra	4:13 pm	Scorpio
26	Scorpio		
27	Scorpio	4:30 pm	Sagittarius
28	Sagittarius		
29	Sagittarius		
30	Sagittarius	3:26 pm	Capricorn

December

1	Capricorn		
2	Capricorn	12:42 pm	Aquarius
3	Aquarius		
4	Aquarius	7:48 pm	Pisces
5	Pisces		
6	Pisces		
7	Pisces	12:11 am	Aries
8	Aries		
9	Aries	1:59 am	Taurus
10	Taurus		
11	Taurus	2:15 am	Gemini
12	Gemini		
13	Gemini	2:49 am	Cancer
14	Cancer		
15	Cancer	5:41 am	Leo
16	Leo		
17	Leo	12:19 pm	Virgo
18	Virgo		
19	Virgo	10:45 pm	Libra
20	Libra		
21	Libra		
22	Libra	11:18 am	Scorpio
23	Scorpio		
24	Scorpio	11:37 pm	Sagittarius
25	Sagittarius		
26	Sagittarius		
27	Sagittarius	10:10 am	Capricorn
28	Capricorn		
29	Capricorn	6:38 pm	Aquarius
30	Aquarius		
31	Aquarius		

MOONPOSITIONS 1990

January

1	Aquarius	1:10 am	Pisces
2	Pisces		
3	Pisces	5:56 am	Aries
4	Aries		
5	Aries	9:04 am	Taurus
6	Taurus		
7	Taurus	11:02 am	Gemini
8	Gemini		
9	Gemini	12:52 pm	Cancer
10	Cancer		
11	Cancer	4:02 pm	Leo
12	Leo		
13	Leo	9:57 pm	Virgo
14	Virgo		
15	Virgo		
16	Virgo	7:17 am	Libra
17	Libra		
18	Libra	7:16 pm	Scorpio
19	Scorpio		
20	Scorpio		
21	Scorpio	7:44 am	Sagittarius
22	Sagittarius		
23	Sagittarius	6:27 pm	Capricorn
24	Capricorn		
25	Capricorn		
26	Capricorn	2:25 am	Aquarius
27	Aquarius		
28	Aquarius	7:51 am	Pisces
29	Pisces		
30	Pisces	11:34 am	Aries
31	Aries		

February

1	Aries	2:27 pm	Taurus
2	Taurus		
3	Taurus	5:12 pm	Gemini
4	Gemini		
5	Gemini	8:27 pm	Cancer
6	Cancer		
7	Cancer		
8	Cancer	12:51 am	Leo
9	Leo		
10	Leo	7:13 am	Virgo
11	Virgo		
12	Virgo	4:09 pm	Libra
13	Libra		
14	Libra		
15	Libra	3:34 am	Scorpio
16	Scorpio		
17	Scorpio	4:07 pm	Sagittarius
18	Sagittarius		
19	Sagittarius		
20	Sagittarius	3:30 am	Capricorn
21	Capricorn		
22	Capricorn	11:52 am	Aquarius
23	Aquarius		
24	Aquarius	4:49 pm	Pisces
25	Pisces		
26	Pisces	7:16 pm	Aries
27	Aries		
28	Aries	8:43 pm	Taurus

March

1	Taurus		
2	Taurus	10:37 pm	Gemini
3	Gemini		
4	Gemini		
5	Gemini	2:02 am	Cancer
6	Cancer		
7	Cancer	7:24 am	Leo
8	Leo		
9	Leo	2:47 pm	Virgo
10	Virgo		
11	Virgo		
12	Virgo	12:09 am	Libra
13	Libra		
14	Libra	11:25 am	Scorpio
15	Scorpio		
16	Scorpio	11:56 pm	Sagittarius
17	Sagittarius		
18	Sagittarius		
19	Sagittarius	12:01 pm	Capricorn
20	Capricorn		
21	Capricorn	9:31 pm	Aquarius
22	Aquarius		
23	Aquarius		
24	Aquarius	3:08 am	Pisces
25	Pisces		
26	Pisces	5:15 am	Aries
27	Aries		
28	Aries	5:26 am	Taurus
29	Taurus		
30	Taurus	5:42 am	Gemini
31	Gemini		

April

1	Gemini	7:50 am	Cancer
2	Cancer		
3	Cancer	12:50 pm	Leo
4	Leo		
5	Leo	8:42 pm	Virgo
6	Virgo		
7	Virgo		
8	Virgo	6:44 am	Libra
9	Libra		
10	Libra	6:18 pm	Scorpio
11	Scorpio		
12	Scorpio		
13	Scorpio	6:48 am	Sagittarius
14	Sagittarius		
15	Sagittarius	7:15 pm	Capricorn
16	Capricorn		
17	Capricorn		
18	Capricorn	5:53 am	Aquarius
19	Aquarius		
20	Aquarius	12:57 pm	Pisces
21	Pisces		
22	Pisces	3:58 pm	Aries
23	Aries		
24	Aries	4:03 pm	Taurus
25	Taurus		
26	Taurus	3:12 pm	Gemini
27	Gemini		
28	Gemini	3:39 pm	Cancer
29	Cancer		
30	Cancer	7:08 pm	Leo

May

1	Leo		
2	Leo		
3	Leo	2:18 am	Virgo
4	Virgo		
5	Virgo	12:28 pm	Libra
6	Libra		
7	Libra		
8	Libra	12:22 am	Scorpio
9	Scorpio		
10	Scorpio	12:56 pm	Sagittarius
11	Sagittarius		
12	Sagittarius		
13	Sagittarius	1:21 am	Capricorn
14	Capricorn		
15	Capricorn	12:30 pm	Aquarius
16	Aquarius		
17	Aquarius	8:54 pm	Pisces
18	Pisces		
19	Pisces		
20	Pisces	1:31 am	Aries
21	Aries		
22	Aries	2:42 am	Taurus
23	Taurus		
24	Taurus	2:00 am	Gemini
25	Gemini		
26	Gemini	1:34 am	Cancer
27	Cancer		
28	Cancer	3:29 am	Leo
29	Leo		
30	Leo	9:08 am	Virgo
31	Virgo		

June

1	Virgo	6:31 pm	Libra
2	Libra		
3	Libra		
4	Libra	6:21 am	Scorpio
5	Scorpio		
6	Scorpio	6:59 pm	Sagittarius
7	Sagittarius		
8	Sagittarius		
9	Sagittarius	7:12 am	Capricorn
10	Capricorn		
11	Capricorn	6:09 pm	Aquarius
12	Aquarius		
13	Aquarius		
14	Aquarius	3:00 am	Pisces
15	Pisces		
16	Pisces	8:55 am	Aries
17	Aries		
18	Aries	11:43 am	Taurus
19	Taurus		
20	Taurus	12:14 pm	Gemini
21	Gemini		
22	Gemini	12:10 pm	Cancer
23	Cancer		
24	Cancer	1:25 pm	Leo
25	Leo		
26	Leo	5:42 pm	Virgo
27	Virgo		
28	Virgo		
29	Virgo	1:47 am	Libra
30	Libra		

MOON POSITIONS 1990

July

1	Libra	1:01 pm	Scorpio
2	Scorpio		
3	Scorpio		
4	Scorpio	1:35 am	Sagittarius
5	Sagittarius		
6	Sagittarius	1:39 pm	Capricorn
7	Capricorn		
8	Capricorn		
9	Capricorn	12:07 am	Aquarius
10	Aquarius		
11	Aquarius	8:29 am	Pisces
12	Pisces		
13	Pisces	2:36 pm	Aries
14	Aries		
15	Aries	6:29 pm	Taurus
16	Taurus		
17	Taurus	8:32 pm	Gemini
18	Gemini		
19	Gemini	9:44 pm	Cancer
20	Cancer		
21	Cancer	11:29 pm	Leo
22	Leo		
23	Leo		
24	Leo	3:17 am	Virgo
25	Virgo		
26	Virgo	10:19 am	Libra
27	Libra		
28	Libra	8:39 pm	Scorpio
29	Scorpio		
30	Scorpio		
31	Scorpio	9:00 am	Sagittarius

August

1	Sagittarius		
2	Sagittarius	9:08 pm	Capricorn
3	Capricorn		
4	Capricorn		
5	Capricorn	7:19 am	Aquarius
6	Aquarius		
7	Aquarius	2:54 pm	Pisces
8	Pisces		
9	Pisces	8:13 pm	Aries
10	Aries		
11	Aries	11:55 pm	Taurus
12	Taurus		
13	Taurus		
14	Taurus	2:41 am	Gemini
15	Gemini		
16	Gemini	5:12 am	Cancer
17	Cancer		
18	Cancer	8:11 am	Leo
19	Leo		
20	Leo	12:33 pm	Virgo
21	Virgo		
22	Virgo	7:17 pm	Libra
23	Libra		
24	Libra		
25	Libra	4:56 am	Scorpio
26	Scorpio		
27	Scorpio	4:57 pm	Sagittarius
28	Sagittarius		
29	Sagittarius		
30	Sagittarius	5:23 am	Capricorn
31	Capricorn		

September

1	Capricorn	3:51 pm	Aquarius
2	Aquarius		
3	Aquarius	11:06 pm	Pisces
4	Pisces		
5	Pisces		
6	Pisces	3:23 am	Aries
7	Aries		
8	Aries	5:55 am	Taurus
9	Taurus		
10	Taurus	8:05 am	Gemini
11	Gemini		
12	Gemini	10:53 am	Cancer
13	Cancer		
14	Cancer	2:52 pm	Leo
15	Leo		
16	Leo	8:19 pm	Virgo
17	Virgo		
18	Virgo		
19	Virgo	3:34 am	Libra
20	Libra		
21	Libra	1:06 pm	Scorpio
22	Scorpio		
23	Scorpio		
24	Scorpio	12:52 am	Sagittarius
25	Sagittarius		
26	Sagittarius	1:36 pm	Capricorn
27	Capricorn		
28	Capricorn		
29	Capricorn	12:54 am	Aquarius
30	Aquarius		

October

1	Aquarius	8:42 am	Pisces
2	Pisces		
3	Pisces	12:42 am	Aries
4	Aries		
5	Aries	2:06 pm	Taurus
6	Taurus		
7	Taurus	2:47 pm	Gemini
8	Gemini		
9	Gemini	4:29 pm	Cancer
10	Cancer		
11	Cancer	8:16 pm	Leo
12	Leo		
13	Leo		
14	Leo	2:21 am	Virgo
15	Virgo		
16	Virgo	10:26 am	Libra
17	Libra		
18	Libra	8:24 pm	Scorpio
19	Scorpio		
20	Scorpio		
21	Scorpio	8:09 am	Sagittarius
22	Sagittarius		
23	Sagittarius	9:03 pm	Capricorn
24	Capricorn		
25	Capricorn		
26	Capricorn	9:14 am	Aquarius
27	Aquarius		
28	Aquarius	6:22 pm	Pisces
29	Pisces		
30	Pisces	11:14 pm	Aries
31	Aries		

November

1	Aries		
2	Aries	12:31 am	Taurus
3	Taurus		
4	Taurus	12:06 am	Gemini
5	Gemini		
6	Gemini	12:07 am	Cancer
7	Cancer		
8	Cancer	2:24 am	Leo
9	Leo		
10	Leo	7:48 am	Virgo
11	Virgo		
12	Virgo	4:08 pm	Libra
13	Libra		
14	Libra		
15	Libra	2:39 am	Scorpio
16	Scorpio		
17	Scorpio	2:39 pm	Sagittarius
18	Sagittarius		
19	Sagittarius		
20	Sagittarius	3:31 am	Capricorn
21	Capricorn		
22	Capricorn	4:07 pm	Aquarius
23	Aquarius		
24	Aquarius		
25	Aquarius	2:32 am	Pisces
26	Pisces		
27	Pisces	9:06 am	Aries
28	Aries		
29	Aries	11:37 am	Taurus
30	Taurus		

December

1	Taurus	11:22 am	Gemini
2	Gemini		
3	Gemini	10:27 am	Cancer
4	Cancer		
5	Cancer	11:00 am	Leo
6	Leo		
7	Leo	2:39 pm	Virgo
8	Virgo		
9	Virgo	10:00 pm	Libra
10	Libra		
11	Libra		
12	Libra	8:28 am	Scorpio
13	Scorpio		
14	Scorpio	8:44 pm	Sagittarius
15	Sagittarius		
16	Sagittarius		
17	Sagittarius	9:35 am	Capricorn
18	Capricorn		
19	Capricorn	9:59 pm	Aquarius
20	Aquarius		
21	Aquarius		
22	Aquarius	8:48 am	Pisces
23	Pisces		
24	Pisces	4:45 pm	Aries
25	Aries		
26	Aries	9:09 pm	Taurus
27	Taurus		
28	Taurus	10:26 pm	Gemini
29	Gemini		
30	Gemini	10:02 pm	Cancer
31	Cancer		

MOON POSITIONS 1991

January

1	Cancer	9:54 pm	Leo
2	Leo		
3	Leo	11:57 pm	Virgo
4	Virgo		
5	Virgo		
6	Virgo	5:33 am	Libra
7	Libra		
8	Libra	2:59 pm	Scorpio
9	Scorpio		
10	Scorpio		
11	Scorpio	3:06 am	Sagittarius
12	Sagittarius		
13	Sagittarius	4:00 pm	Capricorn
14	Capricorn		
15	Capricorn		
16	Capricorn	4:04 am	Aquarius
17	Aquarius		
18	Aquarius	2:23 pm	Pisces
19	Pisces		
20	Pisces	10:28 pm	Aries
21	Aries		
22	Aries		
23	Aries	4:01 am	Taurus
24	Taurus		
25	Taurus	7:06 am	Gemini
26	Gemini		
27	Gemini	8:23 am	Cancer
28	Cancer		
29	Cancer	9:03 am	Leo
30	Leo		
31	Leo	10:44 am	Virgo

February

1	Virgo		
2	Virgo	3:02 pm	Libra
3	Libra		
4	Libra	11:01 pm	Scorpio
5	Scorpio		
6	Scorpio		
7	Scorpio	10:23 am	Sagittarius
8	Sagittarius		
9	Sagittarius	11:16 pm	Capricorn
10	Capricorn		
11	Capricorn		
12	Capricorn	11:16 am	Aquarius
13	Aquarius		
14	Aquarius	8:59 pm	Pisces
15	Pisces		
16	Pisces		
17	Pisces	4:11 am	Aries
18	Aries		
19	Aries	9:24 am	Taurus
20	Taurus		
21	Taurus	1:10 pm	Gemini
22	Gemini		
23	Gemini	3:56 pm	Cancer
24	Cancer		
25	Cancer	6:13 pm	Leo
26	Leo		
27	Leo	8:50 pm	Virgo
28	Virgo		

March

1	Virgo		
2	Virgo	1:03 am	Libra
3	Libra		
4	Libra	8:08 am	Scorpio
5	Scorpio		
6	Scorpio	6:35 pm	Sagittarius
7	Sagittarius		
8	Sagittarius		
9	Sagittarius	7:14 am	Capricorn
10	Capricorn		
11	Capricorn	7:31 pm	Aquarius
12	Aquarius		
13	Aquarius		
14	Aquarius	5:11 am	Pisces
15	Pisces		
16	Pisces	11:37 am	Aries
17	Aries		
18	Aries	3:40 pm	Taurus
19	Taurus		
20	Taurus	6:37 pm	Gemini
21	Gemini		
22	Gemini	9:27 pm	Cancer
23	Cancer		
24	Cancer		
25	Cancer	12:43 am	Leo
26	Leo		
27	Leo	4:41 am	Virgo
28	Virgo		
29	Virgo	9:49 am	Libra
30	Libra		
31	Libra	5:01 pm	Scorpio

April

1	Scorpio		
2	Scorpio		
3	Scorpio	2:59 am	Sagittarius
4	Sagittarius		
5	Sagittarius	3:20 pm	Capricorn
6	Capricorn		
7	Capricorn		
8	Capricorn	4:00 am	Aquarius
9	Aquarius		
10	Aquarius	2:17 pm	Pisces
11	Pisces		
12	Pisces	8:49 pm	Aries
13	Aries		
14	Aries		
15	Aries	12:06 am	Taurus
16	Taurus		
17	Taurus	1:41 am	Gemini
18	Gemini		
19	Gemini	3:17 am	Cancer
20	Cancer		
21	Cancer	6:04 am	Leo
22	Leo		
23	Leo	10:29 am	Virgo
24	Virgo		
25	Virgo	4:36 pm	Libra
26	Libra		
27	Libra		
28	Libra	12:34 am	Scorpio
29	Scorpio		
30	Scorpio	10:42 am	Sagittarius

May

1	Sagittarius		
2	Sagittarius	10:55 pm	Capricorn
3	Capricorn		
4	Capricorn		
5	Capricorn	11:51 am	Aquarius
6	Aquarius		
7	Aquarius	11:04 pm	Pisces
8	Pisces		
9	Pisces		
10	Pisces	6:34 am	Aries
11	Aries		
12	Aries	10:07 am	Taurus
13	Taurus		
14	Taurus	11:02 am	Gemini
15	Gemini		
16	Gemini	11:14 am	Cancer
17	Cancer		
18	Cancer	12:30 pm	Leo
19	Leo		
20	Leo	4:00 pm	Virgo
21	Virgo		
22	Virgo	10:08 pm	Libra
23	Libra		
24	Libra		
25	Libra	6:41 am	Scorpio
26	Scorpio		
27	Scorpio	5:21 pm	Sagittarius
28	Sagittarius		
29	Sagittarius		
30	Sagittarius	5:40 am	Capricorn
31	Capricorn		

June

1	Capricorn	6:42 pm	Aquarius
2	Aquarius		
3	Aquarius		
4	Aquarius	6:36 am	Pisces
5	Pisces		
6	Pisces	3:25 pm	Aries
7	Aries		
8	Aries	8:13 pm	Taurus
9	Taurus		
10	Taurus	9:36 pm	Gemini
11	Gemini		
12	Gemini	9:16 pm	Cancer
13	Cancer		
14	Cancer	9:10 pm	Leo
15	Leo		
16	Leo	11:03 pm	Virgo
17	Virgo		
18	Virgo		
19	Virgo	4:01 am	Libra
20	Libra		
21	Libra	12:18 pm	Scorpio
22	Scorpio		
23	Scorpio	11:16 pm	Sagittarius
24	Sagittarius		
25	Sagittarius		
26	Sagittarius	11:49 am	Capricorn
27	Capricorn		
28	Capricorn		
29	Capricorn	12:47 am	Aquarius
30	Aquarius		

MOON POSITIONS 1991

July

1	Aquarius	12:51 pm	Pisces
2	Pisces		
3	Pisces	10:33 pm	Aries
4	Aries		
5	Aries		
6	Aries	4:52 am	Taurus
7	Taurus		
8	Taurus	7:42 am	Gemini
9	Gemini		
10	Gemini	8:03 am	Cancer
11	Cancer		
12	Cancer	7:35 am	Leo
13	Leo		
14	Leo	8:12 am	Virgo
15	Virgo		
16	Virgo	11:34 am	Libra
17	Libra		
18	Libra	6:41 am	Scorpio
19	Scorpio		
20	Scorpio		
21	Scorpio	5:16 am	Sagittarius
22	Sagittarius		
23	Sagittarius	5:55 am	Capricorn
24	Capricorn		
25	Capricorn		
26	Capricorn	6:49 am	Aquarius
27	Aquarius		
28	Aquarius	6:35 pm	Pisces
29	Pisces		
30	Pisces		
31	Pisces	4:20 am	Aries

August

1	Aries		
2	Aries	11:32 am	Taurus
3	Taurus		
4	Taurus	3:54 pm	Gemini
5	Gemini		
6	Gemini	5:47 pm	Cancer
7	Cancer		
8	Cancer	6:09 pm	Leo
9	Leo		
10	Leo	6:35 pm	Virgo
11	Virgo		
12	Virgo	8:52 pm	Libra
13	Libra		
14	Libra		
15	Libra	2:34 am	Scorpio
16	Scorpio		
17	Scorpio	12:11 pm	Sagittarius
18	Sagittarius		
19	Sagittarius		
20	Sagittarius	12:34 am	Capricorn
21	Capricorn		
22	Capricorn	1:27 pm	Aquarius
23	Aquarius		
24	Aquarius		
25	Aquarius	12:51 am	Pisces
26	Pisces		
27	Pisces	10:01 am	Aries
28	Aries		
29	Aries	5:00 pm	Taurus
30	Taurus		
31	Taurus	10:02 am	Gemini

September

1	Gemini		
2	Gemini		
3	Gemini	1:19 am	Cancer
4	Cancer		
5	Cancer	3:13 am	Leo
6	Leo		
7	Leo	4:35 am	Virgo
8	Virgo		
9	Virgo	6:52 am	Libra
10	Libra		
11	Libra	11:42 am	Scorpio
12	Scorpio		
13	Scorpio	8:14 pm	Sagittarius
14	Sagittarius		
15	Sagittarius		
16	Sagittarius	8:04 am	Capricorn
17	Capricorn		
18	Capricorn	8:58 pm	Aquarius
19	Aquarius		
20	Aquarius		
21	Aquarius	8:20 am	Pisces
22	Pisces		
23	Pisces	4:56 pm	Aries
24	Aries		
25	Aries	10:59 pm	Taurus
26	Taurus		
27	Taurus		
28	Taurus	3:25 am	Gemini
29	Gemini		
30	Gemini	6:58 am	Cancer

October

1	Cancer		
2	Cancer	9:58 am	Leo
3	Leo		
4	Leo	12:45 pm	Virgo
5	Virgo		
6	Virgo	4:00 pm	Libra
7	Libra		
8	Libra	9:00 pm	Scorpio
9	Scorpio		
10	Scorpio		
11	Scorpio	4:58 am	Sagittarius
12	Sagittarius		
13	Sagittarius	4:10 pm	Capricorn
14	Capricorn		
15	Capricorn		
16	Capricorn	5:04 am	Aquarius
17	Aquarius		
18	Aquarius	4:53 pm	Pisces
19	Pisces		
20	Pisces		
21	Pisces	1:33 am	Aries
22	Aries		
23	Aries	6:55 am	Taurus
24	Taurus		
25	Taurus	10:09 am	Gemini
26	Gemini		
27	Gemini	12:37 pm	Cancer
28	Cancer		
29	Cancer	3:20 pm	Leo
30	Leo		
31	Leo	6:47 pm	Virgo

November

1	Virgo		
2	Virgo	11:13 pm	Libra
3	Libra		
4	Libra		
5	Libra	5:09 am	Scorpio
6	Scorpio		
7	Scorpio	1:21 pm	Sagittarius
8	Sagittarius		
9	Sagittarius		
10	Sagittarius	12:16 am	Capricorn
11	Capricorn		
12	Capricorn	1:06 pm	Aquarius
13	Aquarius		
14	Aquarius		
15	Aquarius	1:33 am	Pisces
16	Pisces		
17	Pisces	11:08 am	Aries
18	Aries		
19	Aries	4:49 pm	Taurus
20	Taurus		
21	Taurus	7:22 pm	Gemini
22	Gemini		
23	Gemini	8:25 pm	Cancer
24	Cancer		
25	Cancer	9:37 pm	Leo
26	Leo		
27	Leo		
28	Leo	12:12 am	Virgo
29	Virgo		
30	Virgo	4:47 am	Libra

December

1	Libra		
2	Libra	11:33 am	Scorpio
3	Scorpio		
4	Scorpio	8:32 pm	Sagittarius
5	Sagittarius		
6	Sagittarius		
7	Sagittarius	7:41 am	Capricorn
8	Capricorn		
9	Capricorn	8:27 pm	Aquarius
10	Aquarius		
11	Aquarius		
12	Aquarius	9:19 am	Pisces
13	Pisces		
14	Pisces	8:06 pm	Aries
15	Aries		
16	Aries		
17	Aries	3:10 am	Taurus
18	Taurus		
19	Taurus	6:21 am	Gemini
20	Gemini		
21	Gemini	6:55 am	Cancer
22	Cancer		
23	Cancer	6:38 am	Leo
24	Leo		
25	Leo	7:24 am	Virgo
26	Virgo		
27	Virgo	10:37 am	Libra
28	Libra		
29	Libra	5:03 pm	Scorpio
30	Scorpio		
31	Scorpio		

MOON POSITIONS 1992

January

1	Scorpio	2:30 am	Sagittarius	
2	Sagittarius			
3	Sagittarius	2:09 pm	Capricorn	
4	Capricorn			
5	Capricorn			
6	Capricorn	2:59 am	Aquarius	
7	Aquarius			
8	Aquarius	3:52 pm	Pisces	
9	Pisces			
10	Pisces			
11	Pisces	3:22 am	Aries	
12	Aries			
13	Aries	12:00 pm	Taurus	
14	Taurus			
15	Taurus	4:54 pm	Gemini	
16	Gemini			
17	Gemini	6:26 pm	Cancer	
18	Cancer			
19	Cancer	5:57 pm	Leo	
20	Leo			
21	Leo	5:22 pm	Virgo	
22	Virgo			
23	Virgo	6:42 pm	Libra	
24	Libra			
25	Libra	11:32 pm	Scorpio	
26	Scorpio			
27	Scorpio			
28	Scorpio	8:20 am	Sagittarius	
29	Sagittarius			
30	Sagittarius	8:07 pm	Capricorn	
31	Capricorn			

February

1	Capricorn			
2	Capricorn	9:09 am	Aquarius	
3	Aquarius			
4	Aquarius	9:51 pm	Pisces	
5	Pisces			
6	Pisces			
7	Pisces	9:15 am	Aries	
8	Aries			
9	Aries	6:36 pm	Taurus	
10	Taurus			
11	Taurus			
12	Taurus	1:08 am	Gemini	
13	Gemini			
14	Gemini	4:31 am	Cancer	
15	Cancer			
16	Cancer	5:15 am	Leo	
17	Leo			
18	Leo	4:47 am	Virgo	
19	Virgo			
20	Virgo	5:05 am	Libra	
21	Libra			
22	Libra	8:11 am	Scorpio	
23	Scorpio			
24	Scorpio	3:26 pm	Sagittarius	
25	Sagittarius			
26	Sagittarius			
27	Sagittarius	2:33 am	Capricorn	
28	Capricorn			
29	Capricorn	3:34 pm	Aquarius	

March

1	Aquarius			
2	Aquarius			
3	Aquarius	4:11 am	Pisces	
4	Pisces			
5	Pisces	3:07 pm	Aries	
6	Aries			
7	Aries			
8	Aries	12:05 am	Taurus	
9	Taurus			
10	Taurus	7:03 am	Gemini	
11	Gemini			
12	Gemini	11:50 am	Cancer	
13	Cancer			
14	Cancer	2:20 pm	Leo	
15	Leo			
16	Leo	3:13 pm	Virgo	
17	Virgo			
18	Virgo	3:55 pm	Libra	
19	Libra			
20	Libra	6:20 pm	Scorpio	
21	Scorpio			
22	Scorpio			
23	Scorpio	12:13 pm	Sagittarius	
24	Sagittarius			
25	Sagittarius	10:08 am	Capricorn	
26	Capricorn			
27	Capricorn	10:44 pm	Aquarius	
28	Aquarius			
29	Aquarius			
30	Aquarius	11:23 am	Pisces	
31	Pisces			

April

1	Pisces	10:04 pm	Aries	
2	Aries			
3	Aries			
4	Aries	6:18 am	Taurus	
5	Taurus			
6	Taurus	12:33 pm	Gemini	
7	Gemini			
8	Gemini	5:18 pm	Cancer	
9	Cancer			
10	Cancer	8:46 pm	Leo	
11	Leo			
12	Leo	11:09 pm	Virgo	
13	Virgo			
14	Virgo			
15	Virgo	1:10 am	Libra	
16	Libra			
17	Libra	4:10 am	Scorpio	
18	Scorpio			
19	Scorpio	9:40 am	Sagittarius	
20	Sagittarius			
21	Sagittarius	6:41 pm	Capricorn	
22	Capricorn			
23	Capricorn			
24	Capricorn	6:38 am	Aquarius	
25	Aquarius			
26	Aquarius	7:20 pm	Pisces	
27	Pisces			
28	Pisces			
29	Pisces	6:13 am	Aries	
30	Aries			

May

1	Aries	2:09 pm	Taurus	
2	Taurus			
3	Taurus	7:28 pm	Gemini	
4	Gemini			
5	Gemini	11:09 pm	Cancer	
6	Cancer			
7	Cancer			
8	Cancer	2:07 am	Leo	
9	Leo			
10	Leo	4:56 am	Virgo	
11	Virgo			
12	Virgo	8:05 am	Libra	
13	Libra			
14	Libra	12:15 pm	Scorpio	
15	Scorpio			
16	Scorpio	6:22 pm	Sagittarius	
17	Sagittarius			
18	Sagittarius			
19	Sagittarius	3:13 am	Capricorn	
20	Capricorn			
21	Capricorn	2:43 pm	Aquarius	
22	Aquarius			
23	Aquarius			
24	Aquarius	3:25 am	Pisces	
25	Pisces			
26	Pisces	2:52 pm	Aries	
27	Aries			
28	Aries	11:16 pm	Taurus	
29	Taurus			
30	Taurus			
31	Taurus	4:19 am	Gemini	

June

1	Gemini			
2	Gemini	6:58 am	Cancer	
3	Cancer			
4	Cancer	8:35 am	Leo	
5	Leo			
6	Leo	10:28 am	Virgo	
7	Virgo			
8	Virgo	1:33 pm	Libra	
9	Libra			
10	Libra	6:27 pm	Scorpio	
11	Scorpio			
12	Scorpio			
13	Scorpio	1:29 am	Sagittarius	
14	Sagittarius			
15	Sagittarius	10:50 am	Capricorn	
16	Capricorn			
17	Capricorn	10:19 pm	Aquarius	
18	Aquarius			
19	Aquarius			
20	Aquarius	11:00 am	Pisces	
21	Pisces			
22	Pisces	11:03 pm	Aries	
23	Aries			
24	Aries			
25	Aries	8:28 am	Taurus	
26	Taurus			
27	Taurus	2:14 pm	Gemini	
28	Gemini			
29	Gemini	4:42 pm	Cancer	
30	Cancer			

MOONPOSITIONS 1992

July

1	Cancer	5:15 pm	Leo
2	Leo		
3	Leo	5:37 pm	Virgo
4	Virgo		
5	Virgo	7:27 pm	Libra
6	Libra		
7	Libra	11:53 pm	Scorpio
8	Scorpio		
9	Scorpio		
10	Scorpio	7:17 am	Sagittarius
11	Sagittarius		
12	Sagittarius	5:16 pm	Capricorn
13	Capricorn		
14	Capricorn		
15	Capricorn	5:03 am	Aquarius
16	Aquarius		
17	Aquarius	5:44 pm	Pisces
18	Pisces		
19	Pisces		
20	Pisces	6:07 am	Aries
21	Aries		
22	Aries	4:36 pm	Taurus
23	Taurus		
24	Taurus	11:44 pm	Gemini
25	Gemini		
26	Gemini		
27	Gemini	3:08 am	Cancer
28	Cancer		
29	Cancer	3:39 am	Leo
30	Leo		
31	Leo	3:01 am	Virgo

August

1	Virgo		
2	Virgo	3:17 am	Libra
3	Libra		
4	Libra	6:16 am	Scorpio
5	Scorpio		
6	Scorpio	12:57 pm	Sagittarius
7	Sagittarius		
8	Sagittarius	11:00 pm	Capricorn
9	Capricorn		
10	Capricorn		
11	Capricorn	11:06 am	Aquarius
12	Aquarius		
13	Aquarius	11:51 pm	Pisces
14	Pisces		
15	Pisces		
16	Pisces	12:11 pm	Aries
17	Aries		
18	Aries	11:10 pm	Taurus
19	Taurus		
20	Taurus		
21	Taurus	7:36 am	Gemini
22	Gemini		
23	Gemini	12:36 pm	Cancer
24	Cancer		
25	Cancer	2:15 pm	Leo
26	Leo		
27	Leo	1:46 pm	Virgo
28	Virgo		
29	Virgo	1:11 pm	Libra
30	Libra		
31	Libra	2:38 pm	Scorpio

September

1	Scorpio		
2	Scorpio	7:50 pm	Sagittarius
3	Sagittarius		
4	Sagittarius		
5	Sagittarius	5:06 am	Capricorn
6	Capricorn		
7	Capricorn	5:08 pm	Aquarius
8	Aquarius		
9	Aquarius		
10	Aquarius	5:56 am	Pisces
11	Pisces		
12	Pisces	6:02 pm	Aries
13	Aries		
14	Aries		
15	Aries	4:47 am	Taurus
16	Taurus		
17	Taurus	1:40 pm	Gemini
18	Gemini		
19	Gemini	7:59 pm	Cancer
20	Cancer		
21	Cancer	11:19 pm	Leo
22	Leo		
23	Leo		
24	Leo	12:08 am	Virgo
25	Virgo	11:55 pm	Libra
26	Libra		
27	Libra		
28	Libra	12:44 am	Scorpio
29	Scorpio		
30	Scorpio	4:33 am	Sagittarius

October

1	Sagittarius		
2	Sagittarius	12:29 pm	Capricorn
3	Capricorn		
4	Capricorn	11:53 pm	Aquarius
5	Aquarius		
6	Aquarius		
7	Aquarius	12:38 pm	Pisces
8	Pisces		
9	Pisces		
10	Pisces	12:36 am	Aries
11	Aries		
12	Aries	10:48 am	Taurus
13	Taurus		
14	Taurus	7:08 pm	Gemini
15	Gemini		
16	Gemini		
17	Gemini	1:36 am	Cancer
18	Cancer		
19	Cancer	6:01 am	Leo
20	Leo		
21	Leo	8:27 am	Virgo
22	Virgo		
23	Virgo	9:39 am	Libra
24	Libra		
25	Libra	11:04 am	Scorpio
26	Scorpio		
27	Scorpio	2:29 pm	Sagittarius
28	Sagittarius		
29	Sagittarius	9:18 pm	Capricorn
30	Capricorn		
31	Capricorn		

November

1	Capricorn	7:43 am	Aquarius
2	Aquarius		
3	Aquarius	8:13 pm	Pisces
4	Pisces		
5	Pisces		
6	Pisces	8:19 am	Aries
7	Aries		
8	Aries	6:19 pm	Taurus
9	Taurus		
10	Taurus		
11	Taurus	1:49 am	Gemini
12	Gemini		
13	Gemini	7:19 am	Cancer
14	Cancer		
15	Cancer	11:23 am	Leo
16	Leo		
17	Leo	2:28 pm	Virgo
18	Virgo		
19	Virgo	5:03 pm	Libra
20	Libra		
21	Libra	7:52 pm	Scorpio
22	Scorpio		
23	Scorpio		
24	Scorpio	12:01 am	Sagittarius
25	Sagittarius		
26	Sagittarius	6:38 am	Capricorn
27	Capricorn		
28	Capricorn	4:19 pm	Aquarius
29	Aquarius		
30	Aquarius		

December

1	Aquarius	4:23 am	Pisces
2	Pisces		
3	Pisces	4:49 pm	Aries
4	Aries		
5	Aries		
6	Aries	3:16 am	Taurus
7	Taurus		
8	Taurus	10:37 am	Gemini
9	Gemini		
10	Gemini	3:05 pm	Cancer
11	Cancer		
12	Cancer	5:47 pm	Leo
13	Leo		
14	Leo	7:56 pm	Virgo
15	Virgo		
16	Virgo	10:33 pm	Libra
17	Libra		
18	Libra		
19	Libra	2:20 am	Scorpio
20	Scorpio		
21	Scorpio	7:42 am	Sagittarius
22	Sagittarius		
23	Sagittarius	3:04 pm	Capricorn
24	Capricorn		
25	Capricorn		
26	Capricorn	12:43 am	Aquarius
27	Aquarius		
28	Aquarius	12:28 pm	Pisces
29	Pisces		
30	Pisces		
31	Pisces	1:07 am	Aries

MOONPOSITIONS1993

January

1	Aries		
2	Aries	12:30 pm	Taurus
3	Taurus		
4	Taurus	8:42 pm	Gemini
5	Gemini		
6	Gemini		
7	Gemini	1:10 am	Cancer
8	Cancer		
9	Cancer	2:49 am	Leo
10	Leo		
11	Leo	3:20 am	Virgo
12	Virgo		
13	Virgo	4:30 am	Libra
14	Libra		
15	Libra	7:42 am	Scorpio
16	Scorpio		
17	Scorpio	1:30 pm	Sagittarius
18	Sagittarius		
19	Sagittarius	9:46 pm	Capricorn
20	Capricorn		
21	Capricorn		
22	Capricorn	8:00 am	Aquarius
23	Aquarius		
24	Aquarius	7:47 pm	Pisces
25	Pisces		
26	Pisces		
27	Pisces	8:28 am	Aries
28	Aries		
29	Aries	8:37 pm	Taurus
30	Taurus		
31	Taurus		

February

1	Taurus	6:15 am	Gemini
2	Gemini		
3	Gemini	11:56 am	Cancer
4	Cancer		
5	Cancer	1:51 pm	Leo
6	Leo		
7	Leo	1:29 pm	Virgo
8	Virgo		
9	Virgo	12:58 pm	Libra
10	Libra		
11	Libra	2:24 pm	Scorpio
12	Scorpio		
13	Scorpio	7:08 pm	Sagittarius
14	Sagittarius		
15	Sagittarius		
16	Sagittarius	3:20 am	Capricorn
17	Capricorn		
18	Capricorn	2:05 pm	Aquarius
19	Aquarius		
20	Aquarius		
21	Aquarius	2:12 am	Pisces
22	Pisces		
23	Pisces	2:50 pm	Aries
24	Aries		
25	Aries		
26	Aries	3:11 am	Taurus
27	Taurus		
28	Taurus	1:52 pm	Gemini

March

1	Gemini		
2	Gemini	9:16 pm	Cancer
3	Cancer		
4	Cancer		
5	Cancer	12:40 am	Leo
6	Leo		
7	Leo	12:52 am	Virgo
8	Virgo	11:46 pm	Libra
9	Libra		
10	Libra	11:40 pm	Scorpio
11	Scorpio		
12	Scorpio		
13	Scorpio	2:33 am	Sagittarius
14	Sagittarius		
15	Sagittarius	9:28 am	Capricorn
16	Capricorn		
17	Capricorn	7:52 pm	Aquarius
18	Aquarius		
19	Aquarius		
20	Aquarius	8:11 am	Pisces
21	Pisces		
22	Pisces	8:51 pm	Aries
23	Aries		
24	Aries		
25	Aries	8:59 am	Taurus
26	Taurus		
27	Taurus	7:48 pm	Gemini
28	Gemini		
29	Gemini		
30	Gemini	4:14 am	Cancer
31	Cancer		

April

1	Cancer	9:21 am	Leo
2	Leo		
3	Leo	11:10 am	Virgo
4	Virgo		
5	Virgo	10:54 am	Libra
6	Libra		
7	Libra	10:32 am	Scorpio
8	Scorpio		
9	Scorpio	12:10 pm	Sagittarius
10	Sagittarius		
11	Sagittarius	5:24 pm	Capricorn
12	Capricorn		
13	Capricorn		
14	Capricorn	2:36 am	Aquarius
15	Aquarius		
16	Aquarius	2:32 pm	Pisces
17	Pisces		
18	Pisces		
19	Pisces	3:14 am	Aries
20	Aries		
21	Aries	3:08 pm	Taurus
22	Taurus		
23	Taurus		
24	Taurus	1:27 am	Gemini
25	Gemini		
26	Gemini	9:45 am	Cancer
27	Cancer		
28	Cancer	3:39 pm	Leo
29	Leo		
30	Leo	7:00 pm	Virgo

May

1	Virgo		
2	Virgo	8:20 pm	Libra
3	Libra		
4	Libra	8:57 pm	Scorpio
5	Scorpio		
6	Scorpio	10:34 pm	Sagittarius
7	Sagittarius		
8	Sagittarius		
9	Sagittarius	2:51 am	Capricorn
10	Capricorn		
11	Capricorn	10:44 am	Aquarius
12	Aquarius		
13	Aquarius	9:51 pm	Pisces
14	Pisces		
15	Pisces		
16	Pisces	10:24 am	Aries
17	Aries		
18	Aries	10:16 pm	Taurus
19	Taurus		
20	Taurus		
21	Taurus	8:07 am	Gemini
22	Gemini		
23	Gemini	3:38 pm	Cancer
24	Cancer		
25	Cancer	9:03 pm	Leo
26	Leo		
27	Leo		
28	Leo	12:46 am	Virgo
29	Virgo		
30	Virgo	3:18 am	Libra
31	Libra		

June

1	Libra	5:22 am	Scorpio
2	Scorpio		
3	Scorpio	8:01 am	Sagittarius
4	Sagittarius		
5	Sagittarius	12:26 pm	Capricorn
6	Capricorn		
7	Capricorn	7:39 pm	Aquarius
8	Aquarius		
9	Aquarius		
10	Aquarius	5:57 am	Pisces
11	Pisces		
12	Pisces	6:14 pm	Aries
13	Aries		
14	Aries		
15	Aries	6:19 am	Taurus
16	Taurus		
17	Taurus	4:12 pm	Gemini
18	Gemini		
19	Gemini	11:05 pm	Cancer
20	Cancer		
21	Cancer		
22	Cancer	3:26 am	Leo
23	Leo		
24	Leo	6:18 am	Virgo
25	Virgo		
26	Virgo	8:45 am	Libra
27	Libra		
28	Libra	11:37 am	Scorpio
29	Scorpio		
30	Scorpio	3:28 pm	Sagittarius

MOONPOSITIONS 1993

July

1	Sagittarius		
2	Sagittarius	8:49 pm	Capricorn
3	Capricorn		
4	Capricorn		
5	Capricorn	4:14 am	Aquarius
6	Aquarius		
7	Aquarius	2:10 pm	Pisces
8	Pisces		
9	Pisces		
10	Pisces	2:11 am	Aries
11	Aries		
12	Aries	2:37 pm	Taurus
13	Taurus		
14	Taurus		
15	Taurus	1:07 am	Gemini
16	Gemini		
17	Gemini	8:08 am	Cancer
18	Cancer		
19	Cancer	11:47 am	Leo
20	Leo		
21	Leo	1:24 pm	Virgo
22	Virgo		
23	Virgo	2:39 pm	Libra
24	Libra		
25	Libra	5:00 pm	Scorpio
26	Scorpio		
27	Scorpio	9:13 pm	Sagittarius
28	Sagittarius		
29	Sagittarius		
30	Sagittarius	3:27 am	Capricorn
31	Capricorn		

August

1	Capricorn	11:36 am	Aquarius
2	Aquarius		
3	Aquarius	9:44 pm	Pisces
4	Pisces		
5	Pisces		
6	Pisces	9:39 am	Aries
7	Aries		
8	Aries	10:22 pm	Taurus
9	Taurus		
10	Taurus		
11	Taurus	9:47 am	Gemini
12	Gemini		
13	Gemini	5:46 pm	Cancer
14	Cancer		
15	Cancer	9:43 pm	Leo
16	Leo		
17	Leo	10:41 pm	Virgo
18	Virgo		
19	Virgo	10:35 pm	Libra
20	Libra		
21	Libra	11:27 pm	Scorpio
22	Scorpio		
23	Scorpio		
24	Scorpio	2:45 am	Sagittarius
25	Sagittarius		
26	Sagittarius	8:58 am	Capricorn
27	Capricorn		
28	Capricorn	5:42 pm	Aquarius
29	Aquarius		
30	Aquarius		
31	Aquarius	4:19 am	Pisces

September

1	Pisces		
2	Pisces	4:21 pm	Aries
3	Aries		
4	Aries		
5	Aries	5:09 am	Taurus
6	Taurus		
7	Taurus	5:16 pm	Gemini
8	Gemini		
9	Gemini		
10	Gemini	2:37 am	Cancer
11	Cancer		
12	Cancer	7:51 am	Leo
13	Leo		
14	Leo	9:20 am	Virgo
15	Virgo		
16	Virgo	8:44 am	Libra
17	Libra		
18	Libra	8:15 am	Scorpio
19	Scorpio		
20	Scorpio	9:53 am	Sagittarius
21	Sagittarius		
22	Sagittarius	2:54 pm	Capricorn
23	Capricorn		
24	Capricorn	11:19 pm	Aquarius
25	Aquarius		
26	Aquarius		
27	Aquarius	10:13 am	Pisces
28	Pisces		
29	Pisces	10:29 pm	Aries
30	Aries		

October

1	Aries		
2	Aries	11:13 am	Taurus
3	Taurus		
4	Taurus	11:27 pm	Gemini
5	Gemini		
6	Gemini		
7	Gemini	9:42 am	Cancer
8	Cancer		
9	Cancer	4:34 pm	Leo
10	Leo		
11	Leo	7:36 pm	Virgo
12	Virgo		
13	Virgo	7:47 pm	Libra
14	Libra		
15	Libra	7:01 pm	Scorpio
16	Scorpio		
17	Scorpio	7:23 pm	Sagittarius
18	Sagittarius		
19	Sagittarius	10:42 pm	Capricorn
20	Capricorn		
21	Capricorn		
22	Capricorn	5:49 am	Aquarius
23	Aquarius		
24	Aquarius	4:17 pm	Pisces
25	Pisces		
26	Pisces		
27	Pisces	4:39 am	Aries
28	Aries		
29	Aries	5:20 pm	Taurus
30	Taurus		
31	Taurus		

November

1	Taurus	5:13 am	Gemini
2	Gemini		
3	Gemini	3:25 pm	Cancer
4	Cancer		
5	Cancer	11:06 pm	Leo
6	Leo		
7	Leo		
8	Leo	3:47 am	Virgo
9	Virgo		
10	Virgo	5:42 am	Libra
11	Libra		
12	Libra	6:00 am	Scorpio
13	Scorpio		
14	Scorpio	6:20 am	Sagittarius
15	Sagittarius		
16	Sagittarius	8:34 am	Capricorn
17	Capricorn		
18	Capricorn	2:08 pm	Aquarius
19	Aquarius		
20	Aquarius	11:27 pm	Pisces
21	Pisces		
22	Pisces		
23	Pisces	11:30 am	Aries
24	Aries		
25	Aries		
26	Aries	12:14 am	Taurus
27	Taurus		
28	Taurus	11:48 am	Gemini
29	Gemini		
30	Gemini	9:17 pm	Cancer

December

1	Cancer		
2	Cancer		
3	Cancer	4:33 am	Leo
4	Leo		
5	Leo	9:43 am	Virgo
6	Virgo		
7	Virgo	1:03 pm	Libra
8	Libra		
9	Libra	3:04 pm	Scorpio
10	Scorpio		
11	Scorpio	4:39 pm	Sagittarius
12	Sagittarius		
13	Sagittarius	7:06 pm	Capricorn
14	Capricorn		
15	Capricorn	11:51 pm	Aquarius
16	Aquarius		
17	Aquarius		
18	Aquarius	7:59 am	Pisces
19	Pisces		
20	Pisces	7:19 pm	Aries
21	Aries		
22	Aries		
23	Aries	8:05 am	Taurus
24	Taurus		
25	Taurus	7:46 pm	Gemini
26	Gemini		
27	Gemini		
28	Gemini	4:46 am	Cancer
29	Cancer		
30	Cancer	10:59 am	Leo
31	Leo		

MOON POSITIONS 1994

January

1	Leo	3:15 pm	Virgo
2	Virgo		
3	Virgo	6:31 pm	Libra
4	Libra		
5	Libra	9:29 pm	Scorpio
6	Scorpio		
7	Scorpio		
8	Scorpio	12:34 am	Sagittarius
9	Sagittarius		
10	Sagittarius	4:16 am	Capricorn
11	Capricorn		
12	Capricorn	9:25 am	Aquarius
13	Aquarius		
14	Aquarius	5:04 pm	Pisces
15	Pisces		
16	Pisces		
17	Pisces	3:42 am	Aries
18	Aries		
19	Aries	4:22 pm	Taurus
20	Taurus		
21	Taurus		
22	Taurus	4:35 am	Gemini
23	Gemini		
24	Gemini	1:55 pm	Cancer
25	Cancer		
26	Cancer	7:38 pm	Leo
27	Leo		
28	Leo	10:39 pm	Virgo
29	Virgo		
30	Virgo		
31	Virgo	12:34 am	Libra

February

1	Libra		
2	Libra	2:49 am	Scorpio
3	Scorpio		
4	Scorpio	6:14 am	Sagittarius
5	Sagittarius		
6	Sagittarius	11:02 am	Capricorn
7	Capricorn		
8	Capricorn	5:16 am	Aquarius
9	Aquarius		
10	Aquarius		
11	Aquarius	1:23 pm	Pisces
12	Pisces		
13	Pisces	11:49 am	Aries
14	Aries		
15	Aries		
16	Aries	12:20 pm	Taurus
17	Taurus		
18	Taurus	1:05 pm	Gemini
19	Gemini		
20	Gemini	11:27 am	Cancer
21	Cancer		
22	Cancer		
23	Cancer	5:48 am	Leo
24	Leo		
25	Leo	8:27 am	Virgo
26	Virgo		
27	Virgo	9:06 am	Libra
28	Libra		

March

1	Libra	9:43 am	Scorpio
2	Scorpio		
3	Scorpio	11:54 am	Sagittarius
4	Sagittarius		
5	Sagittarius	4:24 pm	Capricorn
6	Capricorn		
7	Capricorn	11:15 pm	Aquarius
8	Aquarius		
9	Aquarius		
10	Aquarius	8:09 am	Pisces
11	Pisces		
12	Pisces	6:59 pm	Aries
13	Aries		
14	Aries		
15	Aries	7:27 am	Taurus
16	Taurus		
17	Taurus	8:29 am	Gemini
18	Gemini		
19	Gemini		
20	Gemini	7:54 am	Cancer
21	Cancer		
22	Cancer	3:39 pm	Leo
23	Leo		
24	Leo	7:14 pm	Virgo
25	Virgo		
26	Virgo	7:46 pm	Libra
27	Libra		
28	Libra	7:15 pm	Scorpio
29	Scorpio		
30	Scorpio	7:41 pm	Sagittarius
31	Sagittarius		

April

1	Sagittarius	10:38 pm	Capricorn
2	Capricorn		
3	Capricorn		
4	Capricorn	4:45 am	Aquarius
5	Aquarius		
6	Aquarius	1:51 pm	Pisces
7	Pisces		
8	Pisces		
9	Pisces	1:09 am	Aries
10	Aries		
11	Aries	1:48 pm	Taurus
12	Taurus		
13	Taurus		
14	Taurus	2:48 am	Gemini
15	Gemini		
16	Gemini	2:41 pm	Cancer
17	Cancer		
18	Cancer	11:45 pm	Leo
19	Leo		
20	Leo		
21	Leo	4:58 am	Virgo
22	Virgo		
23	Virgo	6:40 am	Libra
24	Libra		
25	Libra	6:18 am	Scorpio
26	Scorpio		
27	Scorpio	5:48 am	Sagittarius
28	Sagittarius		
29	Sagittarius	7:05 am	Capricorn
30	Capricorn		

May

1	Capricorn	11:34 am	Aquarius
2	Aquarius		
3	Aquarius	7:47 pm	Pisces
4	Pisces		
5	Pisces		
6	Pisces	7:01 am	Aries
7	Aries		
8	Aries	7:50 pm	Taurus
9	Taurus		
10	Taurus		
11	Taurus	8:43 am	Gemini
12	Gemini		
13	Gemini	8:27 pm	Cancer
14	Cancer		
15	Cancer		
16	Cancer	5:58 am	Leo
17	Leo		
18	Leo	12:31 pm	Virgo
19	Virgo		
20	Virgo	3:54 pm	Libra
21	Libra		
22	Libra	4:51 pm	Scorpio
23	Scorpio		
24	Scorpio	4:43 pm	Sagittarius
25	Sagittarius		
26	Sagittarius	5:17 pm	Capricorn
27	Capricorn		
28	Capricorn	8:19 pm	Aquarius
29	Aquarius		
30	Aquarius		
31	Aquarius	3:03 am	Pisces

June

1	Pisces		
2	Pisces	1:31 pm	Aries
3	Aries		
4	Aries		
5	Aries	2:14 am	Taurus
6	Taurus		
7	Taurus	3:03 pm	Gemini
8	Gemini		
9	Gemini		
10	Gemini	2:22 am	Cancer
11	Cancer		
12	Cancer	11:29 am	Leo
13	Leo		
14	Leo	6:16 pm	Virgo
15	Virgo		
16	Virgo	10:48 pm	Libra
17	Libra		
18	Libra		
19	Libra	1:20 am	Scorpio
20	Scorpio		
21	Scorpio	2:32 am	Sagittarius
22	Sagittarius		
23	Sagittarius	3:37 am	Capricorn
24	Capricorn		
25	Capricorn	6:10 am	Aquarius
26	Aquarius		
27	Aquarius	11:44 am	Pisces
28	Pisces		
29	Pisces	9:07 pm	Aries
30	Aries		

MOON POSITIONS 1994

July

1	Aries		
2	Aries	9:23 am	Taurus
3	Taurus		
4	Taurus	10:12 pm	Gemini
5	Gemini		
6	Gemini		
7	Gemini	9:17 am	Cancer
8	Cancer		
9	Cancer	5:43 pm	Leo
10	Leo		
11	Leo	11:48 pm	Virgo
12	Virgo		
13	Virgo		
14	Virgo	4:15 am	Libra
15	Libra		
16	Libra	7:35 am	Scorpio
17	Scorpio		
18	Scorpio	10:09 am	Sagittarius
19	Sagittarius		
20	Sagittarius	12:30 pm	Capricorn
21	Capricorn		
22	Capricorn	3:38 pm	Aquarius
23	Aquarius		
24	Aquarius	8:56 pm	Pisces
25	Pisces		
26	Pisces		
27	Pisces	5:31 am	Aries
28	Aries		
29	Aries	5:13 pm	Taurus
30	Taurus		
31	Taurus		

August

1	Taurus	6:05 am	Gemini
2	Gemini		
3	Gemini	5:22 pm	Cancer
4	Cancer		
5	Cancer		
6	Cancer	1:31 am	Leo
7	Leo		
8	Leo	6:42 am	Virgo
9	Virgo		
10	Virgo	10:07 am	Libra
11	Libra		
12	Libra	12:56 pm	Scorpio
13	Scorpio		
14	Scorpio	3:53 pm	Sagittarius
15	Sagittarius		
16	Sagittarius	7:18 pm	Capricorn
17	Capricorn		
18	Capricorn	11:34 pm	Aquarius
19	Aquarius		
20	Aquarius		
21	Aquarius	5:27 am	Pisces
22	Pisces		
23	Pisces	1:55 pm	Aries
24	Aries		
25	Aries		
26	Aries	1:13 am	Taurus
27	Taurus		
28	Taurus	2:07 pm	Gemini
29	Gemini		
30	Gemini		
31	Gemini	2:00 am	Cancer

September

1	Cancer		
2	Cancer	10:37 am	Leo
3	Leo		
4	Leo	3:33 pm	Virgo
5	Virgo		
6	Virgo	5:57 pm	Libra
7	Libra		
8	Libra	7:26 pm	Scorpio
9	Scorpio		
10	Scorpio	9:25 pm	Sagittarius
11	Sagittarius		
12	Sagittarius		
13	Sagittarius	12:44 am	Capricorn
14	Capricorn		
15	Capricorn	5:42 am	Aquarius
16	Aquarius		
17	Aquarius	12:31 pm	Pisces
18	Pisces		
19	Pisces	9:30 pm	Aries
20	Aries		
21	Aries		
22	Aries	8:47 am	Taurus
23	Taurus		
24	Taurus	9:41 pm	Gemini
25	Gemini		
26	Gemini		
27	Gemini	10:12 am	Cancer
28	Cancer		
29	Cancer	7:55 pm	Leo
30	Leo		

October

1	Leo		
2	Leo	1:39 am	Virgo
3	Virgo		
4	Virgo	3:56 am	Libra
5	Libra		
6	Libra	4:22 am	Scorpio
7	Scorpio		
8	Scorpio	4:47 am	Sagittarius
9	Sagittarius		
10	Sagittarius	6:44 am	Capricorn
11	Capricorn		
12	Capricorn	11:09 am	Aquarius
13	Aquarius		
14	Aquarius	6:18 pm	Pisces
15	Pisces		
16	Pisces		
17	Pisces	3:56 am	Aries
18	Aries		
19	Aries	3:34 pm	Taurus
20	Taurus		
21	Taurus		
22	Taurus	4:28 am	Gemini
23	Gemini		
24	Gemini	5:15 pm	Cancer
25	Cancer		
26	Cancer		
27	Cancer	4:05 am	Leo
28	Leo		
29	Leo	11:21 am	Virgo
30	Virgo		
31	Virgo	2:46 pm	Libra

November

1	Libra		
2	Libra	3:19 pm	Scorpio
3	Scorpio		
4	Scorpio	2:46 pm	Sagittarius
5	Sagittarius		
6	Sagittarius	3:02 pm	Capricorn
7	Capricorn		
8	Capricorn	5:48 pm	Aquarius
9	Aquarius		
10	Aquarius		
11	Aquarius	12:04 am	Pisces
12	Pisces		
13	Pisces	9:44 am	Aries
14	Aries		
15	Aries	9:44 pm	Taurus
16	Taurus		
17	Taurus		
18	Taurus	10:41 am	Gemini
19	Gemini		
20	Gemini	11:21 pm	Cancer
21	Cancer		
22	Cancer		
23	Cancer	10:33 am	Leo
24	Leo		
25	Leo	7:09 pm	Virgo
26	Virgo		
27	Virgo		
28	Virgo	12:22 am	Libra
29	Libra		
30	Libra	2:21 am	Scorpio

December

1	Scorpio		
2	Scorpio	2:13 am	Sagittarius
3	Sagittarius		
4	Sagittarius	1:42 am	Capricorn
5	Capricorn		
6	Capricorn	2:51 am	Aquarius
7	Aquarius		
8	Aquarius	7:24 am	Pisces
9	Pisces		
10	Pisces	4:03 pm	Aries
11	Aries		
12	Aries		
13	Aries	3:56 am	Taurus
14	Taurus		
15	Taurus	5:00 pm	Gemini
16	Gemini		
17	Gemini		
18	Gemini	5:25 am	Cancer
19	Cancer		
20	Cancer	4:13 pm	Leo
21	Leo		
22	Leo		
23	Leo	1:01 am	Virgo
24	Virgo		
25	Virgo	7:27 am	Libra
26	Libra		
27	Libra	11:17 am	Scorpio
28	Scorpio		
29	Scorpio	12:45 pm	Sagittarius
30	Sagittarius		
31	Sagittarius	12:57 pm	Capricorn

MOON POSITIONS 1995

January

1	Capricorn		
2	Capricorn	1:39 pm	Aquarius
3	Aquarius		
4	Aquarius	4:49 pm	Pisces
5	Pisces		
6	Pisces	11:56 pm	Aries
7	Aries		
8	Aries		
9	Aries	10:58 am	Taurus
10	Taurus		
11	Taurus	11:57 pm	Gemini
12	Gemini		
13	Gemini		
14	Gemini	12:20 pm	Cancer
15	Cancer		
16	Cancer	10:36 pm	Leo
17	Leo		
18	Leo		
19	Leo	6:39 am	Virgo
20	Virgo		
21	Virgo	12:54 pm	Libra
22	Libra		
23	Libra	5:32 pm	Scorpio
24	Scorpio		
25	Scorpio	8:37 pm	Sagittarius
26	Sagittarius		
27	Sagittarius	10:26 pm	Capricorn
28	Capricorn		
29	Capricorn		
30	Capricorn	12:03 am	Aquarius
31	Aquarius		

February

1	Aquarius	3:05 am	Pisces
2	Pisces		
3	Pisces	9:12 am	Aries
4	Aries		
5	Aries	7:09 pm	Taurus
6	Taurus		
7	Taurus		
8	Taurus	7:44 am	Gemini
9	Gemini		
10	Gemini	8:17 pm	Cancer
11	Cancer		
12	Cancer		
13	Cancer	6:31 am	Leo
14	Leo		
15	Leo	1:52 pm	Virgo
16	Virgo		
17	Virgo	7:00 pm	Libra
18	Libra		
19	Libra	10:55 pm	Scorpio
20	Scorpio		
21	Scorpio		
22	Scorpio	2:13 am	Sagittarius
23	Sagittarius		
24	Sagittarius	5:11 am	Capricorn
25	Capricorn		
26	Capricorn	8:14 am	Aquarius
27	Aquarius		
28	Aquarius	12:16 pm	Pisces

March

1	Pisces		
2	Pisces	6:30 pm	Aries
3	Aries		
4	Aries		
5	Aries	3:50 am	Taurus
6	Taurus		
7	Taurus	3:55 pm	Gemini
8	Gemini		
9	Gemini		
10	Gemini	4:40 am	Cancer
11	Cancer		
12	Cancer	3:28 pm	Leo
13	Leo		
14	Leo	10:54 pm	Virgo
15	Virgo		
16	Virgo		
17	Virgo	3:18 am	Libra
18	Libra		
19	Libra	5:52 am	Scorpio
20	Scorpio		
21	Scorpio	7:57 am	Sagittarius
22	Sagittarius		
23	Sagittarius	10:31 am	Capricorn
24	Capricorn		
25	Capricorn	2:10 pm	Aquarius
26	Aquarius		
27	Aquarius	7:18 pm	Pisces
28	Pisces		
29	Pisces		
30	Pisces	2:26 am	Aries
31	Aries		

April

1	Aries	11:59 am	Taurus
2	Taurus		
3	Taurus	11:49 pm	Gemini
4	Gemini		
5	Gemini		
6	Gemini	12:40 pm	Cancer
7	Cancer		
8	Cancer		
9	Cancer	12:16 am	Leo
10	Leo		
11	Leo	8:39 am	Virgo
12	Virgo		
13	Virgo	1:20 pm	Libra
14	Libra		
15	Libra	3:13 pm	Scorpio
16	Scorpio		
17	Scorpio	3:52 pm	Sagittarius
18	Sagittarius		
19	Sagittarius	4:54 pm	Capricorn
20	Capricorn		
21	Capricorn	7:38 pm	Aquarius
22	Aquarius		
23	Aquarius		
24	Aquarius	12:51 am	Pisces
25	Pisces		
26	Pisces	8:41 am	Aries
27	Aries		
28	Aries	6:53 pm	Taurus
29	Taurus		
30	Taurus		

May

1	Taurus	6:53 am	Gemini
2	Gemini		
3	Gemini	7:45 pm	Cancer
4	Cancer		
5	Cancer		
6	Cancer	7:55 am	Leo
7	Leo		
8	Leo	5:33 pm	Virgo
9	Virgo		
10	Virgo	11:30 pm	Libra
11	Libra		
12	Libra		
13	Libra	1:53 am	Scorpio
14	Scorpio		
15	Scorpio	1:58 am	Sagittarius
16	Sagittarius		
17	Sagittarius	1:36 am	Capricorn
18	Capricorn		
19	Capricorn	2:39 am	Aquarius
20	Aquarius		
21	Aquarius	6:40 am	Pisces
22	Pisces		
23	Pisces	2:13 pm	Aries
24	Aries		
25	Aries		
26	Aries	12:46 am	Taurus
27	Taurus		
28	Taurus	1:07 pm	Gemini
29	Gemini		
30	Gemini		
31	Gemini	1:59 am	Cancer

June

1	Cancer		
2	Cancer	2:17 pm	Leo
3	Leo		
4	Leo		
5	Leo	12:46 am	Virgo
6	Virgo		
7	Virgo	8:13 am	Libra
8	Libra		
9	Libra	12:03 pm	Scorpio
10	Scorpio		
11	Scorpio	12:50 pm	Sagittarius
12	Sagittarius		
13	Sagittarius	12:05 pm	Capricorn
14	Capricorn		
15	Capricorn	11:52 am	Aquarius
16	Aquarius		
17	Aquarius	2:13 pm	Pisces
18	Pisces		
19	Pisces	8:29 pm	Aries
20	Aries		
21	Aries		
22	Aries	6:35 am	Taurus
23	Taurus		
24	Taurus	7:02 pm	Gemini
25	Gemini		
26	Gemini		
27	Gemini	7:56 am	Cancer
28	Cancer		
29	Cancer	8:02 pm	Leo
30	Leo		

MOON POSITIONS 1995

July

1	Leo		
2	Leo	6:35 am	Virgo
3	Virgo		
4	Virgo	2:55 pm	Libra
5	Libra		
6	Libra	8:19 pm	Scorpio
7	Scorpio		
8	Scorpio	10:37 am	Sagittarius
9	Sagittarius		
10	Sagittarius	10:43 pm	Capricorn
11	Capricorn		
12	Capricorn	10:21 pm	Aquarius
13	Aquarius		
14	Aquarius	11:37 pm	Pisces
15	Pisces		
16	Pisces		
17	Pisces	4:23 am	Aries
18	Aries		
19	Aries	1:20 pm	Taurus
20	Taurus		
21	Taurus		
22	Taurus	1:23 am	Gemini
23	Gemini		
24	Gemini	2:16 pm	Cancer
25	Cancer		
26	Cancer		
27	Cancer	2:07 am	Leo
28	Leo		
29	Leo	12:12 pm	Virgo
30	Virgo		
31	Virgo	8:23 pm	Libra

August

1	Libra		
2	Libra		
3	Libra	2:29 am	Scorpio
4	Scorpio		
5	Scorpio	6:14 am	Sagittarius
6	Sagittarius		
7	Sagittarius	7:52 am	Capricorn
8	Capricorn		
9	Capricorn	8:28 am	Aquarius
10	Aquarius		
11	Aquarius	9:46 am	Pisces
12	Pisces		
13	Pisces	1:41 pm	Aries
14	Aries		
15	Aries	9:25 pm	Taurus
16	Taurus		
17	Taurus		
18	Taurus	8:40 am	Gemini
19	Gemini		
20	Gemini	9:24 pm	Cancer
21	Cancer		
22	Cancer		
23	Cancer	9:13 am	Leo
24	Leo		
25	Leo	6:50 pm	Virgo
26	Virgo		
27	Virgo		
28	Virgo	2:15 am	Libra
29	Libra		
30	Libra	7:51 am	Scorpio
31	Scorpio		

September

1	Scorpio	11:57 am	Sagittarius
2	Sagittarius		
3	Sagittarius	2:45 pm	Capricorn
4	Capricorn		
5	Capricorn	4:47 pm	Aquarius
6	Aquarius		
7	Aquarius	7:08 pm	Pisces
8	Pisces		
9	Pisces	11:14 pm	Aries
10	Aries		
11	Aries		
12	Aries	6:21 am	Taurus
13	Taurus		
14	Taurus	4:48 pm	Gemini
15	Gemini		
16	Gemini		
17	Gemini	5:16 am	Cancer
18	Cancer		
19	Cancer	5:19 pm	Leo
20	Leo		
21	Leo		
22	Leo	3:01 am	Virgo
23	Virgo		
24	Virgo	9:50 am	Libra
25	Libra		
26	Libra	2:20 pm	Scorpio
27	Scorpio		
28	Scorpio	5:30 pm	Sagittarius
29	Sagittarius		
30	Sagittarius	8:10 pm	Capricorn

October

1	Capricorn		
2	Capricorn	10:59 pm	Aquarius
3	Aquarius		
4	Aquarius		
5	Aquarius	2:35 am	Pisces
6	Pisces		
7	Pisces	7:42 am	Aries
8	Aries		
9	Aries	3:05 pm	Taurus
10	Taurus		
11	Taurus		
12	Taurus	1:10 am	Gemini
13	Gemini		
14	Gemini	1:20 pm	Cancer
15	Cancer		
16	Cancer		
17	Cancer	1:46 am	Leo
18	Leo		
19	Leo	12:11 pm	Virgo
20	Virgo		
21	Virgo	7:15 pm	Libra
22	Libra		
23	Libra	11:06 pm	Scorpio
24	Scorpio		
25	Scorpio		
26	Scorpio	12:56 am	Sagittarius
27	Sagittarius		
28	Sagittarius	2:15 am	Capricorn
29	Capricorn		
30	Capricorn	4:23 am	Aquarius
31	Aquarius		

November

1	Aquarius	8:17 am	Pisces
2	Pisces		
3	Pisces	2:21 pm	Aries
4	Aries		
5	Aries	10:35 pm	Taurus
6	Taurus		
7	Taurus		
8	Taurus	8:55 am	Gemini
9	Gemini		
10	Gemini	8:57 pm	Cancer
11	Cancer		
12	Cancer		
13	Cancer	9:37 am	Leo
14	Leo		
15	Leo	9:02 pm	Virgo
16	Virgo		
17	Virgo		
18	Virgo	5:18 am	Libra
19	Libra		
20	Libra	9:40 am	Scorpio
21	Scorpio		
22	Scorpio	10:56 am	Sagittarius
23	Sagittarius		
24	Sagittarius	10:48 am	Capricorn
25	Capricorn		
26	Capricorn	11:15 am	Aquarius
27	Aquarius		
28	Aquarius	1:59 pm	Pisces
29	Pisces		
30	Pisces	7:51 pm	Aries

December

1	Aries		
2	Aries		
3	Aries	4:40 am	Taurus
4	Taurus		
5	Taurus	3:35 pm	Gemini
6	Gemini		
7	Gemini		
8	Gemini	3:44 am	Cancer
9	Cancer		
10	Cancer	4:24 pm	Leo
11	Leo		
12	Leo		
13	Leo	4:26 am	Virgo
14	Virgo		
15	Virgo	2:09 pm	Libra
16	Libra		
17	Libra	8:07 pm	Scorpio
18	Scorpio		
19	Scorpio	10:13 pm	Sagittarius
20	Sagittarius		
21	Sagittarius	9:46 pm	Capricorn
22	Capricorn		
23	Capricorn	8:52 pm	Aquarius
24	Aquarius		
25	Aquarius	9:45 pm	Pisces
26	Pisces		
27	Pisces		
28	Pisces	2:06 am	Aries
29	Aries		
30	Aries	10:21 am	Taurus
31	Taurus		

MOON POSITIONS 1996

January

1	Taurus	9:29 pm	Gemini
2	Gemini		
3	Gemini		
4	Gemini	9:56 am	Cancer
5	Cancer		
6	Cancer	10:30 pm	Leo
7	Leo		
8	Leo		
9	Leo	10:29 am	Virgo
10	Virgo		
11	Virgo	8:55 pm	Libra
12	Libra		
13	Libra		
14	Libra	4:30 am	Scorpio
15	Scorpio		
16	Scorpio	8:25 am	Sagittarius
17	Sagittarius		
18	Sagittarius	9:07 am	Capricorn
19	Capricorn		
20	Capricorn	8:15 am	Aquarius
21	Aquarius		
22	Aquarius	8:02 am	Pisces
23	Pisces		
24	Pisces	10:37 am	Aries
25	Aries		
26	Aries	5:16 pm	Taurus
27	Taurus		
28	Taurus		
29	Taurus	3:42 am	Gemini
30	Gemini		
31	Gemini	4:11 pm	Cancer

February

1	Cancer		
2	Cancer		
3	Cancer	4:46 am	Leo
4	Leo		
5	Leo	4:22 pm	Virgo
6	Virgo		
7	Virgo		
8	Virgo	2:30 am	Libra
9	Libra		
10	Libra	10:35 am	Scorpio
11	Scorpio		
12	Scorpio	3:58 pm	Sagittarius
13	Sagittarius		
14	Sagittarius	6:29 pm	Capricorn
15	Capricorn		
16	Capricorn	7:00 pm	Aquarius
17	Aquarius		
18	Aquarius	7:09 pm	Pisces
19	Pisces		
20	Pisces	8:58 pm	Aries
21	Aries		
22	Aries		
23	Aries	2:08 am	Taurus
24	Taurus		
25	Taurus	11:14 am	Gemini
26	Gemini		
27	Gemini	11:10 pm	Cancer
28	Cancer		
29	Cancer		

March

1	Cancer	11:47 am	Leo
2	Leo		
3	Leo	11:13 pm	Virgo
4	Virgo		
5	Virgo		
6	Virgo	8:40 am	Libra
7	Libra		
8	Libra	4:05 pm	Scorpio
9	Scorpio		
10	Scorpio	9:32 pm	Sagittarius
11	Sagittarius		
12	Sagittarius		
13	Sagittarius	1:08 am	Capricorn
14	Capricorn		
15	Capricorn	3:15 am	Aquarius
16	Aquarius		
17	Aquarius	4:50 am	Pisces
18	Pisces		
19	Pisces	7:15 am	Aries
20	Aries		
21	Aries	11:59 am	Taurus
22	Taurus		
23	Taurus	7:59 pm	Gemini
24	Gemini		
25	Gemini		
26	Gemini	7:06 am	Cancer
27	Cancer		
28	Cancer	7:37 pm	Leo
29	Leo		
30	Leo		
31	Leo	7:15 am	Virgo

April

1	Virgo		
2	Virgo	4:26 pm	Libra
3	Libra		
4	Libra	10:57 pm	Scorpio
5	Scorpio		
6	Scorpio		
7	Scorpio	3:21 am	Sagittarius
8	Sagittarius		
9	Sagittarius	6:30 am	Capricorn
10	Capricorn		
11	Capricorn	9:09 am	Aquarius
12	Aquarius		
13	Aquarius	12:00 pm	Pisces
14	Pisces		
15	Pisces	3:43 pm	Aries
16	Aries		
17	Aries	9:05 pm	Taurus
18	Taurus		
19	Taurus		
20	Taurus	4:54 am	Gemini
21	Gemini		
22	Gemini	3:25 pm	Cancer
23	Cancer		
24	Cancer		
25	Cancer	3:44 am	Leo
26	Leo		
27	Leo	3:49 pm	Virgo
28	Virgo		
29	Virgo		
30	Virgo	1:27 am	Libra

May

1	Libra		
2	Libra	7:42 am	Scorpio
3	Scorpio		
4	Scorpio	11:05 am	Sagittarius
5	Sagittarius		
6	Sagittarius	12:54 pm	Capricorn
7	Capricorn		
8	Capricorn	2:39 pm	Aquarius
9	Aquarius		
10	Aquarius	5:29 pm	Pisces
11	Pisces		
12	Pisces	10:00 pm	Aries
13	Aries		
14	Aries		
15	Aries	4:25 am	Taurus
16	Taurus		
17	Taurus	12:48 pm	Gemini
18	Gemini		
19	Gemini	11:16 pm	Cancer
20	Cancer		
21	Cancer		
22	Cancer	11:28 am	Leo
23	Leo		
24	Leo	11:58 pm	Virgo
25	Virgo		
26	Virgo		
27	Virgo	10:33 am	Libra
28	Libra		
29	Libra	5:30 pm	Scorpio
30	Scorpio		
31	Scorpio	8:43 pm	Sagittarius

June

1	Sagittarius		
2	Sagittarius	9:29 pm	Capricorn
3	Capricorn		
4	Capricorn	9:45 pm	Aquarius
5	Aquarius		
6	Aquarius	11:19 pm	Pisces
7	Pisces		
8	Pisces		
9	Pisces	3:23 am	Aries
10	Aries		
11	Aries	10:11 am	Taurus
12	Taurus		
13	Taurus	7:16 pm	Gemini
14	Gemini		
15	Gemini		
16	Gemini	6:08 am	Cancer
17	Cancer		
18	Cancer	6:22 pm	Leo
19	Leo		
20	Leo		
21	Leo	7:07 am	Virgo
22	Virgo		
23	Virgo	6:37 pm	Libra
24	Libra		
25	Libra		
26	Libra	2:53 am	Scorpio
27	Scorpio		
28	Scorpio	7:01 am	Sagittarius
29	Sagittarius		
30	Sagittarius	7:47 am	Capricorn

MOON POSITIONS 1996

July

1	Capricorn		
2	Capricorn	7:05 am	Aquarius
3	Aquarius		
4	Aquarius	7:07 am	Pisces
5	Pisces		
6	Pisces	9:42 am	Aries
7	Aries		
8	Aries	3:43 pm	Taurus
9	Taurus		
10	Taurus		
11	Taurus	12:52 am	Gemini
12	Gemini		
13	Gemini	12:08 pm	Cancer
14	Cancer		
15	Cancer		
16	Cancer	12:31 am	Leo
17	Leo		
18	Leo	1:16 pm	Virgo
19	Virgo		
20	Virgo		
21	Virgo	1:14 am	Libra
22	Libra		
23	Libra	10:43 am	Scorpio
24	Scorpio		
25	Scorpio	4:24 pm	Sagittarius
26	Sagittarius		
27	Sagittarius	6:17 pm	Capricorn
28	Capricorn		
29	Capricorn	5:47 pm	Aquarius
30	Aquarius		
31	Aquarius	5:01 pm	Pisces

August

1	Pisces		
2	Pisces	6:05 pm	Aries
3	Aries		
4	Aries	10:33 pm	Taurus
5	Taurus		
6	Taurus		
7	Taurus	6:49 am	Gemini
8	Gemini		
9	Gemini	5:57 pm	Cancer
10	Cancer		
11	Cancer		
12	Cancer	6:29 am	Leo
13	Leo		
14	Leo	7:07 pm	Virgo
15	Virgo		
16	Virgo		
17	Virgo	6:55 am	Libra
18	Libra		
19	Libra	4:50 pm	Scorpio
20	Scorpio		
21	Scorpio	11:48 pm	Sagittarius
22	Sagittarius		
23	Sagittarius		
24	Sagittarius	3:22 am	Capricorn
25	Capricorn		
26	Capricorn	4:10 am	Aquarius
27	Aquarius		
28	Aquarius	3:49 am	Pisces
29	Pisces		
30	Pisces	4:15 am	Aries
31	Aries		

September

1	Aries	7:19 am	Taurus
2	Taurus		
3	Taurus	2:08 pm	Gemini
4	Gemini		
5	Gemini		
6	Gemini	12:29 am	Cancer
7	Cancer		
8	Cancer	12:54 pm	Leo
9	Leo		
10	Leo		
11	Leo	1:28 am	Virgo
12	Virgo		
13	Virgo	12:51 pm	Libra
14	Libra		
15	Libra	10:20 pm	Scorpio
16	Scorpio		
17	Scorpio		
18	Scorpio	5:31 am	Sagittarius
19	Sagittarius		
20	Sagittarius	10:12 am	Capricorn
21	Capricorn		
22	Capricorn	12:39 pm	Aquarius
23	Aquarius		
24	Aquarius	1:43 pm	Pisces
25	Pisces		
26	Pisces	2:46 pm	Aries
27	Aries		
28	Aries	5:24 pm	Taurus
29	Taurus		
30	Taurus	11:01 pm	Gemini

October

1	Gemini		
2	Gemini		
3	Gemini	8:14 am	Cancer
4	Cancer		
5	Cancer	8:12 pm	Leo
6	Leo		
7	Leo		
8	Leo	8:49 am	Virgo
9	Virgo		
10	Virgo	8:00 pm	Libra
11	Libra		
12	Libra		
13	Libra	4:46 am	Scorpio
14	Scorpio		
15	Scorpio	11:07 am	Sagittarius
16	Sagittarius		
17	Sagittarius	3:37 pm	Capricorn
18	Capricorn		
19	Capricorn	6:51 pm	Aquarius
20	Aquarius		
21	Aquarius	9:22 pm	Pisces
22	Pisces		
23	Pisces	11:50 pm	Aries
24	Aries		
25	Aries		
26	Aries	3:11 am	Taurus
27	Taurus		
28	Taurus	8:35 am	Gemini
29	Gemini		
30	Gemini	4:56 pm	Cancer
31	Cancer		

November

1	Cancer		
2	Cancer	4:16 am	Leo
3	Leo		
4	Leo	4:57 pm	Virgo
5	Virgo		
6	Virgo		
7	Virgo	4:29 am	Libra
8	Libra		
9	Libra	1:02 pm	Scorpio
10	Scorpio		
11	Scorpio	6:26 pm	Sagittarius
12	Sagittarius		
13	Sagittarius	9:44 pm	Capricorn
14	Capricorn		
15	Capricorn		
16	Capricorn	12:14 am	Aquarius
17	Aquarius		
18	Aquarius	3:00 am	Pisces
19	Pisces		
20	Pisces	6:34 am	Aries
21	Aries		
22	Aries	11:12 am	Taurus
23	Taurus		
24	Taurus	5:20 pm	Gemini
25	Gemini		
26	Gemini		
27	Gemini	1:37 am	Cancer
28	Cancer		
29	Cancer	12:30 pm	Leo
30	Leo		

December

1	Leo		
2	Leo	1:11 am	Virgo
3	Virgo		
4	Virgo	1:23 pm	Libra
5	Libra		
6	Libra	10:39 pm	Scorpio
7	Scorpio		
8	Scorpio		
9	Scorpio	3:58 am	Sagittarius
10	Sagittarius		
11	Sagittarius	6:15 am	Capricorn
12	Capricorn		
13	Capricorn	7:14 am	Aquarius
14	Aquarius		
15	Aquarius	8:44 am	Pisces
16	Pisces		
17	Pisces	11:55 am	Aries
18	Aries		
19	Aries	5:10 pm	Taurus
20	Taurus		
21	Taurus		
22	Taurus	12:17 am	Gemini
23	Gemini		
24	Gemini	9:14 am	Cancer
25	Cancer		
26	Cancer	8:09 pm	Leo
27	Leo		
28	Leo		
29	Leo	8:45 am	Virgo
30	Virgo		
31	Virgo	9:32 pm	Libra

MOON POSITIONS 1997

January

1	Libra		
2	Libra		
3	Libra	8:02 am	Scorpio
4	Scorpio		
5	Scorpio	2:27 pm	Sagittarius
6	Sagittarius		
7	Sagittarius	4:55 pm	Capricorn
8	Capricorn		
9	Capricorn	5:00 pm	Aquarius
10	Aquarius		
11	Aquarius	4:51 pm	Pisces
12	Pisces		
13	Pisces	6:22 pm	Aries
14	Aries		
15	Aries	10:40 pm	Taurus
16	Taurus		
17	Taurus		
18	Taurus	5:53 am	Gemini
19	Gemini		
20	Gemini	3:29 pm	Cancer
21	Cancer		
22	Cancer		
23	Cancer	2:50 am	Leo
24	Leo		
25	Leo	3:26 pm	Virgo
26	Virgo		
27	Virgo		
28	Virgo	4:21 am	Libra
29	Libra		
30	Libra	3:48 pm	Scorpio
31	Scorpio		

February

1	Scorpio	11:51 pm	Sagittarius
2	Sagittarius		
3	Sagittarius		
4	Sagittarius	3:44 am	Capricorn
5	Capricorn		
6	Capricorn	4:21 am	Aquarius
7	Aquarius		
8	Aquarius	3:34 am	Pisces
9	Pisces		
10	Pisces	3:29 am	Aries
11	Aries		
12	Aries	5:56 am	Taurus
13	Taurus		
14	Taurus	11:53 am	Gemini
15	Gemini		
16	Gemini	9:13 pm	Cancer
17	Cancer		
18	Cancer		
19	Cancer	8:52 am	Leo
20	Leo		
21	Leo	9:38 pm	Virgo
22	Virgo		
23	Virgo		
24	Virgo	10:23 am	Libra
25	Libra		
26	Libra	9:57 pm	Scorpio
27	Scorpio		
28	Scorpio		

March

1	Scorpio	7:01 am	Sagittarius
2	Sagittarius		
3	Sagittarius	12:38 pm	Capricorn
4	Capricorn		
5	Capricorn	2:54 pm	Aquarius
6	Aquarius		
7	Aquarius	2:57 pm	Pisces
8	Pisces		
9	Pisces	2:33 pm	Aries
10	Aries		
11	Aries	3:37 pm	Taurus
12	Taurus		
13	Taurus	7:48 pm	Gemini
14	Gemini		
15	Gemini		
16	Gemini	3:51 am	Cancer
17	Cancer		
18	Cancer	3:08 pm	Leo
19	Leo		
20	Leo		
21	Leo	3:59 am	Virgo
22	Virgo		
23	Virgo	4:35 pm	Libra
24	Libra		
25	Libra		
26	Libra	3:42 am	Scorpio
27	Scorpio		
28	Scorpio	12:40 pm	Sagittarius
29	Sagittarius		
30	Sagittarius	7:07 pm	Capricorn
31	Capricorn		

April

1	Capricorn	10:59 pm	Aquarius
2	Aquarius		
3	Aquarius		
4	Aquarius	12:42 am	Pisces
5	Pisces		
6	Pisces	1:19 am	Aries
7	Aries		
8	Aries	2:20 am	Taurus
9	Taurus		
10	Taurus	5:28 am	Gemini
11	Gemini		
12	Gemini	12:03 pm	Cancer
13	Cancer		
14	Cancer	10:22 pm	Leo
15	Leo		
16	Leo		
17	Leo	11:00 am	Virgo
18	Virgo		
19	Virgo	11:36 pm	Libra
20	Libra		
21	Libra		
22	Libra	10:19 am	Scorpio
23	Scorpio		
24	Scorpio	6:32 pm	Sagittarius
25	Sagittarius		
26	Sagittarius		
27	Sagittarius	12:32 am	Capricorn
28	Capricorn		
29	Capricorn	4:50 am	Aquarius
30	Aquarius		

May

1	Aquarius	7:50 am	Pisces
2	Pisces		
3	Pisces	9:59 am	Aries
4	Aries		
5	Aries	12:04 pm	Taurus
6	Taurus		
7	Taurus	3:21 pm	Gemini
8	Gemini		
9	Gemini	9:13 pm	Cancer
10	Cancer		
11	Cancer		
12	Cancer	6:33 am	Leo
13	Leo		
14	Leo	6:43 pm	Virgo
15	Virgo		
16	Virgo		
17	Virgo	7:27 am	Libra
18	Libra		
19	Libra	6:11 pm	Scorpio
20	Scorpio		
21	Scorpio		
22	Scorpio	1:51 am	Sagittarius
23	Sagittarius		
24	Sagittarius	6:51 am	Capricorn
25	Capricorn		
26	Capricorn	10:20 am	Aquarius
27	Aquarius		
28	Aquarius	1:18 pm	Pisces
29	Pisces		
30	Pisces	4:18 pm	Aries
31	Aries		

June

1	Aries	7:39 pm	Taurus
2	Taurus		
3	Taurus	11:55 pm	Gemini
4	Gemini		
5	Gemini		
6	Gemini	6:02 am	Cancer
7	Cancer		
8	Cancer	2:58 pm	Leo
9	Leo		
10	Leo		
11	Leo	2:43 am	Virgo
12	Virgo		
13	Virgo	3:35 pm	Libra
14	Libra		
15	Libra		
16	Libra	2:51 am	Scorpio
17	Scorpio		
18	Scorpio	10:39 am	Sagittarius
19	Sagittarius		
20	Sagittarius	3:02 pm	Capricorn
21	Capricorn		
22	Capricorn	5:20 pm	Aquarius
23	Aquarius		
24	Aquarius	7:09 pm	Pisces
25	Pisces		
26	Pisces	9:38 pm	Aries
27	Aries		
28	Aries		
29	Aries	1:23 am	Taurus
30	Taurus		

MOON POSITIONS 1997

July

1	Taurus	6:35 am	Gemini
2	Gemini		
3	Gemini	1:33 pm	Cancer
4	Cancer		
5	Cancer	10:45 pm	Leo
6	Leo		
7	Leo		
8	Leo	10:22 am	Virgo
9	Virgo		
10	Virgo	11:21 pm	Libra
11	Libra		
12	Libra		
13	Libra	11:20 am	Scorpio
14	Scorpio		
15	Scorpio	8:02 pm	Sagittarius
16	Sagittarius		
17	Sagittarius		
18	Sagittarius	12:45 am	Capricorn
19	Capricorn		
20	Capricorn	2:29 am	Aquarius
21	Aquarius		
22	Aquarius	3:00 am	Pisces
23	Pisces		
24	Pisces	4:03 am	Aries
25	Aries		
26	Aries	6:53 am	Taurus
27	Taurus		
28	Taurus	12:04 pm	Gemini
29	Gemini		
30	Gemini	7:38 pm	Cancer
31	Cancer		

August

1	Cancer		
2	Cancer	5:27 am	Leo
3	Leo		
4	Leo	5:15 pm	Virgo
5	Virgo		
6	Virgo		
7	Virgo	6:17 am	Libra
8	Libra		
9	Libra	6:50 pm	Scorpio
10	Scorpio		
11	Scorpio		
12	Scorpio	4:45 am	Sagittarius
13	Sagittarius		
14	Sagittarius	10:42 am	Capricorn
15	Capricorn		
16	Capricorn	12:58 pm	Aquarius
17	Aquarius		
18	Aquarius	1:01 pm	Pisces
19	Pisces		
20	Pisces	12:45 pm	Aries
21	Aries		
22	Aries	1:57 pm	Taurus
23	Taurus		
24	Taurus	5:56 pm	Gemini
25	Gemini		
26	Gemini		
27	Gemini	1:11 am	Cancer
28	Cancer		
29	Cancer	11:19 am	Leo
30	Leo		
31	Leo	11:27 pm	Virgo

September

1	Virgo		
2	Virgo		
3	Virgo	12:30 pm	Libra
4	Libra		
5	Libra		
6	Libra	1:10 am	Scorpio
7	Scorpio		
8	Scorpio	11:54 am	Sagittarius
9	Sagittarius		
10	Sagittarius	7:23 pm	Capricorn
11	Capricorn		
12	Capricorn	11:10 pm	Aquarius
13	Aquarius		
14	Aquarius	11:59 pm	Pisces
15	Pisces		
16	Pisces	11:25 pm	Aries
17	Aries		
18	Aries	11:21 pm	Taurus
19	Taurus		
20	Taurus		
21	Taurus	1:38 am	Gemini
22	Gemini		
23	Gemini	7:33 am	Cancer
24	Cancer		
25	Cancer	5:12 pm	Leo
26	Leo		
27	Leo		
28	Leo	5:27 am	Virgo
29	Virgo		
30	Virgo	6:32 pm	Libra

October

1	Libra		
2	Libra		
3	Libra	6:57 am	Scorpio
4	Scorpio		
5	Scorpio	5:43 pm	Sagittarius
6	Sagittarius		
7	Sagittarius		
8	Sagittarius	2:04 am	Capricorn
9	Capricorn		
10	Capricorn	7:29 am	Aquarius
11	Aquarius		
12	Aquarius	9:59 am	Pisces
13	Pisces		
14	Pisces	10:25 am	Aries
15	Aries		
16	Aries	10:16 am	Taurus
17	Taurus		
18	Taurus	11:26 am	Gemini
19	Gemini		
20	Gemini	3:45 pm	Cancer
21	Cancer		
22	Cancer		
23	Cancer	12:10 am	Leo
24	Leo		
25	Leo	11:59 am	Virgo
26	Virgo		
27	Virgo		
28	Virgo	1:05 am	Libra
29	Libra		
30	Libra	1:15 pm	Scorpio
31	Scorpio		

November

1	Scorpio	11:27 pm	Sagittarius
2	Sagittarius		
3	Sagittarius		
4	Sagittarius	7:31 am	Capricorn
5	Capricorn		
6	Capricorn	1:33 pm	Aquarius
7	Aquarius		
8	Aquarius	5:34 pm	Pisces
9	Pisces		
10	Pisces	7:44 pm	Aries
11	Aries		
12	Aries	8:45 pm	Taurus
13	Taurus		
14	Taurus	10:05 pm	Gemini
15	Gemini		
16	Gemini		
17	Gemini	1:32 am	Cancer
18	Cancer		
19	Cancer	8:38 am	Leo
20	Leo		
21	Leo	7:33 pm	Virgo
22	Virgo		
23	Virgo		
24	Virgo	8:29 am	Libra
25	Libra		
26	Libra	8:43 pm	Scorpio
27	Scorpio		
28	Scorpio		
29	Scorpio	6:28 am	Sagittarius
30	Sagittarius		

December

1	Sagittarius	1:38 pm	Capricorn
2	Capricorn		
3	Capricorn	6:58 pm	Aquarius
4	Aquarius		
5	Aquarius	11:07 pm	Pisces
6	Pisces		
7	Pisces		
8	Pisces	2:24 am	Aries
9	Aries		
10	Aries	5:00 am	Taurus
11	Taurus		
12	Taurus	7:35 am	Gemini
13	Gemini		
14	Gemini	11:25 am	Cancer
15	Cancer		
16	Cancer	5:58 pm	Leo
17	Leo		
18	Leo		
19	Leo	4:00 am	Virgo
20	Virgo		
21	Virgo	4:35 pm	Libra
22	Libra		
23	Libra		
24	Libra	5:07 am	Scorpio
25	Scorpio		
26	Scorpio	3:07 pm	Sagittarius
27	Sagittarius		
28	Sagittarius	9:48 pm	Capricorn
29	Capricorn		
30	Capricorn		
31	Capricorn	1:58 am	Aquarius

MOON POSITIONS 1998

January

1	Aquarius		
2	Aquarius	4:56 am	Pisces
3	Pisces		
4	Pisces	7:43 am	Aries
5	Aries		
6	Aries	10:52 am	Taurus
7	Taurus		
8	Taurus	2:42 pm	Gemini
9	Gemini		
10	Gemini	7:43 pm	Cancer
11	Cancer		
12	Cancer		
13	Cancer	2:45 am	Leo
14	Leo		
15	Leo	12:31 pm	Virgo
16	Virgo		
17	Virgo		
18	Virgo	12:44 am	Libra
19	Libra		
20	Libra	1:34 pm	Scorpio
21	Scorpio		
22	Scorpio		
23	Scorpio	12:25 am	Sagittarius
24	Sagittarius		
25	Sagittarius	7:39 am	Capricorn
26	Capricorn		
27	Capricorn	11:27 am	Aquarius
28	Aquarius		
29	Aquarius	1:08 pm	Pisces
30	Pisces		
31	Pisces	2:21 pm	Aries

February

1	Aries		
2	Aries	4:25 pm	Taurus
3	Taurus		
4	Taurus	8:09 pm	Gemini
5	Gemini		
6	Gemini		
7	Gemini	1:57 am	Cancer
8	Cancer		
9	Cancer	9:57 am	Leo
10	Leo		
11	Leo	8:09 pm	Virgo
12	Virgo		
13	Virgo		
14	Virgo	8:17 am	Libra
15	Libra		
16	Libra	9:13 pm	Scorpio
17	Scorpio		
18	Scorpio		
19	Scorpio	8:56 am	Sagittarius
20	Sagittarius		
21	Sagittarius	5:29 pm	Capricorn
22	Capricorn		
23	Capricorn	10:10 pm	Aquarius
24	Aquarius		
25	Aquarius	11:42 pm	Pisces
26	Pisces		
27	Pisces	11:42 pm	Aries
28	Aries		

March

1	Aries		
2	Aries	12:00 am	Taurus
3	Taurus		
4	Taurus	2:15 am	Gemini
5	Gemini		
6	Gemini	7:27 am	Cancer
7	Cancer		
8	Cancer	3:46 pm	Leo
9	Leo		
10	Leo		
11	Leo	2:35 am	Virgo
12	Virgo		
13	Virgo	2:58 pm	Libra
14	Libra		
15	Libra		
16	Libra	3:51 am	Scorpio
17	Scorpio		
18	Scorpio	3:56 pm	Sagittarius
19	Sagittarius		
20	Sagittarius		
21	Sagittarius	1:43 am	Capricorn
22	Capricorn		
23	Capricorn	8:01 am	Aquarius
24	Aquarius		
25	Aquarius	10:43 am	Pisces
26	Pisces		
27	Pisces	10:49 am	Aries
28	Aries		
29	Aries	10:06 am	Taurus
30	Taurus		
31	Taurus	10:38 am	Gemini

April

1	Gemini		
2	Gemini	2:10 pm	Cancer
3	Cancer		
4	Cancer	9:36 pm	Leo
5	Leo		
6	Leo		
7	Leo	8:25 am	Virgo
8	Virgo		
9	Virgo	9:04 pm	Libra
10	Libra		
11	Libra		
12	Libra	9:56 am	Scorpio
13	Scorpio		
14	Scorpio	9:52 pm	Sagittarius
15	Sagittarius		
16	Sagittarius		
17	Sagittarius	8:05 am	Capricorn
18	Capricorn		
19	Capricorn	3:41 pm	Aquarius
20	Aquarius		
21	Aquarius	8:06 pm	Pisces
22	Pisces		
23	Pisces	9:30 pm	Aries
24	Aries		
25	Aries	9:09 pm	Taurus
26	Taurus		
27	Taurus	8:55 pm	Gemini
28	Gemini		
29	Gemini	10:57 pm	Cancer
30	Cancer		

May

1	Cancer		
2	Cancer	4:49 am	Leo
3	Leo		
4	Leo	2:47 pm	Virgo
5	Virgo		
6	Virgo		
7	Virgo	3:19 am	Libra
8	Libra		
9	Libra	4:10 pm	Scorpio
10	Scorpio		
11	Scorpio		
12	Scorpio	3:48 am	Sagittarius
13	Sagittarius		
14	Sagittarius	1:39 pm	Capricorn
15	Capricorn		
16	Capricorn	9:30 pm	Aquarius
17	Aquarius		
18	Aquarius		
19	Aquarius	3:03 am	Pisces
20	Pisces		
21	Pisces	6:06 am	Aries
22	Aries		
23	Aries	7:06 am	Taurus
24	Taurus		
25	Taurus	7:25 am	Gemini
26	Gemini		
27	Gemini	8:58 am	Cancer
28	Cancer		
29	Cancer	1:38 pm	Leo
30	Leo		
31	Leo	10:21 pm	Virgo

June

1	Virgo		
2	Virgo		
3	Virgo	10:17 am	Libra
4	Libra		
5	Libra	11:06 pm	Scorpio
6	Scorpio		
7	Scorpio		
8	Scorpio	10:34 am	Sagittarius
9	Sagittarius		
10	Sagittarius	7:50 pm	Capricorn
11	Capricorn		
12	Capricorn		
13	Capricorn	3:03 am	Aquarius
14	Aquarius		
15	Aquarius	8:31 am	Pisces
16	Pisces		
17	Pisces	12:23 pm	Aries
18	Aries		
19	Aries	2:47 pm	Taurus
20	Taurus		
21	Taurus	4:26 pm	Gemini
22	Gemini		
23	Gemini	6:39 pm	Cancer
24	Cancer		
25	Cancer	11:04 pm	Leo
26	Leo		
27	Leo		
28	Leo	6:54 am	Virgo
29	Virgo		
30	Virgo	6:05 pm	Libra

MOON POSITIONS 1998

July

1	Libra		
2	Libra		
3	Libra	6:45 am	Scorpio
4	Scorpio		
5	Scorpio	6:24 pm	Sagittarius
6	Sagittarius		
7	Sagittarius		
8	Sagittarius	3:27 am	Capricorn
9	Capricorn		
10	Capricorn	9:52 am	Aquarius
11	Aquarius		
12	Aquarius	2:22 pm	Pisces
13	Pisces		
14	Pisces	5:45 pm	Aries
15	Aries		
16	Aries	8:33 pm	Taurus
17	Taurus		
18	Taurus	11:18 pm	Gemini
19	Gemini		
20	Gemini		
21	Gemini	2:43 am	Cancer
22	Cancer		
23	Cancer	7:48 am	Leo
24	Leo		
25	Leo	3:34 pm	Virgo
26	Virgo		
27	Virgo		
28	Virgo	2:14 am	Libra
29	Libra		
30	Libra	2:44 pm	Scorpio
31	Scorpio		

August

1	Scorpio		
2	Scorpio	2:48 am	Sagittarius
3	Sagittarius		
4	Sagittarius	12:18 pm	Capricorn
5	Capricorn		
6	Capricorn	6:31 pm	Aquarius
7	Aquarius		
8	Aquarius	10:04 pm	Pisces
9	Pisces		
10	Pisces		
11	Pisces	12:10 am	Aries
12	Aries		
13	Aries	2:04 am	Taurus
14	Taurus		
15	Taurus	4:46 am	Gemini
16	Gemini		
17	Gemini	8:55 am	Cancer
18	Cancer		
19	Cancer	3:01 pm	Leo
20	Leo		
21	Leo	11:21 pm	Virgo
22	Virgo		
23	Virgo		
24	Virgo	10:02 am	Libra
25	Libra		
26	Libra	10:25 pm	Scorpio
27	Scorpio		
28	Scorpio		
29	Scorpio	10:55 am	Sagittarius
30	Sagittarius		
31	Sagittarius	9:23 pm	Capricorn

September

1	Capricorn		
2	Capricorn		
3	Capricorn	4:21 am	Aquarius
4	Aquarius		
5	Aquarius	7:48 am	Pisces
6	Pisces		
7	Pisces	8:52 am	Aries
8	Aries		
9	Aries	9:16 am	Taurus
10	Taurus		
11	Taurus	10:40 am	Gemini
12	Gemini		
13	Gemini	2:20 pm	Cancer
14	Cancer		
15	Cancer	8:48 pm	Leo
16	Leo		
17	Leo		
18	Leo	5:52 am	Virgo
19	Virgo		
20	Virgo	4:57 pm	Libra
21	Libra		
22	Libra		
23	Libra	5:22 am	Scorpio
24	Scorpio		
25	Scorpio	6:05 pm	Sagittarius
26	Sagittarius		
27	Sagittarius		
28	Sagittarius	5:30 am	Capricorn
29	Capricorn		
30	Capricorn	1:53 pm	Aquarius

October

1	Aquarius		
2	Aquarius	6:23 pm	Pisces
3	Pisces		
4	Pisces	7:32 pm	Aries
5	Aries		
6	Aries	6:57 pm	Taurus
7	Taurus		
8	Taurus	6:44 pm	Gemini
9	Gemini		
10	Gemini	8:48 pm	Cancer
11	Cancer		
12	Cancer		
13	Cancer	2:25 am	Leo
14	Leo		
15	Leo	11:32 am	Virgo
16	Virgo		
17	Virgo	11:02 pm	Libra
18	Libra		
19	Libra		
20	Libra	11:36 am	Scorpio
21	Scorpio		
22	Scorpio		
23	Scorpio	12:16 am	Sagittarius
24	Sagittarius		
25	Sagittarius	12:05 pm	Capricorn
26	Capricorn		
27	Capricorn	9:44 pm	Aquarius
28	Aquarius		
29	Aquarius		
30	Aquarius	3:58 am	Pisces
31	Pisces		

November

1	Pisces	6:27 am	Aries
2	Aries		
3	Aries	6:12 am	Taurus
4	Taurus		
5	Taurus	5:11 am	Gemini
6	Gemini		
7	Gemini	5:39 am	Cancer
8	Cancer		
9	Cancer	9:33 am	Leo
10	Leo		
11	Leo	5:37 pm	Virgo
12	Virgo		
13	Virgo		
14	Virgo	4:58 am	Libra
15	Libra		
16	Libra	5:41 pm	Scorpio
17	Scorpio		
18	Scorpio		
19	Scorpio	6:13 am	Sagittarius
20	Sagittarius		
21	Sagittarius	5:45 pm	Capricorn
22	Capricorn		
23	Capricorn		
24	Capricorn	3:43 am	Aquarius
25	Aquarius		
26	Aquarius	11:14 am	Pisces
27	Pisces		
28	Pisces	3:34 pm	Aries
29	Aries		
30	Aries	4:52 pm	Taurus

December

1	Taurus		
2	Taurus	4:30 pm	Gemini
3	Gemini		
4	Gemini	4:28 pm	Cancer
5	Cancer		
6	Cancer	6:55 pm	Leo
7	Leo		
8	Leo		
9	Leo	1:21 am	Virgo
10	Virgo		
11	Virgo	11:43 am	Libra
12	Libra		
13	Libra		
14	Libra	12:16 am	Scorpio
15	Scorpio		
16	Scorpio	12:47 pm	Sagittarius
17	Sagittarius		
18	Sagittarius	11:55 pm	Capricorn
19	Capricorn		
20	Capricorn		
21	Capricorn	9:17 am	Aquarius
22	Aquarius		
23	Aquarius	4:45 pm	Pisces
24	Pisces		
25	Pisces	10:04 pm	Aries
26	Aries		
27	Aries		
28	Aries	1:05 am	Taurus
29	Taurus		
30	Taurus	2:22 am	Gemini
31	Gemini		

MOONPOSITIONS 1999

January

1	Gemini	3:15 am	Cancer
2	Cancer		
3	Cancer	5:31 am	Leo
4	Leo		
5	Leo	10:49 am	Virgo
6	Virgo		
7	Virgo	7:53 pm	Libra
8	Libra		
9	Libra		
10	Libra	7:49 am	Scorpio
11	Scorpio		
12	Scorpio	8:23 pm	Sagittarius
13	Sagittarius		
14	Sagittarius		
15	Sagittarius	7:28 am	Capricorn
16	Capricorn		
17	Capricorn	4:11 pm	Aquarius
18	Aquarius		
19	Aquarius	10:40 pm	Pisces
20	Pisces		
21	Pisces		
22	Pisces	3:25 am	Aries
23	Aries		
24	Aries	6:52 am	Taurus
25	Taurus		
26	Taurus	9:29 am	Gemini
27	Gemini		
28	Gemini	11:57 am	Cancer
29	Cancer		
30	Cancer	3:16 pm	Leo
31	Leo		

February

1	Leo	8:37 pm	Virgo
2	Virgo		
3	Virgo		
4	Virgo	4:56 am	Libra
5	Libra		
6	Libra	4:06 pm	Scorpio
7	Scorpio		
8	Scorpio		
9	Scorpio	4:38 am	Sagittarius
10	Sagittarius		
11	Sagittarius	4:10 pm	Capricorn
12	Capricorn		
13	Capricorn		
14	Capricorn	12:57 am	Aquarius
15	Aquarius		
16	Aquarius	6:40 am	Pisces
17	Pisces		
18	Pisces	10:06 am	Aries
19	Aries		
20	Aries	12:29 pm	Taurus
21	Taurus		
22	Taurus	2:54 pm	Gemini
23	Gemini		
24	Gemini	6:09 am	Cancer
25	Cancer		
26	Cancer	10:44 pm	Leo
27	Leo		
28	Leo		

March

1	Leo	5:05 am	Virgo
2	Virgo		
3	Virgo	1:34 pm	Libra
4	Libra		
5	Libra		
6	Libra	12:22 am	Scorpio
7	Scorpio		
8	Scorpio	12:46 pm	Sagittarius
9	Sagittarius		
10	Sagittarius		
11	Sagittarius	12:54 am	Capricorn
12	Capricorn		
13	Capricorn	10:32 am	Aquarius
14	Aquarius		
15	Aquarius	4:30 pm	Pisces
16	Pisces		
17	Pisces	7:13 pm	Aries
18	Aries		
19	Aries	8:09 pm	Taurus
20	Taurus		
21	Taurus	9:05 pm	Gemini
22	Gemini		
23	Gemini	11:33 pm	Cancer
24	Cancer		
25	Cancer		
26	Cancer	4:22 am	Leo
27	Leo		
28	Leo	11:34 am	Virgo
29	Virgo		
30	Virgo	8:49 pm	Libra
31	Libra		

April

1	Libra		
2	Libra	7:49 am	Scorpio
3	Scorpio		
4	Scorpio	8:07 pm	Sagittarius
5	Sagittarius		
6	Sagittarius		
7	Sagittarius	8:39 pm	Capricorn
8	Capricorn		
9	Capricorn	7:24 pm	Aquarius
10	Aquarius		
11	Aquarius		
12	Aquarius	2:35 am	Pisces
13	Pisces		
14	Pisces	5:46 am	Aries
15	Aries		
16	Aries	6:07 am	Taurus
17	Taurus		
18	Taurus	5:39 am	Gemini
19	Gemini		
20	Gemini	6:27 am	Cancer
21	Cancer		
22	Cancer	10:06 am	Leo
23	Leo		
24	Leo	5:04 pm	Virgo
25	Virgo		
26	Virgo		
27	Virgo	2:46 am	Libra
28	Libra		
29	Libra	2:12 pm	Scorpio
30	Scorpio		

May

1	Scorpio		
2	Scorpio	2:36 am	Sagittarius
3	Sagittarius		
4	Sagittarius	3:12 pm	Capricorn
5	Capricorn		
6	Capricorn		
7	Capricorn	2:40 am	Aquarius
8	Aquarius		
9	Aquarius	11:16 am	Pisces
10	Pisces		
11	Pisces	3:53 pm	Aries
12	Aries		
13	Aries	4:56 pm	Taurus
14	Taurus		
15	Taurus	4:07 pm	Gemini
16	Gemini		
17	Gemini	3:39 pm	Cancer
18	Cancer		
19	Cancer	5:37 pm	Leo
20	Leo		
21	Leo	11:15 pm	Virgo
22	Virgo		
23	Virgo		
24	Virgo	8:29 am	Libra
25	Libra		
26	Libra	8:05 pm	Scorpio
27	Scorpio		
28	Scorpio		
29	Scorpio	8:37 am	Sagittarius
30	Sagittarius		
31	Sagittarius	9:06 pm	Capricorn

June

1	Capricorn		
2	Capricorn		
3	Capricorn	8:37 am	Aquarius
4	Aquarius		
5	Aquarius	6:00 pm	Pisces
6	Pisces		
7	Pisces		
8	Pisces	12:08 am	Aries
9	Aries		
10	Aries	2:44 am	Taurus
11	Taurus		
12	Taurus	2:48 am	Gemini
13	Gemini		
14	Gemini	2:14 am	Cancer
15	Cancer		
16	Cancer	3:07 am	Leo
17	Leo		
18	Leo	7:12 am	Virgo
19	Virgo		
20	Virgo	3:10 pm	Libra
21	Libra		
22	Libra		
23	Libra	2:18 am	Scorpio
24	Scorpio		
25	Scorpio	2:51 pm	Sagittarius
26	Sagittarius		
27	Sagittarius		
28	Sagittarius	3:12 am	Capricorn
29	Capricorn		
30	Capricorn	2:19 pm	Aquarius

MOONPOSITIONS1999

July

1	Aquarius		
2	Aquarius	11:34 pm	Pisces
3	Pisces		
4	Pisces		
5	Pisces	6:21 am	Aries
6	Aries		
7	Aries	10:22 am	Taurus
8	Taurus		
9	Taurus	12:00 pm	Gemini
10	Gemini		
11	Gemini	12:27 pm	Cancer
12	Cancer		
13	Cancer	1:26 pm	Leo
14	Leo		
15	Leo	4:39 pm	Virgo
16	Virgo		
17	Virgo	11:19 pm	Libra
18	Libra		
19	Libra		
20	Libra	9:30 am	Scorpio
21	Scorpio		
22	Scorpio	9:48 pm	Sagittarius
23	Sagittarius		
24	Sagittarius		
25	Sagittarius	10:08 am	Capricorn
26	Capricorn		
27	Capricorn	8:54 pm	Aquarius
28	Aquarius		
29	Aquarius		
30	Aquarius	5:27 am	Pisces
31	Pisces		

August

1	Pisces	11:47 am	Aries
2	Aries		
3	Aries	4:09 pm	Taurus
4	Taurus		
5	Taurus	6:57 pm	Gemini
6	Gemini		
7	Gemini	8:52 pm	Cancer
8	Cancer		
9	Cancer	10:55 pm	Leo
10	Leo		
11	Leo		
12	Leo	2:22 am	Virgo
13	Virgo		
14	Virgo	8:24 am	Libra
15	Libra		
16	Libra	5:40 pm	Scorpio
17	Scorpio		
18	Scorpio		
19	Scorpio	5:32 am	Sagittarius
20	Sagittarius		
21	Sagittarius	5:59 pm	Capricorn
22	Capricorn		
23	Capricorn		
24	Capricorn	4:49 am	Aquarius
25	Aquarius		
26	Aquarius	12:50 pm	Pisces
27	Pisces		
28	Pisces	6:09 pm	Aries
29	Aries		
30	Aries	9:41 pm	Taurus
31	Taurus		

September

1	Taurus		
2	Taurus	12:25 am	Gemini
3	Gemini		
4	Gemini	3:10 am	Cancer
5	Cancer		
6	Cancer	6:29 am	Leo
7	Leo		
8	Leo	10:57 am	Virgo
9	Virgo		
10	Virgo	5:16 pm	Libra
11	Libra		
12	Libra		
13	Libra	2:08 am	Scorpio
14	Scorpio		
15	Scorpio	1:35 pm	Sagittarius
16	Sagittarius		
17	Sagittarius		
18	Sagittarius	2:13 am	Capricorn
19	Capricorn		
20	Capricorn	1:38 pm	Aquarius
21	Aquarius		
22	Aquarius	9:51 pm	Pisces
23	Pisces		
24	Pisces		
25	Pisces	2:34 am	Aries
26	Aries		
27	Aries	4:51 am	Taurus
28	Taurus		
29	Taurus	6:21 am	Gemini
30	Gemini		

October

1	Gemini	8:31 am	Cancer
2	Cancer		
3	Cancer	12:13 pm	Leo
4	Leo		
5	Leo	5:40 pm	Virgo
6	Virgo		
7	Virgo		
8	Virgo	12:52 am	Libra
9	Libra		
10	Libra	10:01 am	Scorpio
11	Scorpio		
12	Scorpio	9:18 pm	Sagittarius
13	Sagittarius		
14	Sagittarius		
15	Sagittarius	10:04 am	Capricorn
16	Capricorn		
17	Capricorn	10:17 pm	Aquarius
18	Aquarius		
19	Aquarius		
20	Aquarius	7:33 am	Pisces
21	Pisces		
22	Pisces	12:41 pm	Aries
23	Aries		
24	Aries	2:25 pm	Taurus
25	Taurus		
26	Taurus	2:33 pm	Gemini
27	Gemini		
28	Gemini	3:09 pm	Cancer
29	Cancer		
30	Cancer	5:47 pm	Leo
31	Leo		

November

1	Leo	11:07 pm	Virgo
2	Virgo		
3	Virgo		
4	Virgo	6:57 am	Libra
5	Libra		
6	Libra	4:46 pm	Scorpio
7	Scorpio		
8	Scorpio		
9	Scorpio	4:15 pm	Sagittarius
10	Sagittarius		
11	Sagittarius	5:00 pm	Capricorn
12	Capricorn		
13	Capricorn		
14	Capricorn	5:46 am	Aquarius
15	Aquarius		
16	Aquarius	4:21 pm	Pisces
17	Pisces		
18	Pisces	10:57 pm	Aries
19	Aries		
20	Aries		
21	Aries	1:26 am	Taurus
22	Taurus		
23	Taurus	1:14 am	Gemini
24	Gemini		
25	Gemini	12:29 am	Cancer
26	Cancer		
27	Cancer	1:19 am	Leo
28	Leo		
29	Leo	5:11 am	Virgo
30	Virgo		

December

1	Virgo	12:29 pm	Libra
2	Libra		
3	Libra	10:35 pm	Scorpio
4	Scorpio		
5	Scorpio		
6	Scorpio	10:27 pm	Sagittarius
7	Sagittarius		
8	Sagittarius	11:14 pm	Capricorn
9	Capricorn		
10	Capricorn		
11	Capricorn	11:59 am	Aquarius
12	Aquarius		
13	Aquarius	11:18 pm	Pisces
14	Pisces		
15	Pisces		
16	Pisces	7:30 am	Aries
17	Aries		
18	Aries	11:45 am	Taurus
19	Taurus		
20	Taurus	12:39 pm	Gemini
21	Gemini		
22	Gemini	11:52 am	Cancer
23	Cancer		
24	Cancer	11:32 am	Leo
25	Leo		
26	Leo	1:34 pm	Virgo
27	Virgo		
28	Virgo	7:14 pm	Libra
29	Libra		
30	Libra		
31	Libra	4:36 am	Scorpio

MOON POSITIONS 2000

January

1	Scorpio		
2	Scorpio	4:32 pm	Sagittarius
3	Sagittarius		
4	Sagittarius		
5	Sagittarius	5:24 am	Capricorn
6	Capricorn		
7	Capricorn	5:53 pm	Aquarius
8	Aquarius		
9	Aquarius		
10	Aquarius	4:59 am	Pisces
11	Pisces		
12	Pisces	1:48 pm	Aries
13	Aries		
14	Aries	7:38 pm	Taurus
15	Taurus		
16	Taurus	10:25 pm	Gemini
17	Gemini		
18	Gemini	11:01 pm	Cancer
19	Cancer		
20	Cancer	10:58 pm	Leo
21	Leo		
22	Leo		
23	Leo	12:07 am	Virgo
24	Virgo		
25	Virgo	4:09 am	Libra
26	Libra		
27	Libra	12:01 pm	Scorpio
28	Scorpio		
29	Scorpio	11:17 pm	Sagittarius
30	Sagittarius		
31	Sagittarius		

February

1	Sagittarius	12:10 pm	Capricorn
2	Capricorn		
3	Capricorn		
4	Capricorn	12:31 am	Aquarius
5	Aquarius		
6	Aquarius	11:02 am	Pisces
7	Pisces		
8	Pisces	7:17 pm	Aries
9	Aries		
10	Aries		
11	Aries	1:21 am	Taurus
12	Taurus		
13	Taurus	5:23 am	Gemini
14	Gemini		
15	Gemini	7:45 am	Cancer
16	Cancer		
17	Cancer	9:11 am	Leo
18	Leo		
19	Leo	10:53 am	Virgo
20	Virgo		
21	Virgo	2:21 pm	Libra
22	Libra		
23	Libra	8:58 pm	Scorpio
24	Scorpio		
25	Scorpio		
26	Scorpio	7:10 am	Sagittarius
27	Sagittarius		
28	Sagittarius	7:45 pm	Capricorn
29	Capricorn		

March

1	Capricorn		
2	Capricorn	8:14 am	Aquarius
3	Aquarius		
4	Aquarius	6:30 pm	Pisces
5	Pisces		
6	Pisces		
7	Pisces	1:54 am	Aries
8	Aries		
9	Aries	7:01 am	Taurus
10	Taurus		
11	Taurus	10:46 am	Gemini
12	Gemini		
13	Gemini	1:51 pm	Cancer
14	Cancer		
15	Cancer	4:43 pm	Leo
16	Leo		
17	Leo	7:48 pm	Virgo
18	Virgo		
19	Virgo	11:57 pm	Libra
20	Libra		
21	Libra		
22	Libra	6:17 am	Scorpio
23	Scorpio		
24	Scorpio	3:43 pm	Sagittarius
25	Sagittarius		
26	Sagittarius		
27	Sagittarius	3:51 am	Capricorn
28	Capricorn		
29	Capricorn	4:34 pm	Aquarius
30	Aquarius		
31	Aquarius		

April

1	Aquarius	3:12 am	Pisces
2	Pisces		
3	Pisces	10:22 am	Aries
4	Aries		
5	Aries	2:29 pm	Taurus
6	Taurus		
7	Taurus	4:58 pm	Gemini
8	Gemini		
9	Gemini	7:16 pm	Cancer
10	Cancer		
11	Cancer	10:16 pm	Leo
12	Leo		
13	Leo		
14	Leo	2:19 am	Virgo
15	Virgo		
16	Virgo	7:36 am	Libra
17	Libra		
18	Libra	2:35 pm	Scorpio
19	Scorpio		
20	Scorpio	11:58 pm	Sagittarius
21	Sagittarius		
22	Sagittarius		
23	Sagittarius	11:47 am	Capricorn
24	Capricorn		
25	Capricorn		
26	Capricorn	12:42 am	Aquarius
27	Aquarius		
28	Aquarius	12:06 pm	Pisces
29	Pisces		
30	Pisces	7:55 pm	Aries

May

1	Aries		
2	Aries	11:54 pm	Taurus
3	Taurus		
4	Taurus		
5	Taurus	1:23 am	Gemini
6	Gemini		
7	Gemini	2:14 am	Cancer
8	Cancer		
9	Cancer	4:01 am	Leo
10	Leo		
11	Leo	7:41 am	Virgo
12	Virgo		
13	Virgo	1:27 pm	Libra
14	Libra		
15	Libra	9:16 pm	Scorpio
16	Scorpio		
17	Scorpio		
18	Scorpio	7:09 am	Sagittarius
19	Sagittarius		
20	Sagittarius	7:01 pm	Capricorn
21	Capricorn		
22	Capricorn		
23	Capricorn	8:00 am	Aquarius
24	Aquarius		
25	Aquarius	8:07 pm	Pisces
26	Pisces		
27	Pisces		
28	Pisces	5:08 am	Aries
29	Aries		
30	Aries	10:02 am	Taurus
31	Taurus		

June

1	Taurus	11:34 am	Gemini
2	Gemini		
3	Gemini	11:30 am	Cancer
4	Cancer		
5	Cancer	11:46 am	Leo
6	Leo		
7	Leo	1:57 pm	Virgo
8	Virgo		
9	Virgo	6:59 pm	Libra
10	Libra		
11	Libra		
12	Libra	2:55 am	Scorpio
13	Scorpio		
14	Scorpio	1:18 pm	Sagittarius
15	Sagittarius		
16	Sagittarius		
17	Sagittarius	1:26 am	Capricorn
18	Capricorn		
19	Capricorn	2:26 pm	Aquarius
20	Aquarius		
21	Aquarius		
22	Aquarius	2:52 am	Pisces
23	Pisces		
24	Pisces	12:55 pm	Aries
25	Aries		
26	Aries	7:19 pm	Taurus
27	Taurus		
28	Taurus	9:59 pm	Gemini
29	Gemini		
30	Gemini	10:09 pm	Cancer

MOONPOSITIONS2000

July

1	Cancer		
2	Cancer	9:38 pm	Leo
3	Leo		
4	Leo	10:19 pm	Virgo
5	Virgo		
6	Virgo		
7	Virgo	1:47 am	Libra
8	Libra		
9	Libra	8:48 am	Scorpio
10	Scorpio		
11	Scorpio	7:06 pm	Sagittarius
12	Sagittarius		
13	Sagittarius		
14	Sagittarius	7:28 am	Capricorn
15	Capricorn		
16	Capricorn	8:27 pm	Aquarius
17	Aquarius		
18	Aquarius		
19	Aquarius	8:44 am	Pisces
20	Pisces		
21	Pisces	7:09 pm	Aries
22	Aries		
23	Aries		
24	Aries	2:44 am	Taurus
25	Taurus		
26	Taurus	7:01 am	Gemini
27	Gemini		
28	Gemini	8:30 am	Cancer
29	Cancer		
30	Cancer	8:24 am	Leo
31	Leo		

August

1	Leo	8:27 am	Virgo
2	Virgo		
3	Virgo	10:31 am	Libra
4	Libra		
5	Libra	4:04 pm	Scorpio
6	Scorpio		
7	Scorpio		
8	Scorpio	1:30 am	Sagittarius
9	Sagittarius		
10	Sagittarius	1:44 pm	Capricorn
11	Capricorn		
12	Capricorn		
13	Capricorn	2:43 am	Aquarius
14	Aquarius		
15	Aquarius	2:41 pm	Pisces
16	Pisces		
17	Pisces		
18	Pisces	12:44 am	Aries
19	Aries		
20	Aries	8:31 am	Taurus
21	Taurus		
22	Taurus	1:55 pm	Gemini
23	Gemini		
24	Gemini	5:00 pm	Cancer
25	Cancer		
26	Cancer	6:17 pm	Leo
27	Leo		
28	Leo	6:55 pm	Virgo
29	Virgo		
30	Virgo	8:33 pm	Libra
31	Libra		

September

1	Libra		
2	Libra	12:55 am	Scorpio
3	Scorpio		
4	Scorpio	9:08 am	Sagittarius
5	Sagittarius		
6	Sagittarius	8:47 pm	Capricorn
7	Capricorn		
8	Capricorn		
9	Capricorn	9:44 am	Aquarius
10	Aquarius		
11	Aquarius	9:34 pm	Pisces
12	Pisces		
13	Pisces		
14	Pisces	7:00 am	Aries
15	Aries		
16	Aries	2:05 pm	Taurus
17	Taurus		
18	Taurus	7:22 pm	Gemini
19	Gemini		
20	Gemini	11:16 pm	Cancer
21	Cancer		
22	Cancer		
23	Cancer	2:00 am	Leo
24	Leo		
25	Leo	4:02 am	Virgo
26	Virgo		
27	Virgo	6:22 am	Libra
28	Libra		
29	Libra	10:30 am	Scorpio
30	Scorpio		

October

1	Scorpio	5:50 pm	Sagittarius
2	Sagittarius		
3	Sagittarius		
4	Sagittarius	4:42 am	Capricorn
5	Capricorn		
6	Capricorn	5:33 pm	Aquarius
7	Aquarius		
8	Aquarius		
9	Aquarius	5:36 am	Pisces
10	Pisces		
11	Pisces	2:51 pm	Aries
12	Aries		
13	Aries	9:06 pm	Taurus
14	Taurus		
15	Taurus		
16	Taurus	1:19 am	Gemini
17	Gemini		
18	Gemini	4:37 am	Cancer
19	Cancer		
20	Cancer	7:42 am	Leo
21	Leo		
22	Leo	10:52 am	Virgo
23	Virgo		
24	Virgo	2:30 pm	Libra
25	Libra		
26	Libra	7:23 pm	Scorpio
27	Scorpio		
28	Scorpio		
29	Scorpio	2:40 am	Sagittarius
30	Sagittarius		
31	Sagittarius	1.02 pm	Capricorn

November

1	Capricorn		
2	Capricorn		
3	Capricorn	1:41 am	Aquarius
4	Aquarius		
5	Aquarius	2:13 pm	Pisces
6	Pisces		
7	Pisces		
8	Pisces	12:02 am	Aries
9	Aries		
10	Aries	6:12 am	Taurus
11	Taurus		
12	Taurus	9:27 am	Gemini
13	Gemini		
14	Gemini	11:21 am	Cancer
15	Cancer		
16	Cancer	1:19 pm	Leo
17	Leo		
18	Leo	4:15 pm	Virgo
19	Virgo		
20	Virgo	8:35 pm	Libra
21	Libra		
22	Libra		
23	Libra	2:33 am	Scorpio
24	Scorpio		
25	Scorpio	10:33 am	Sagittarius
26	Sagittarius		
27	Sagittarius	8:57 pm	Capricorn
28	Capricorn		
29	Capricorn		
30	Capricorn	9:26 am	Aquarius

December

1	Aquarius		
2	Aquarius	10:23 pm	Pisces
3	Pisces		
4	Pisces		
5	Pisces	9:17 am	Aries
6	Aries		
7	Aries	4:27 pm	Taurus
8	Taurus		
9	Taurus	7:50 pm	Gemini
10	Gemini		
11	Gemini	8:48 pm	Cancer
12	Cancer		
13	Cancer	9:09 pm	Leo
14	Leo		
15	Leo	10:30 pm	Virgo
16	Virgo		
17	Virgo		
18	Virgo	2:01 am	Libra
19	Libra		
20	Libra	8:12 am	Scorpio
21	Scorpio		
22	Scorpio	4:57 pm	Sagittarius
23	Sagittarius		
24	Sagittarius		
25	Sagittarius	3:54 am	Capricorn
26	Capricorn		
27	Capricorn	4:25 pm	Aquarius
28	Aquarius		
29	Aquarius		
30	Aquarius	5:27 am	Pisces
31	Pisces		

MOONPOSITIONS2001

January

1	Pisces	5:14 pm	Aries
2	Aries		
3	Aries		
4	Aries	1:57 am	Taurus
5	Taurus		
6	Taurus	6:44 am	Gemini
7	Gemini		
8	Gemini	8: 9 am	Cancer
9	Cancer		
10	Cancer	7:44 am	Leo
11	Leo		
12	Leo	7:26 am	Virgo
13	Virgo		
14	Virgo	9: 5 am	Libra
15	Libra		
16	Libra	2: 2 pm	Scorpio
17	Scorpio		
18	Scorpio	10:35 pm	Sagittarius
19	Sagittarius		
20	Sagittarius		
21	Sagittarius	9:57 am	Capricorn
22	Capricorn		
23	Capricorn	10:43 pm	Aquarius
24	Aquarius		
25	Aquarius		
26	Aquarius	11:39 am	Pisces
27	Pisces		
28	Pisces	11:35 pm	Aries
29	Aries		
30	Aries		
31	Aries	9:21 am	Taurus

February

1	Taurus		
2	Taurus	3:55 pm	Gemini
3	Gemini		
4	Gemini	7: 0 pm	Cancer
5	Cancer		
6	Cancer	7:21 pm	Leo
7	Leo		
8	Leo	6:35 pm	Virgo
9	Virgo		
10	Virgo	6:46 pm	Libra
11	Libra		
12	Libra	9:51 pm	Scorpio
13	Scorpio		
14	Scorpio		
15	Scorpio	5: 2 am	Sagittarius
16	Sagittarius		
17	Sagittarius	3:59 pm	Capricorn
18	Capricorn		
19	Capricorn		
20	Capricorn	4:53 am	Aquarius
21	Aquarius		
22	Aquarius	5:45 pm	Pisces
23	Pisces		
24	Pisces		
25	Pisces	5:20 am	Aries
26	Aries		
27	Aries	3: 6 pm	Taurus
28	Taurus		

March

1	Taurus	10:36 pm	Gemini
2	Gemini		
3	Gemini		
4	Gemini	3:24 am	Cancer
5	Cancer		
6	Cancer	5:30 am	Leo
7	Leo		
8	Leo	5:44 am	Virgo
9	Virgo		
10	Virgo	5:47 am	Libra
11	Libra		
12	Libra	7:43 am	Scorpio
13	Scorpio		
14	Scorpio	1:17 pm	Sagittarius
15	Sagittarius		
16	Sagittarius	11: 2 pm	Capricorn
17	Capricorn		
18	Capricorn		
19	Capricorn	11:36 am	Aquarius
20	Aquarius		
21	Aquarius		
22	Aquarius	12:28 am	Pisces
23	Pisces		
24	Pisces	11:43 am	Aries
25	Aries		
26	Aries	8:50 pm	Taurus
27	Taurus		
28	Taurus		
29	Taurus	4: 1 am	Gemini
30	Gemini		
31	Gemini	9:23 am	Cancer

April

1	Cancer		
2	Cancer	12:54 pm	Leo
3	Leo		
4	Leo	2:46 pm	Virgo
5	Virgo		
6	Virgo	3:57 pm	Libra
7	Libra		
8	Libra	6: 1 pm	Scorpio
9	Scorpio		
10	Scorpio	10:47 pm	Sagittarius
11	Sagittarius		
12	Sagittarius		
13	Sagittarius	7:21 am	Capricorn
14	Capricorn		
15	Capricorn	7:11 pm	Aquarius
16	Aquarius		
17	Aquarius		
18	Aquarius	8: 0 am	Pisces
19	Pisces		
20	Pisces	7:18 pm	Aries
21	Aries		
22	Aries		
23	Aries	3:56 am	Taurus
24	Taurus		
25	Taurus	10:11 am	Gemini
26	Gemini		
27	Gemini	2:49 pm	Cancer
28	Cancer		
29	Cancer	6:25 pm	Leo
30	Leo		

May

1	Leo	9:16 pm	Virgo
2	Virgo		
3	Virgo	11:50 pm	Libra
4	Libra		
5	Libra		
6	Libra	3: 0 am	Scorpio
7	Scorpio		
8	Scorpio	8: 5 am	Sagittarius
9	Sagittarius		
10	Sagittarius	4:10 pm	Capricorn
11	Capricorn		
12	Capricorn		
13	Capricorn	3:20 am	Aquarius
14	Aquarius		
15	Aquarius	4: 1 pm	Pisces
16	Pisces		
17	Pisces		
18	Pisces	3:41 am	Aries
19	Aries		
20	Aries	12:29 pm	Taurus
21	Taurus		
22	Taurus	6:12 pm	Gemini
23	Gemini		
24	Gemini	9:42 pm	Cancer
25	Cancer		
26	Cancer		
27	Cancer	12:12 am	Leo
28	Leo		
29	Leo	2:38 am	Virgo
30	Virgo		
31	Virgo	5:41 am	Libra

June

1	Libra		
2	Libra	9:56 am	Scorpio
3	Scorpio		
4	Scorpio	3:58 pm	Sagittarius
5	Sagittarius		
6	Sagittarius		
7	Sagittarius	12:23 am	Capricorn
8	Capricorn		
9	Capricorn	11:20 am	Aquarius
10	Aquarius		
11	Aquarius	11:53 pm	Pisces
12	Pisces		
13	Pisces		
14	Pisces	12: 3 pm	Aries
15	Aries		
16	Aries	9:39 pm	Taurus
17	Taurus		
18	Taurus		
19	Taurus	3:42 am	Gemini
20	Gemini		
21	Gemini	6:40 am	Cancer
22	Cancer		
23	Cancer	7:55 am	Leo
24	Leo		
25	Leo	8:57 am	Virgo
26	Virgo		
27	Virgo	11:11 am	Libra
28	Libra		
29	Libra	3:28 pm	Scorpio
30	Scorpio		

MOONPOSITIONS 2001

July

1	Scorpio	10:13 pm	Sagittarius
2	Sagittarius		
3	Sagittarius		
4	Sagittarius	7:21 am	Capricorn
5	Capricorn		
6	Capricorn	6:33 pm	Aquarius
7	Aquarius		
8	Aquarius		
9	Aquarius	7: 5 am	Pisces
10	Pisces		
11	Pisces	7:36 pm	Aries
12	Aries		
13	Aries		
14	Aries	6:13 am	Taurus
15	Taurus		
16	Taurus	1:25 pm	Gemini
17	Gemini		
18	Gemini	4:56 pm	Cancer
19	Cancer		
20	Cancer	5:43 pm	Leo
21	Leo		
22	Leo	5:29 pm	Virgo
23	Virgo		
24	Virgo	6: 8 pm	Libra
25	Libra		
26	Libra	9:17 pm	Scorpio
27	Scorpio		
28	Scorpio		
29	Scorpio	3:44 am	Sagittarius
30	Sagittarius		
31	Sagittarius	1:16 pm	Capricorn

August

1	Capricorn		
2	Capricorn		
3	Capricorn	12:53 am	Aquarius
4	Aquarius		
5	Aquarius	1:30 pm	Pisces
6	Pisces		
7	Pisces		
8	Pisces	2: 5 am	Aries
9	Aries		
10	Aries	1:23 pm	Taurus
11	Taurus		
12	Taurus	9:59 pm	Gemini
13	Gemini		
14	Gemini		
15	Gemini	2:55 am	Cancer
16	Cancer		
17	Cancer	4:25 am	Leo
18	Leo		
19	Leo	3:53 am	Virgo
20	Virgo		
21	Virgo	3:19 am	Libra
22	Libra		
23	Libra	4:50 am	Scorpio
24	Scorpio		
25	Scorpio	9:59 am	Sagittarius
26	Sagittarius		
27	Sagittarius	7: 2 pm	Capricorn
28	Capricorn		
29	Capricorn		
30	Capricorn	6:47 am	Aquarius
31	Aquarius		

September

1	Aquarius	7:32 pm	Pisces
2	Pisces		
3	Pisces		
4	Pisces	7:58 am	Aries
5	Aries		
6	Aries	7:18 pm	Taurus
7	Taurus		
8	Taurus		
9	Taurus	4:41 am	Gemini
10	Gemini		
11	Gemini	11: 9 am	Cancer
12	Cancer		
13	Cancer	2:16 pm	Leo
14	Leo		
15	Leo	2:39 pm	Virgo
16	Virgo		
17	Virgo	2: 0 pm	Libra
18	Libra		
19	Libra	2:27 pm	Scorpio
20	Scorpio		
21	Scorpio	6: 2 pm	Sagittarius
22	Sagittarius		
23	Sagittarius		
24	Sagittarius	1:48 am	Capricorn
25	Capricorn		
26	Capricorn	1: 5 pm	Aquarius
27	Aquarius		
28	Aquarius		
29	Aquarius	1:50 pm	Pisces
30	Pisces		

October

1	Pisces	2: 8 pm	Aries
2	Aries		
3	Aries		
4	Aries	1: 1 am	Taurus
5	Taurus		
6	Taurus	10:12 am	Gemini
7	Gemini		
8	Gemini	5:19 pm	Cancer
9	Cancer		
10	Cancer	9:54 pm	Leo
11	Leo		
12	Leo	11:58 pm	Virgo
13	Virgo		
14	Virgo		
15	Virgo	12:26 am	Libra
16	Libra		
17	Libra	1: 2 am	Scorpio
18	Scorpio		
19	Scorpio	3:47 am	Sagittarius
20	Sagittarius		
21	Sagittarius	10:11 am	Capricorn
22	Capricorn		
23	Capricorn	8:26 pm	Aquarius
24	Aquarius		
25	Aquarius		
26	Aquarius	8:56 am	Pisces
27	Pisces		
28	Pisces	9:15 am	Aries
29	Aries		
30	Aries		
31	Aries	7:48 am	Taurus

November

1	Taurus		
2	Taurus	4:12 pm	Gemini
3	Gemini		
4	Gemini	10:44 pm	Cancer
5	Cancer		
6	Cancer		
7	Cancer	3:34 am	Leo
8	Leo		
9	Leo	6:49 am	Virgo
10	Virgo		
11	Virgo	8:53 am	Libra
12	Libra		
13	Libra	10:44 am	Scorpio
14	Scorpio		
15	Scorpio	1:51 pm	Sagittarius
16	Sagittarius		
17	Sagittarius	7:40 pm	Capricorn
18	Capricorn		
19	Capricorn		
20	Capricorn	4:55 am	Aquarius
21	Aquarius		
22	Aquarius	4:52 pm	Pisces
23	Pisces		
24	Pisces		
25	Pisces	5:21 am	Aries
26	Aries		
27	Aries	4: 6 pm	Taurus
28	Taurus		
29	Taurus		
30	Taurus	12: 4 am	Gemini

December

1	Gemini		
2	Gemini	5:30 am	Cancer
3	Cancer		
4	Cancer	9:15 am	Leo
5	Leo		
6	Leo	12:11 pm	Virgo
7	Virgo		
8	Virgo	2:57 pm	Libra
9	Libra		
10	Libra	6: 9 pm	Scorpio
11	Scorpio		
12	Scorpio	10:30 pm	Sagittarius
13	Sagittarius		
14	Sagittarius		
15	Sagittarius	4:48 am	Capricorn
16	Capricorn		
17	Capricorn	1:43 pm	Aquarius
18	Aquarius		
19	Aquarius		
20	Aquarius	1: 9 am	Pisces
21	Pisces		
22	Pisces	1:45 pm	Aries
23	Aries		
24	Aries		
25	Aries	1:12 am	Taurus
26	Taurus		
27	Taurus	9:39 am	Gemini
28	Gemini		
29	Gemini	2:40 pm	Cancer
30	Cancer		
31	Cancer	5: 9 pm	Leo

MOON POSITIONS 2002

January

1	Leo		
2	Leo	6:34 pm	Virgo
3	Virgo		
4	Virgo	8:23 pm	Libra
5	Libra		
6	Libra	11:41 pm	Scorpio
7	Scorpio		
8	Scorpio		
9	Scorpio	4:57 am	Sagittarius
10	Sagittarius		
11	Sagittarius	12:18 pm	Capricorn
12	Capricorn		
13	Capricorn	9:41 pm	Aquarius
14	Aquarius		
15	Aquarius		
16	Aquarius	9: 0 am	Pisces
17	Pisces		
18	Pisces	9:35 pm	Aries
19	Aries		
20	Aries		
21	Aries	9:47 am	Taurus
22	Taurus		
23	Taurus	7:28 pm	Gemini
24	Gemini		
25	Gemini		
26	Gemini	1:17 am	Cancer
27	Cancer		
28	Cancer	3:31 am	Leo
29	Leo		
30	Leo	3:40 am	Virgo
31	Virgo		

February

1	Virgo	3:44 am	Libra
2	Libra		
3	Libra	5:35 am	Scorpio
4	Scorpio		
5	Scorpio	10:21 am	Sagittarius
6	Sagittarius		
7	Sagittarius	6: 8 pm	Capricorn
8	Capricorn		
9	Capricorn		
10	Capricorn	4:15 am	Aquarius
11	Aquarius		
12	Aquarius	3:53 pm	Pisces
13	Pisces		
14	Pisces		
15	Pisces	4:26 am	Aries
16	Aries		
17	Aries	4:58 pm	Taurus
18	Taurus		
19	Taurus		
20	Taurus	3:50 am	Gemini
21	Gemini		
22	Gemini	11:16 am	Cancer
23	Cancer		
24	Cancer	2:36 pm	Leo
25	Leo		
26	Leo	2:47 pm	Virgo
27	Virgo		
28	Virgo	1:47 pm	Libra

March

1	Libra		
2	Libra	1:51 pm	Scorpio
3	Scorpio		
4	Scorpio	4:55 pm	Sagittarius
5	Sagittarius		
6	Sagittarius	11:48 pm	Capricorn
7	Capricorn		
8	Capricorn		
9	Capricorn	9:56 am	Aquarius
10	Aquarius		
11	Aquarius	9:56 pm	Pisces
12	Pisces		
13	Pisces		
14	Pisces	10:34 am	Aries
15	Aries		
16	Aries	11: 1 pm	Taurus
17	Taurus		
18	Taurus		
19	Taurus	10:20 am	Gemini
20	Gemini		
21	Gemini	7: 6 pm	Cancer
22	Cancer		
23	Cancer		
24	Cancer	12:13 am	Leo
25	Leo		
26	Leo	1:44 am	Virgo
27	Virgo		
28	Virgo	1: 4 am	Libra
29	Libra		
30	Libra	12:21 am	Scorpio
31	Scorpio		

April

1	Scorpio	1:48 am	Sagittarius
2	Sagittarius		
3	Sagittarius	6:58 am	Capricorn
4	Capricorn		
5	Capricorn	4: 7 pm	Aquarius
6	Aquarius		
7	Aquarius		
8	Aquarius	3:57 am	Pisces
9	Pisces		
10	Pisces	4:40 pm	Aries
11	Aries		
12	Aries		
13	Aries	4:55 am	Taurus
14	Taurus		
15	Taurus	3:56 pm	Gemini
16	Gemini		
17	Gemini		
18	Gemini	1: 1 am	Cancer
19	Cancer		
20	Cancer	7:20 am	Leo
21	Leo		
22	Leo	10:35 am	Virgo
23	Virgo		
24	Virgo	11:22 am	Libra
25	Libra		
26	Libra	11:15 am	Scorpio
27	Scorpio		
28	Scorpio	12:13 pm	Sagittarius
29	Sagittarius		
30	Sagittarius	4: 3 pm	Capricorn

May

1	Capricorn		
2	Capricorn	11:43 pm	Aquarius
3	Aquarius		
4	Aquarius		
5	Aquarius	10:46 am	Pisces
6	Pisces		
7	Pisces	11:22 pm	Aries
8	Aries		
9	Aries		
10	Aries	11:32 am	Taurus
11	Taurus		
12	Taurus	10: 4 pm	Gemini
13	Gemini		
14	Gemini		
15	Gemini	6:33 am	Cancer
16	Cancer		
17	Cancer	12:52 pm	Leo
18	Leo		
19	Leo	5: 1 pm	Virgo
20	Virgo		
21	Virgo	7:19 pm	Libra
22	Libra		
23	Libra	8:38 pm	Scorpio
24	Scorpio		
25	Scorpio	10:20 pm	Sagittarius
26	Sagittarius		
27	Sagittarius		
28	Sagittarius	1:54 am	Capricorn
29	Capricorn		
30	Capricorn	8:35 am	Aquarius
31	Aquarius		

June

1	Aquarius	6:37 pm	Pisces
2	Pisces		
3	Pisces		
4	Pisces	6:51 am	Aries
5	Aries		
6	Aries	7: 6 pm	Taurus
7	Taurus		
8	Taurus		
9	Taurus	5:29 am	Gemini
10	Gemini		
11	Gemini	1:15 pm	Cancer
12	Cancer		
13	Cancer	6:39 pm	Leo
14	Leo		
15	Leo	10:23 pm	Virgo
16	Virgo		
17	Virgo		
18	Virgo	1:11 am	Libra
19	Libra		
20	Libra	3:42 am	Scorpio
21	Scorpio		
22	Scorpio	6:42 am	Sagittarius
23	Sagittarius		
24	Sagittarius	11: 1 am	Capricorn
25	Capricorn		
26	Capricorn	5:36 pm	Aquarius
27	Aquarius		
28	Aquarius		
29	Aquarius	3: 0 am	Pisces
30	Pisces		

MOONPOSITIONS2002

July

1	Pisces	2:49 pm	Aries
2	Aries		
3	Aries		
4	Aries	3:16 am	Taurus
5	Taurus		
6	Taurus	2: 1 pm	Gemini
7	Gemini		
8	Gemini	9:36 pm	Cancer
9	Cancer		
10	Cancer		
11	Cancer	2: 8 am	Leo
12	Leo		
13	Leo	4:41 am	Virgo
14	Virgo		
15	Virgo	6:39 am	Libra
16	Libra		
17	Libra	9:13 am	Scorpio
18	Scorpio		
19	Scorpio	1: 2 pm	Sagittarius
20	Sagittarius		
21	Sagittarius	6:26 pm	Capricorn
22	Capricorn		
23	Capricorn		
24	Capricorn	1:40 am	Aquarius
25	Aquarius		
26	Aquarius	11: 4 am	Pisces
27	Pisces		
28	Pisces	10:38 pm	Aries
29	Aries		
30	Aries		
31	Aries	11:17 am	Taurus

August

1	Taurus		
2	Taurus	10:46 pm	Gemini
3	Gemini		
4	Gemini		
5	Gemini	7: 2 am	Cancer
6	Cancer		
7	Cancer	11:27 am	Leo
8	Leo		
9	Leo	1: 3 pm	Virgo
10	Virgo		
11	Virgo	1:38 pm	Libra
12	Libra		
13	Libra	3: 1 pm	Scorpio
14	Scorpio		
15	Scorpio	6:25 pm	Sagittarius
16	Sagittarius		
17	Sagittarius		
18	Sagittarius	12:15 am	Capricorn
19	Capricorn		
20	Capricorn	8:16 am	Aquarius
21	Aquarius		
22	Aquarius	6:11 pm	Pisces
23	Pisces		
24	Pisces		
25	Pisces	5:47 am	Aries
26	Aries		
27	Aries	6:31 pm	Taurus
28	Taurus		
29	Taurus		
30	Taurus	6:45 am	Gemini
31	Gemini		

September

1	Gemini	4:14 pm	Cancer
2	Cancer		
3	Cancer	9:36 pm	Leo
4	Leo		
5	Leo	11:16 pm	Virgo
6	Virgo		
7	Virgo	10:57 pm	Libra
8	Libra		
9	Libra	10:48 pm	Scorpio
10	Scorpio		
11	Scorpio		
12	Scorpio	12:44 am	Sagittarius
13	Sagittarius		
14	Sagittarius	5:47 am	Capricorn
15	Capricorn		
16	Capricorn	1:54 pm	Aquarius
17	Aquarius		
18	Aquarius		
19	Aquarius	12:18 am	Pisces
20	Pisces		
21	Pisces	12:11 pm	Aries
22	Aries		
23	Aries		
24	Aries	12:54 am	Taurus
25	Taurus		
26	Taurus	1:26 pm	Gemini
27	Gemini		
28	Gemini		
29	Gemini	12: 1 am	Cancer
30	Cancer		

October

1	Cancer	6:58 am	Leo
2	Leo		
3	Leo	9:52 am	Virgo
4	Virgo		
5	Virgo	9:51 am	Libra
6	Libra		
7	Libra	8:57 am	Scorpio
8	Scorpio		
9	Scorpio	9:21 am	Sagittarius
10	Sagittarius		
11	Sagittarius	12:45 pm	Capricorn
12	Capricorn		
13	Capricorn	7:51 pm	Aquarius
14	Aquarius		
15	Aquarius		
16	Aquarius	6: 7 am	Pisces
17	Pisces		
18	Pisces	6:13 pm	Aries
19	Aries		
20	Aries		
21	Aries	6:57 am	Taurus
22	Taurus		
23	Taurus	7:17 pm	Gemini
24	Gemini		
25	Gemini		
26	Gemini	6:10 am	Cancer
27	Cancer		
28	Cancer	2:20 pm	Leo
29	Leo		
30	Leo	6:59 pm	Virgo
31	Virgo		

November

1	Virgo	8:28 pm	Libra
2	Libra		
3	Libra	8:10 pm	Scorpio
4	Scorpio		
5	Scorpio	8: 1 pm	Sagittarius
6	Sagittarius		
7	Sagittarius	9:59 pm	Capricorn
8	Capricorn		
9	Capricorn		
10	Capricorn	3:27 am	Aquarius
11	Aquarius		
12	Aquarius	12:42 pm	Pisces
13	Pisces		
14	Pisces		
15	Pisces	12:38 am	Aries
16	Aries		
17	Aries	1:23 pm	Taurus
18	Taurus		
19	Taurus		
20	Taurus	1:25 am	Gemini
21	Gemini		
22	Gemini	11:48 am	Cancer
23	Cancer		
24	Cancer	8: 0 pm	Leo
25	Leo		
26	Leo		
27	Leo	1:42 am	Virgo
28	Virgo		
29	Virgo	4:54 am	Libra
30	Libra		

December

1	Libra	6:15 am	Scorpio
2	Scorpio		
3	Scorpio	6:58 am	Sagittarius
4	Sagittarius		
5	Sagittarius	8:39 am	Capricorn
6	Capricorn		
7	Capricorn	12:54 pm	Aquarius
8	Aquarius		
9	Aquarius	8:46 pm	Pisces
10	Pisces		
11	Pisces		
12	Pisces	7:58 am	Aries
13	Aries		
14	Aries	8:43 pm	Taurus
15	Taurus		
16	Taurus		
17	Taurus	8:43 am	Gemini
18	Gemini		
19	Gemini	6:30 pm	Cancer
20	Cancer		
21	Cancer		
22	Cancer	1:48 am	Leo
23	Leo		
24	Leo	7: 5 am	Virgo
25	Virgo		
26	Virgo	10:53 am	Libra
27	Libra		
28	Libra	1:41 pm	Scorpio
29	Scorpio		
30	Scorpio	4: 1 pm	Sagittarius
31	Sagittarius		

MOON POSITIONS 2003

January

1	Sagittarius	6:42 pm	Capricorn
2	Capricorn		
3	Capricorn	10:56 pm	Aquarius
4	Aquarius		
5	Aquarius		
6	Aquarius	5:57 am	Pisces
7	Pisces		
8	Pisces	4:15 pm	Aries
9	Aries		
10	Aries		
11	Aries	4:48 am	Taurus
12	Taurus		
13	Taurus	5: 8 pm	Gemini
14	Gemini		
15	Gemini		
16	Gemini	2:56 am	Cancer
17	Cancer		
18	Cancer	9:29 am	Leo
19	Leo		
20	Leo	1:32 pm	Virgo
21	Virgo		
22	Virgo	4:23 pm	Libra
23	Libra		
24	Libra	7: 9 pm	Scorpio
25	Scorpio		
26	Scorpio	10:26 pm	Sagittarius
27	Sagittarius		
28	Sagittarius		
29	Sagittarius	2:30 am	Capricorn
30	Capricorn		
31	Capricorn	7:44 am	Aquarius

February

1	Aquarius		
2	Aquarius	2:54 pm	Pisces
3	Pisces		
4	Pisces		
5	Pisces	12:44 am	Aries
6	Aries		
7	Aries	12:59 pm	Taurus
8	Taurus		
9	Taurus		
10	Taurus	1:45 am	Gemini
11	Gemini		
12	Gemini	12:19 pm	Cancer
13	Cancer		
14	Cancer	7: 4 pm	Leo
15	Leo		
16	Leo	10:22 pm	Virgo
17	Virgo		
18	Virgo	11:48 pm	Libra
19	Libra		
20	Libra		
21	Libra	1: 9 am	Scorpio
22	Scorpio		
23	Scorpio	3:46 am	Sagittarius
24	Sagittarius		
25	Sagittarius	8:11 am	Capricorn
26	Capricorn		
27	Capricorn	2:24 pm	Aquarius
28	Aquarius		

March

1	Aquarius	10:26 pm	Pisces
2	Pisces		
3	Pisces		
4	Pisces	8:30 am	Aries
5	Aries		
6	Aries	8:36 am	Taurus
7	Taurus		
8	Taurus		
9	Taurus	9:38 am	Gemini
10	Gemini		
11	Gemini	9:12 pm	Cancer
12	Cancer		
13	Cancer		
14	Cancer	5: 6 am	Leo
15	Leo		
16	Leo	8:52 am	Virgo
17	Virgo		
18	Virgo	9:43 am	Libra
19	Libra		
20	Libra	9:38 am	Scorpio
21	Scorpio		
22	Scorpio	10:33 am	Sagittarius
23	Sagittarius		
24	Sagittarius	1:48 pm	Capricorn
25	Capricorn		
26	Capricorn	7:51 pm	Aquarius
27	Aquarius		
28	Aquarius		
29	Aquarius	4:26 am	Pisces
30	Pisces		
31	Pisces	3: 4 pm	Aries

April

1	Aries		
2	Aries		
3	Aries	3:20 am	Taurus
4	Taurus		
5	Taurus	4:24 pm	Gemini
6	Gemini		
7	Gemini		
8	Gemini	4:36 am	Cancer
9	Cancer		
10	Cancer	1:54 pm	Leo
11	Leo		
12	Leo	7: 7 pm	Virgo
13	Virgo		
14	Virgo	8:42 pm	Libra
15	Libra		
16	Libra	8:16 pm	Scorpio
17	Scorpio		
18	Scorpio	7:51 pm	Sagittarius
19	Sagittarius		
20	Sagittarius	9:20 pm	Capricorn
21	Capricorn		
22	Capricorn		
23	Capricorn	1:58 am	Aquarius
24	Aquarius		
25	Aquarius	10: 2 am	Pisces
26	Pisces		
27	Pisces	8:54 pm	Aries
28	Aries		
29	Aries		
30	Aries	9:26 am	Taurus

May

1	Taurus		
2	Taurus	10:27 pm	Gemini
3	Gemini		
4	Gemini		
5	Gemini	10:42 am	Cancer
6	Cancer		
7	Cancer	8:46 pm	Leo
8	Leo		
9	Leo		
10	Leo	3:31 am	Virgo
11	Virgo		
12	Virgo	6:42 am	Libra
13	Libra		
14	Libra	7:13 am	Scorpio
15	Scorpio		
16	Scorpio	6:43 am	Sagittarius
17	Sagittarius		
18	Sagittarius	7: 3 am	Capricorn
19	Capricorn		
20	Capricorn	10: 1 am	Aquarius
21	Aquarius		
22	Aquarius	4:41 pm	Pisces
23	Pisces		
24	Pisces		
25	Pisces	2:59 am	Aries
26	Aries		
27	Aries	3:32 pm	Taurus
28	Taurus		
29	Taurus		
30	Taurus	4:32 am	Gemini
31	Gemini		

June

1	Gemini	4:27 pm	Cancer
2	Cancer		
3	Cancer		
4	Cancer	2:25 am	Leo
5	Leo		
6	Leo	9:51 am	Virgo
7	Virgo		
8	Virgo	2:30 pm	Libra
9	Libra		
10	Libra	4:39 pm	Scorpio
11	Scorpio		
12	Scorpio	5:12 pm	Sagittarius
13	Sagittarius		
14	Sagittarius	5:38 pm	Capricorn
15	Capricorn		
16	Capricorn	7:41 pm	Aquarius
17	Aquarius		
18	Aquarius		
19	Aquarius	12:57 am	Pisces
20	Pisces		
21	Pisces	10: 6 am	Aries
22	Aries		
23	Aries	10:15 pm	Taurus
24	Taurus		
25	Taurus		
26	Taurus	11:13 am	Gemini
27	Gemini		
28	Gemini	10:52 pm	Cancer
29	Cancer		
30	Cancer		

MOONPOSITIONS 2003

July

1	Cancer	8:13 am	Leo
2	Leo		
3	Leo	3:16 pm	Virgo
4	Virgo		
5	Virgo	8:20 pm	Libra
6	Libra		
7	Libra	11:43 pm	Scorpio
8	Scorpio		
9	Scorpio		
10	Scorpio	1:48 am	Sagittarius
11	Sagittarius		
12	Sagittarius	3:21 pm	Capricorn
13	Capricorn		
14	Capricorn	5:38 am	Aquarius
15	Aquarius		
16	Aquarius	10:14 am	Pisces
17	Pisces		
18	Pisces	6:20 pm	Aries
19	Aries		
20	Aries		
21	Aries	5:48 am	Taurus
22	Taurus		
23	Taurus	6:42 pm	Gemini
24	Gemini		
25	Gemini		
26	Gemini	6:23 am	Cancer
27	Cancer		
28	Cancer	3:17 pm	Leo
29	Leo		
30	Leo	9:27 pm	Virgo
31	Virgo		

August

1	Virgo		
2	Virgo	1:48 am	Libra
3	Libra		
4	Libra	5:12 am	Scorpio
5	Scorpio		
6	Scorpio	8:11 am	Sagittarius
7	Sagittarius		
8	Sagittarius	11: 2 am	Capricorn
9	Capricorn		
10	Capricorn	2:23 pm	Aquarius
11	Aquarius		
12	Aquarius	7:19 pm	Pisces
13	Pisces		
14	Pisces		
15	Pisces	3: 0 am	Aries
16	Aries		
17	Aries	1:52 am	Taurus
18	Taurus		
19	Taurus		
20	Taurus	2:41 am	Gemini
21	Gemini		
22	Gemini	2:44 pm	Cancer
23	Cancer		
24	Cancer	11:48 pm	Leo
25	Leo		
26	Leo		
27	Leo	5:27 am	Virgo
28	Virgo		
29	Virgo	8:41 am	Libra
30	Libra		
31	Libra	11: 0 am	Scorpio

September

1	Scorpio		
2	Scorpio	1:32 pm	Sagittarius
3	Sagittarius		
4	Sagittarius	4:51 pm	Capricorn
5	Capricorn		
6	Capricorn	9:15 pm	Aquarius
7	Aquarius		
8	Aquarius		
9	Aquarius	3: 7 am	Pisces
10	Pisces		
11	Pisces	11: 9 am	Aries
12	Aries		
13	Aries	9:50 pm	Taurus
14	Taurus		
15	Taurus		
16	Taurus	10:32 am	Gemini
17	Gemini		
18	Gemini	11: 7 pm	Cancer
19	Cancer		
20	Cancer		
21	Cancer	9: 2 am	Leo
22	Leo		
23	Leo	3: 4 pm	Virgo
24	Virgo		
25	Virgo	5:49 pm	Libra
26	Libra		
27	Libra	6:52 pm	Scorpio
28	Scorpio		
29	Scorpio	7:57 pm	Sagittarius
30	Sagittarius		

October

1	Sagittarius	10:21 pm	Capricorn
2	Capricorn		
3	Capricorn		
4	Capricorn	2:45 am	Aquarius
5	Aquarius		
6	Aquarius	9:20 am	Pisces
7	Pisces		
8	Pisces	6: 7 pm	Aries
9	Aries		
10	Aries		
11	Aries	5: 5 am	Taurus
12	Taurus		
13	Taurus	5:45 pm	Gemini
14	Gemini		
15	Gemini		
16	Gemini	6:41 am	Cancer
17	Cancer		
18	Cancer	5:41 pm	Leo
19	Leo		
20	Leo		
21	Leo	1: 1 am	Virgo
22	Virgo		
23	Virgo	4:27 am	Libra
24	Libra		
25	Libra	5: 8 am	Scorpio
26	Scorpio		
27	Scorpio	4:55 am	Sagittarius
28	Sagittarius		
29	Sagittarius	5:37 am	Capricorn
30	Capricorn		
31	Capricorn	8:41 am	Aquarius

November

1	Aquarius		
2	Aquarius	2:52 pm	Pisces
3	Pisces		
4	Pisces		
5	Pisces	12: 2 am	Aries
6	Aries		
7	Aries	11:29 am	Taurus
8	Taurus		
9	Taurus		
10	Taurus	12:14 am	Gemini
11	Gemini		
12	Gemini	1:10 pm	Cancer
13	Cancer		
14	Cancer		
15	Cancer	12:48 am	Leo
16	Leo		
17	Leo	9:36 am	Virgo
18	Virgo		
19	Virgo	2:42 pm	Libra
20	Libra		
21	Libra	4:23 pm	Scorpio
22	Scorpio		
23	Scorpio	4: 2 pm	Sagittarius
24	Sagittarius		
25	Sagittarius	3:31 pm	Capricorn
26	Capricorn		
27	Capricorn	4:48 pm	Aquarius
28	Aquarius		
29	Aquarius	9:25 pm	Pisces
30	Pisces		

December

1	Pisces		
2	Pisces	5:56 am	Aries
3	Aries		
4	Aries	5:30 pm	Taurus
5	Taurus		
6	Taurus		
7	Taurus	6:26 am	Gemini
8	Gemini		
9	Gemini	7:11 pm	Cancer
10	Cancer		
11	Cancer		
12	Cancer	6:40 am	Leo
13	Leo		
14	Leo	4: 7 pm	Virgo
15	Virgo		
16	Virgo	10:46 pm	Libra
17	Libra		
18	Libra		
19	Libra	2:20 am	Scorpio
20	Scorpio		
21	Scorpio	3:16 am	Sagittarius
22	Sagittarius		
23	Sagittarius	2:55 am	Capricorn
24	Capricorn		
25	Capricorn	3:13 am	Aquarius
26	Aquarius		
27	Aquarius	6:10 am	Pisces
28	Pisces		
29	Pisces	1: 8 pm	Aries
30	Aries		
31	Aries		

MOONPOSITIONS2004

January

1	Aries	12: 1 am	Taurus
2	Taurus		
3	Taurus	12:58 pm	Gemini
4	Gemini		
5	Gemini		
6	Gemini	1:38 am	Cancer
7	Cancer		
8	Cancer	12:38 pm	Leo
9	Leo		
10	Leo	9:37 pm	Virgo
11	Virgo		
12	Virgo		
13	Virgo	4:38 am	Libra
14	Libra		
15	Libra	9:32 am	Scorpio
16	Scorpio		
17	Scorpio	12:18 pm	Sagittarius
18	Sagittarius		
19	Sagittarius	1:24 am	Capricorn
20	Capricorn		
21	Capricorn	2:10 pm	Aquarius
22	Aquarius		
23	Aquarius	4:29 pm	Pisces
24	Pisces		
25	Pisces	10: 6 pm	Aries
26	Aries		
27	Aries		
28	Aries	7:46 am	Taurus
29	Taurus		
30	Taurus	8:18 pm	Gemini
31	Gemini		

February

1	Gemini		
2	Gemini	9: 3 am	Cancer
3	Cancer		
4	Cancer	7:50 pm	Leo
5	Leo		
6	Leo		
7	Leo	4: 3 am	Virgo
8	Virgo		
9	Virgo	10:12 am	Libra
10	Libra		
11	Libra	2:57 pm	Scorpio
12	Scorpio		
13	Scorpio	6:35 pm	Sagittarius
14	Sagittarius		
15	Sagittarius	9:14 pm	Capricorn
16	Capricorn		
17	Capricorn	11:27 pm	Aquarius
18	Aquarius		
19	Aquarius		
20	Aquarius	2:26 am	Pisces
21	Pisces		
22	Pisces	7:45 am	Aries
23	Aries		
24	Aries	4:30 pm	Taurus
25	Taurus		
26	Taurus		
27	Taurus	4:22 am	Gemini
28	Gemini		
29	Gemini	5:12 pm	Cancer

March

1	Cancer		
2	Cancer		
3	Cancer	4:18 am	Leo
4	Leo		
5	Leo	12:18 pm	Virgo
6	Virgo		
7	Virgo	5:31 pm	Libra
8	Libra		
9	Libra	9: 3 pm	Scorpio
10	Scorpio		
11	Scorpio	11:57 pm	Sagittarius
12	Sagittarius		
13	Sagittarius		
14	Sagittarius	2:51 am	Capricorn
15	Capricorn		
16	Capricorn	6:10 am	Aquarius
17	Aquarius		
18	Aquarius	10:26 am	Pisces
19	Pisces		
20	Pisces	4:29 pm	Aries
21	Aries		
22	Aries		
23	Aries	1: 9 am	Taurus
24	Taurus		
25	Taurus	12:35 pm	Gemini
26	Gemini		
27	Gemini		
28	Gemini	1:23 am	Cancer
29	Cancer		
30	Cancer	1: 7 pm	Leo
31	Leo		

April

1	Leo	9:45 pm	Virgo
2	Virgo		
3	Virgo		
4	Virgo	2:52 am	Libra
5	Libra		
6	Libra	5:24 am	Scorpio
7	Scorpio		
8	Scorpio	6:50 am	Sagittarius
9	Sagittarius		
10	Sagittarius	8:33 am	Capricorn
11	Capricorn		
12	Capricorn	11:33 am	Aquarius
13	Aquarius		
14	Aquarius	4:24 pm	Pisces
15	Pisces		
16	Pisces	11:24 pm	Aries
17	Aries		
18	Aries		
19	Aries	8:42 am	Taurus
20	Taurus		
21	Taurus	8:10 pm	Gemini
22	Gemini		
23	Gemini		
24	Gemini	8:56 am	Cancer
25	Cancer		
26	Cancer	9:14 pm	Leo
27	Leo		
28	Leo		
29	Leo	7: 0 am	Virgo
30	Virgo		

May

1	Virgo	1: 2 pm	Libra
2	Libra		
3	Libra	3:38 pm	Scorpio
4	Scorpio		
5	Scorpio	4: 8 pm	Sagittarius
6	Sagittarius		
7	Sagittarius	4:17 pm	Capricorn
8	Capricorn		
9	Capricorn	5:46 pm	Aquarius
10	Aquarius		
11	Aquarius	9:52 pm	Pisces
12	Pisces		
13	Pisces		
14	Pisces	5: 2 am	Aries
15	Aries		
16	Aries	2:57 pm	Taurus
17	Taurus		
18	Taurus		
19	Taurus	2:47 am	Gemini
20	Gemini		
21	Gemini	3:35 pm	Cancer
22	Cancer		
23	Cancer		
24	Cancer	4: 7 am	Leo
25	Leo		
26	Leo	2:52 pm	Virgo
27	Virgo		
28	Virgo	10:22 pm	Libra
29	Libra		
30	Libra		
31	Libra	2: 8 am	Scorpio

June

1	Scorpio		
2	Scorpio	2:52 am	Sagittarius
3	Sagittarius		
4	Sagittarius	2:12 am	Capricorn
5	Capricorn		
6	Capricorn	2:10 am	Aquarius
7	Aquarius		
8	Aquarius	4:38 am	Pisces
9	Pisces		
10	Pisces	10:49 am	Aries
11	Aries		
12	Aries	8:37 pm	Taurus
13	Taurus		
14	Taurus		
15	Taurus	8:44 am	Gemini
16	Gemini		
17	Gemini	9:37 pm	Cancer
18	Cancer		
19	Cancer		
20	Cancer	10: 5 am	Leo
21	Leo		
22	Leo	9:10 pm	Virgo
23	Virgo		
24	Virgo		
25	Virgo	5:50 am	Libra
26	Libra		
27	Libra	11:13 am	Scorpio
28	Scorpio		
29	Scorpio	1:15 pm	Sagittarius
30	Sagittarius		

MOONPOSITIONS 2004

July

1	Sagittarius	1: 1 pm	Capricorn
2	Capricorn		
3	Capricorn	12:22 pm	Aquarius
4	Aquarius		
5	Aquarius	1:26 pm	Pisces
6	Pisces		
7	Pisces	6: 3 pm	Aries
8	Aries		
9	Aries		
10	Aries	2:50 am	Taurus
11	Taurus		
12	Taurus	2:45 pm	Gemini
13	Gemini		
14	Gemini		
15	Gemini	3:40 am	Cancer
16	Cancer		
17	Cancer	3:56 pm	Leo
18	Leo		
19	Leo		
20	Leo	2:44 am	Virgo
21	Virgo		
22	Virgo	11:39 am	Libra
23	Libra		
24	Libra	6: 8 pm	Scorpio
25	Scorpio		
26	Scorpio	9:48 pm	Sagittarius
27	Sagittarius		
28	Sagittarius	10:57 pm	Capricorn
29	Capricorn		
30	Capricorn	10:54 pm	Aquarius
31	Aquarius		

August

1	Aquarius	11:34 pm	Pisces
2	Pisces		
3	Pisces		
4	Pisces	2:59 am	Aries
5	Aries		
6	Aries	10:26 am	Taurus
7	Taurus		
8	Taurus	9:33 pm	Gemini
9	Gemini		
10	Gemini		
11	Gemini	10:20 am	Cancer
12	Cancer		
13	Cancer	10:30 pm	Leo
14	Leo		
15	Leo		
16	Leo	8:49 am	Virgo
17	Virgo		
18	Virgo	5: 9 pm	Libra
19	Libra		
20	Libra	11:37 pm	Scorpio
21	Scorpio		
22	Scorpio		
23	Scorpio	4: 8 am	Sagittarius
24	Sagittarius		
25	Sagittarius	6:46 am	Capricorn
26	Capricorn		
27	Capricorn	8: 8 am	Aquarius
28	Aquarius		
29	Aquarius	9:33 am	Pisces
30	Pisces		
31	Pisces	12:46 am	Aries

September

1	Aries		
2	Aries	7:16 pm	Taurus
3	Taurus		
4	Taurus		
5	Taurus	5:24 am	Gemini
6	Gemini		
7	Gemini	5:50 pm	Cancer
8	Cancer		
9	Cancer		
10	Cancer	6: 6 am	Leo
11	Leo		
12	Leo	4:16 pm	Virgo
13	Virgo		
14	Virgo	11:53 pm	Libra
15	Libra		
16	Libra		
17	Libra	5:25 am	Scorpio
18	Scorpio		
19	Scorpio	9:30 am	Sagittarius
20	Sagittarius		
21	Sagittarius	12:35 pm	Capricorn
22	Capricorn		
23	Capricorn	3: 9 pm	Aquarius
24	Aquarius		
25	Aquarius	5:55 pm	Pisces
26	Pisces		
27	Pisces	9:57 pm	Aries
28	Aries		
29	Aries		
30	Aries	4:24 am	Taurus

October

1	Taurus		
2	Taurus	1:55 pm	Gemini
3	Gemini		
4	Gemini		
5	Gemini	1:54 am	Cancer
6	Cancer		
7	Cancer	2:23 pm	Leo
8	Leo		
9	Leo		
10	Leo	1: 0 am	Virgo
11	Virgo		
12	Virgo	8:32 am	Libra
13	Libra		
14	Libra	1:10 pm	Scorpio
15	Scorpio		
16	Scorpio	3:58 pm	Sagittarius
17	Sagittarius		
18	Sagittarius	6: 7 pm	Capricorn
19	Capricorn		
20	Capricorn	8:37 pm	Aquarius
21	Aquarius		
22	Aquarius		
23	Aquarius	12:13 am	Pisces
24	Pisces		
25	Pisces	5:24 am	Aries
26	Aries		
27	Aries	12:37 pm	Taurus
28	Taurus		
29	Taurus	10:11 pm	Gemini
30	Gemini		
31	Gemini		

November

1	Gemini	9:53 am	Cancer
2	Cancer		
3	Cancer	10:32 pm	Leo
4	Leo		
5	Leo		
6	Leo	10: 0 am	Virgo
7	Virgo		
8	Virgo	6:23 pm	Libra
9	Libra		
10	Libra	11: 5 pm	Scorpio
11	Scorpio		
12	Scorpio		
13	Scorpio	12:56 am	Sagittarius
14	Sagittarius		
15	Sagittarius	1:33 am	Capricorn
16	Capricorn		
17	Capricorn	2:39 am	Aquarius
18	Aquarius		
19	Aquarius	5:38 am	Pisces
20	Pisces		
21	Pisces	11:11 am	Aries
22	Aries		
23	Aries	7:16 pm	Taurus
24	Taurus		
25	Taurus		
26	Taurus	5:25 am	Gemini
27	Gemini		
28	Gemini	5:10 pm	Cancer
29	Cancer		
30	Cancer		

December

1	Cancer	5:50 am	Leo
2	Leo		
3	Leo	6: 0 pm	Virgo
4	Virgo		
5	Virgo		
6	Virgo	3:46 am	Libra
7	Libra		
8	Libra	9:43 am	Scorpio
9	Scorpio		
10	Scorpio	11:54 am	Sagittarius
11	Sagittarius		
12	Sagittarius	11:41 am	Capricorn
13	Capricorn		
14	Capricorn	11:10 am	Aquarius
15	Aquarius		
16	Aquarius	12:24 pm	Pisces
17	Pisces		
18	Pisces	4:52 pm	Aries
19	Aries		
20	Aries		
21	Aries	12:52 am	Taurus
22	Taurus		
23	Taurus	11:32 am	Gemini
24	Gemini		
25	Gemini	11:38 am	Cancer
26	Cancer		
27	Cancer		
28	Cancer	12:14 pm	Leo
29	Leo		
30	Leo		
31	Leo	12:33 am	Virgo

MOONPOSITIONS 2005

January

1	Virgo		
2	Virgo	11:19 am	Libra
3	Libra		
4	Libra	6:59 pm	Scorpio
5	Scorpio		
6	Scorpio	10:44 pm	Sagittarius
7	Sagittarius		
8	Sagittarius	11:11 pm	Capricorn
9	Capricorn		
10	Capricorn	10: 7 pm	Aquarius
11	Aquarius		
12	Aquarius	9:50 pm	Pisces
13	Pisces		
14	Pisces		
15	Pisces	12:27 am	Aries
16	Aries		
17	Aries	7: 6 am	Taurus
18	Taurus		
19	Taurus	5:24 pm	Gemini
20	Gemini		
21	Gemini		
22	Gemini	5:42 am	Cancer
23	Cancer		
24	Cancer	6:21 pm	Leo
25	Leo		
26	Leo		
27	Leo	6:24 am	Virgo
28	Virgo		
29	Virgo	5:13 pm	Libra
30	Libra		
31	Libra		

February

1	Libra	1:51 am	Scorpio
2	Scorpio		
3	Scorpio	7:21 am	Sagittarius
4	Sagittarius		
5	Sagittarius	9:32 am	Capricorn
6	Capricorn		
7	Capricorn	9:26 am	Aquarius
8	Aquarius		
9	Aquarius	8:59 am	Pisces
10	Pisces		
11	Pisces	10:21 am	Aries
12	Aries		
13	Aries	3:18 pm	Taurus
14	Taurus		
15	Taurus		
16	Taurus	12:18 am	Gemini
17	Gemini		
18	Gemini	12:13 pm	Cancer
19	Cancer		
20	Cancer		
21	Cancer	12:54 am	Leo
22	Leo		
23	Leo	12:44 pm	Virgo
24	Virgo		
25	Virgo	10:59 pm	Libra
26	Libra		
27	Libra		
28	Libra	7:20 am	Scorpio

March

1	Scorpio		
2	Scorpio	1:29 pm	Sagittarius
3	Sagittarius		
4	Sagittarius	5:11 pm	Capricorn
5	Capricorn		
6	Capricorn	6:49 pm	Aquarius
7	Aquarius		
8	Aquarius	7:32 pm	Pisces
9	Pisces		
10	Pisces	9: 3 pm	Aries
11	Aries		
12	Aries		
13	Aries	1: 5 am	Taurus
14	Taurus		
15	Taurus	8:44 am	Gemini
16	Gemini		
17	Gemini	7:44 pm	Cancer
18	Cancer		
19	Cancer		
20	Cancer	8:17 am	Leo
21	Leo		
22	Leo	8:10 pm	Virgo
23	Virgo		
24	Virgo		
25	Virgo	6: 0 am	Libra
26	Libra		
27	Libra	1:29 pm	Scorpio
28	Scorpio		
29	Scorpio	6:56 pm	Sagittarius
30	Sagittarius		
31	Sagittarius	10:48 pm	Capricorn

April

1	Capricorn		
2	Capricorn		
3	Capricorn	1:31 am	Aquarius
4	Aquarius		
5	Aquarius	3:45 am	Pisces
6	Pisces		
7	Pisces	6:28 am	Aries
8	Aries		
9	Aries	10:50 am	Taurus
10	Taurus		
11	Taurus	5:54 pm	Gemini
12	Gemini		
13	Gemini		
14	Gemini	4: 3 am	Cancer
15	Cancer		
16	Cancer	4:17 pm	Leo
17	Leo		
18	Leo		
19	Leo	4:27 am	Virgo
20	Virgo		
21	Virgo	2:27 pm	Libra
22	Libra		
23	Libra	9:25 pm	Scorpio
24	Scorpio		
25	Scorpio		
26	Scorpio	1:46 am	Sagittarius
27	Sagittarius		
28	Sagittarius	4:32 am	Capricorn
29	Capricorn		
30	Capricorn	6:54 am	Aquarius

May

1	Aquarius		
2	Aquarius	9:43 am	Pisces
3	Pisces		
4	Pisces	1:36 pm	Aries
5	Aries		
6	Aries	7: 1 pm	Taurus
7	Taurus		
8	Taurus		
9	Taurus	2:29 am	Gemini
10	Gemini		
11	Gemini	12:20 pm	Cancer
12	Cancer		
13	Cancer		
14	Cancer	12:17 am	Leo
15	Leo		
16	Leo	12:46 pm	Virgo
17	Virgo		
18	Virgo	11:30 pm	Libra
19	Libra		
20	Libra		
21	Libra	6:48 am	Scorpio
22	Scorpio		
23	Scorpio	10:38 am	Sagittarius
24	Sagittarius		
25	Sagittarius	12:11 pm	Capricorn
26	Capricorn		
27	Capricorn	!:10 pm	Aquarius
28	Aquarius		
29	Aquarius	3: 9 pm	Pisces
30	Pisces		
31	Pisces	7: 7 pm	Aries

June

1	Aries		
2	Aries		
3	Aries	1:20 am	Taurus
4	Taurus		
5	Taurus	9:36 am	Gemini
6	Gemini		
7	Gemini	7:46 pm	Cancer
8	Cancer		
9	Cancer		
10	Cancer	7:39 am	Leo
11	Leo		
12	Leo	8:22 pm	Virgo
13	Virgo		
14	Virgo		
15	Virgo	7:59 am	Libra
16	Libra		
17	Libra	4:23 pm	Scorpio
18	Scorpio		
19	Scorpio	8:45 pm	Sagittarius
20	Sagittarius		
21	Sagittarius	9:52 pm	Capricorn
22	Capricorn		
23	Capricorn	9:36 pm	Aquarius
24	Aquarius		
25	Aquarius	10: 3 pm	Pisces
26	Pisces		
27	Pisces		
28	Pisces	12:51 am	Aries
29	Aries		
30	Aries	6:45 am	Taurus

MOON POSITIONS 2005

July

1	Taurus		
2	Taurus	3:26 pm	Gemini
3	Gemini		
4	Gemini		
5	Gemini	2: 7 am	Cancer
6	Cancer		
7	Cancer	2:11 pm	Leo
8	Leo		
9	Leo		
10	Leo	2:57 am	Virgo
11	Virgo		
12	Virgo	3: 9 pm	Libra
13	Libra		
14	Libra		
15	Libra	12:51 am	Scorpio
16	Scorpio		
17	Scorpio	6:35 am	Sagittarius
18	Sagittarius		
19	Sagittarius	8:26 am	Capricorn
20	Capricorn		
21	Capricorn	7:55 am	Aquarius
22	Aquarius		
23	Aquarius	7:11 am	Pisces
24	Pisces		
25	Pisces	8:23 am	Aries
26	Aries		
27	Aries	12:54 pm	Taurus
28	Taurus		
29	Taurus	9: 2 pm	Gemini
30	Gemini		
31	Gemini		

August

1	Gemini	7:52 am	Cancer
2	Cancer		
3	Cancer	8:10 pm	Leo
4	Leo		
5	Leo		
6	Leo	8:54 am	Virgo
7	Virgo		
8	Virgo	9: 8 pm	Libra
9	Libra		
10	Libra		
11	Libra	7:35 am	Scorpio
12	Scorpio		
13	Scorpio	2:47 pm	Sagittarius
14	Sagittarius		
15	Sagittarius	6:13 pm	Capricorn
16	Capricorn		
17	Capricorn	6:38 pm	Aquarius
18	Aquarius		
19	Aquarius	5:52 pm	Pisces
20	Pisces		
21	Pisces	6: 1 pm	Aries
22	Aries		
23	Aries	8:58 pm	Taurus
24	Taurus		
25	Taurus		
26	Taurus	3:42 am	Gemini
27	Gemini		
28	Gemini	1:57 pm	Cancer
29	Cancer		
30	Cancer		
31	Cancer	2:14 am	Leo

September

1	Leo		
2	Leo	2:56 pm	Virgo
3	Virgo		
4	Virgo		
5	Virgo	2:52 am	Libra
6	Libra		
7	Libra	1:10 pm	Scorpio
8	Scorpio		
9	Scorpio	9: 3 pm	Sagittarius
10	Sagittarius		
11	Sagittarius		
12	Sagittarius	1:56 am	Capricorn
13	Capricorn		
14	Capricorn	4: 2 am	Aquarius
15	Aquarius		
16	Aquarius	4:24 am	Pisces
17	Pisces		
18	Pisces	4:43 am	Aries
19	Aries		
20	Aries	6:47 am	Taurus
21	Taurus		
22	Taurus	12: 7 pm	Gemini
23	Gemini		
24	Gemini	9:10 pm	Cancer
25	Cancer		
26	Cancer		
27	Cancer	9: 2 am	Leo
28	Leo		
29	Leo	9:44 pm	Virgo
30	Virgo		

October

1	Virgo		
2	Virgo	9:24 am	Libra
3	Libra		
4	Libra	7: 3 pm	Scorpio
5	Scorpio		
6	Scorpio		
7	Scorpio	2:28 am	Sagittarius
8	Sagittarius		
9	Sagittarius	7:43 am	Capricorn
10	Capricorn		
11	Capricorn	11: 5 am	Aquarius
12	Aquarius		
13	Aquarius	1: 5 pm	Pisces
14	Pisces		
15	Pisces	2:39 pm	Aries
16	Aries		
17	Aries	5: 4 pm	Taurus
18	Taurus		
19	Taurus	9:44 pm	Gemini
20	Gemini		
21	Gemini		
22	Gemini	5:41 am	Cancer
23	Cancer		
24	Cancer	4:48 pm	Leo
25	Leo		
26	Leo		
27	Leo	5:28 am	Virgo
28	Virgo		
29	Virgo	5:15 pm	Libra
30	Libra		
31	Libra		

November

1	Libra	2:29 am	Scorpio
2	Scorpio		
3	Scorpio	8:55 am	Sagittarius
4	Sagittarius		
5	Sagittarius	1:17 pm	Capricorn
6	Capricorn		
7	Capricorn	4:31 pm	Aquarius
8	Aquarius		
9	Aquarius	7:22 pm	Pisces
10	Pisces		
11	Pisces	10:22 pm	Aries
12	Aries		
13	Aries		
14	Aries	2: 2 am	Taurus
15	Taurus		
16	Taurus	7:10 am	Gemini
17	Gemini		
18	Gemini	2:42 pm	Cancer
19	Cancer		
20	Cancer		
21	Cancer	1:10 am	Leo
22	Leo		
23	Leo	1:41 pm	Virgo
24	Virgo		
25	Virgo		
26	Virgo	1:58 am	Libra
27	Libra		
28	Libra	11:33 am	Scorpio
29	Scorpio		
30	Scorpio	5:32 pm	Sagittarius

December

1	Sagittarius		
2	Sagittarius	8:42 pm	Capricorn
3	Capricorn		
4	Capricorn	10:36 pm	Aquarius
5	Aquarius		
6	Aquarius		
7	Aquarius	12:44 am	Pisces
8	Pisces		
9	Pisces	4: 2 am	Aries
10	Aries		
11	Aries	8:46 am	Taurus
12	Taurus		
13	Taurus	2:59 pm	Gemini
14	Gemini		
15	Gemini	11: 1 pm	Cancer
16	Cancer		
17	Cancer		
18	Cancer	9:18 am	Leo
19	Leo		
20	Leo	9:39 pm	Virgo
21	Virgo		
22	Virgo		
23	Virgo	10:26 am	Libra
24	Libra		
25	Libra	9: 4 pm	Scorpio
26	Scorpio		
27	Scorpio		
28	Scorpio	3:43 am	Sagittarius
29	Sagittarius		
30	Sagittarius	6:35 am	Capricorn
31	Capricorn		

MERCURY POSITIONS 1985 – 2005

1985

Jan 11	1:25 pm	Capricorn
Feb 1	2:43 am	Aquarius
Feb 18	6:41 pm	Pisces
Mar 6	7:07 pm	Aries
May 13	9:10 pm	Taurus
May 30	2:44 pm	Gemini
Jun 13	11:11 am	Cancer
Jun 29	2:34 pm	Leo
Sep 6	2:39 pm	Virgo
Sep 22	6:13 pm	Libra
Oct 10	1:50 pm	Scorpio
Oct 31	11:44 am	Sagittarius
Dec 4	2:23 pm	Scorpio
Dec 12	6:05 am	Sagittarius

1986

Jan 5	3:42 pm	Capricorn
Jan 24	7:33 pm	Aquarius
Feb 11	12:21 am	Pisces
Mar 3	2:22 am	Aries
Mar 11	12:36 pm	Pisces
Apr 17	7:33 am	Aries
May 7	7:33 am	Taurus
May 22	2:26 am	Gemini
Jun 5	9:06 am	Cancer
Jun 26	9:15 am	Leo
Jul 23	4:51 pm	Cancer
Aug 11	4:09 pm	Leo
Aug 29	10:28 pm	Virgo
Sep 14	9:28 pm	Libra
Oct 3	7:19 pm	Scorpio
Dec 9	7:34 am	Sagittarius
Dec 29	6:09 pm	Capricorn

1987

Jan 17	8:08 am	Aquarius
Feb 3	9:31 pm	Pisces
Mar 11	4:55 pm	Aquarius
Mar 13	4:09 pm	Pisces
Apr 12	3:23 pm	Aries
Apr 29	10:39 am	Taurus
May 13	12:50 pm	Gemini
May 29	11:21 pm	Cancer
Aug 6	4:20 pm	Leo
Aug 21	4:36 pm	Virgo
Sep 7	8:52 am	Libra
Sep 28	12:21 pm	Scorpio
Oct 31	8:57 pm	Libra
Nov 11	4:57 pm	Scorpio
Dec 3	8:33 am	Sagittarius
Dec 22	12:40 pm	Capricorn

1988

Jan 10	12:28 am	Aquarius
Mar 16	5:09 am	Pisces
Apr 4	5:04 am	Aries
Apr 20	1:42 am	Taurus
May 4	2:40 pm	Gemini

Jul 12	1:42 am	Cancer
Jul 28	4:19 pm	Leo
Aug 12	12:29 pm	Virgo
Aug 30	3:25 pm	Libra
Nov 6	9:57 am	Scorpio
Nov 25	5:04 am	Sagittarius
Dec 14	6:53 am	Capricorn

1989

Jan 2	2:41 pm	Aquarius
Jan 28	11:06 pm	Capricorn
Feb 14	1:11 pm	Aquarius
Mar 10	1:07 pm	Pisces
Mar 27	10:16 pm	Aries
Apr 11	4:36 pm	Taurus
Apr 29	2:53 pm	Gemini
May 28	5:53 pm	Taurus
Jun 12	3:56 am	Gemini
Jul 5	7:55 pm	Cancer
Jul 20	4:04 am	Leo
Aug 4	7:54 pm	Virgo
Aug 26	1:14 am	Libra
Sep 26	10:28 am	Virgo
Oct 11	1:11 am	Libra
Oct 30	8:53 am	Scorpio
Nov 17	10:10 pm	Sagittarius
Dec 7	9:30 am	Capricorn

1990

Feb 11	8:11 pm	Aquarius
Mar 3	12:14 pm	Pisces
Mar 19	7:04 pm	Aries
Apr 4	2:35 am	Taurus
Jun 11	7:29 pm	Gemini
Jun 27	3:46 pm	Cancer
Jul 11	6:48 pm	Leo
Jul 29	6:10 pm	Virgo
Oct 5	12:44 pm	Libra
Oct 22	8:46 pm	Scorpio
Nov 10	7:06 pm	Sagittarius
Dec 1	7:13 pm	Capricorn
Dec 25	5:57 pm	Sagittarius

1991

Jan 14	3:02 am	Capricorn
Feb 5	5:20 pm	Aquarius
Feb 23	9:35 pm	Pisces
Mar 11	5:40 pm	Aries
May 16	5:45 pm	Taurus
Jun 4	9:24 pm	Gemini
Jun 19	12:40 am	Cancer
Jul 4	1:05 am	Leo
Jul 26	8:00 am	Virgo
Aug 19	4:40 pm	Leo
Sep 10	12:14 pm	Virgo
Sep 27	10:26 pm	Libra
Oct 15	9:01 am	Scorpio
Nov 4	5:41 am	Sagittarius

1992

Jan 9	8:46 pm	Capricorn
Jan 29	4:15 pm	Aquarius
Feb 16	2:04 am	Pisces
Mar 3	4:45 pm	Aries
Apr 3	6:52 pm	Pisces
Apr 14	12:35 pm	Aries
May 10	11:10 pm	Taurus
May 26	4:16 pm	Gemini
Jun 9	1:27 pm	Cancer
Jun 27	12:11 am	Leo
Sep 3	3:03 am	Virgo
Sep 19	12:41 am	Libra
Oct 7	5:13 am	Scorpio
Oct 29	12:02 pm	Sagittarius
Nov 21	2:44 pm	Scorpio
Dec 12	3:05 am	Sagittarius

1993

Jan 2	9:47 am	Capricorn
Jan 21	6:25 am	Aquarius
Feb 7	11:19 am	Pisces
Apr 15	10:18 am	Aries
May 3	4:54 pm	Taurus
May 18	1:53 am	Gemini
Jun 1	10:54 pm	Cancer
Aug 10	12:51 am	Leo
Aug 26	2:06 am	Virgo
Sep 11	6:18 am	Libra
Sep 30	9:09 pm	Scorpio
Dec 6	8:04 pm	Sagittarius
Dec 26	7:47 am	Capricorn

1994

Jan 13	7:25 pm	Aquarius
Feb 1	5:28 am	Pisces
Feb 21	10:15 am	Aquarius
Mar 18	7:04 am	Pisces
Apr 9	11:30 am	Aries
Apr 25	1:27 pm	Taurus
May 9	4:08 pm	Gemini
May 28	9:52 am	Cancer
Jul 2	6:18 pm	Gemini
Jul 10	7:41 am	Cancer
Aug 3	1:09 am	Leo
Aug 17	7:44 pm	Virgo
Sep 3	11:55 pm	Libra
Sep 27	3:51 am	Scorpio
Oct 19	1:19 am	Libra
Nov 10	7:46 pm	Scorpio
Nov 29	11:38 pm	Sagittarius
Dec 19	1:26 am	Capricorn

1995

Jan 6	5:17 pm	Aquarius
Mar 14	4:35 pm	Pisces
Apr 2	2:29 am	Aries
Apr 17	2:54 am	Taurus

MERCURY POSITIONS 1985 – 2005

May 2	10:18 am	Gemini
Jul 10	11:58 am	Cancer
Jul 25	5:19 pm	Leo
Aug 9	7:13 pm	Virgo
Aug 28	9:07 pm	Libra
Nov 4	3:50 am	Scorpio
Nov 22	5:46 pm	Sagittarius
Dec 11	9:57 pm	Capricorn

1996

Jan 1	1:06 pm	Aquarius
Jan 17	4:37 am	Capricorn
Feb 14	9:44 pm	Aquarius
Mar 7	6:53 am	Pisces
Mar 24	3:03 am	Aries
Apr 7	10:16 pm	Taurus
Jun 13	4:45 pm	Gemini
Jul 2	2:37 am	Cancer
Jul 16	4:56 am	Leo
Aug 1	11:17 am	Virgo
Aug 26	12:17 am	Libra
Sep 12	4:32 am	Virgo
Oct 8	10:13 pm	Libra
Oct 26	8:01 pm	Scorpio
Nov 14	11:36 am	Sagittarius
Dec 4	8:48 am	Capricorn

1997

Feb 9	12:53 am	Aquarius
Feb 27	10:54 pm	Pisces
Mar 15	11:13 pm	Aries
Apr 1	8:45 am	Taurus
May 4	8:48 pm	Aries
May 12	5:25 am	Taurus
Jun 8	6:25 pm	Gemini
Jun 23	3:41 pm	Cancer
Jul 8	12:28 am	Leo
Jul 26	7:42 pm	Virgo
Oct 2	12:38 am	Libra
Oct 19	7:08 am	Scorpio
Nov 7	12:42 pm	Sagittarius
Nov 30	2:11 pm	Capricorn
Dec 13	1:06 pm	Sagittarius

1998

Jan 12	11:20 am	Capricorn
Feb 2	10:15 am	Aquarius
Feb 20	5:22 am	Pisces
Mar 8	3:28 am	Aries
May 14	9:10 pm	Taurus
Jun 1	3:07 am	Gemini
Jun 15	12:33 am	Cancer
Jun 30	6:52 pm	Leo
Sep 7	8:58 pm	Virgo
Sep 24	5:13 am	Libra
Oct 11	9:45 pm	Scorpio
Nov 1	11:03 am	Sagittarius

1999

Jan 6	9:04 pm	Capricorn

Jan 26	4:32 am	Aquarius
Feb 12	10:28 am	Pisces
Mar 2	5:50 am	Aries
Mar 18	4:23 am	Pisces
Apr 17	5:09 pm	Aries
May 8	4:22 pm	Taurus
May 23	4:22 pm	Gemini
Jun 6	7:18 pm	Cancer
Jun 26	10:39 am	Leo
Jul 31	1:44 am	Cancer
Aug 10	11:25 pm	Leo
Aug 31	10:15 am	Virgo
Sep 16	7:53 am	Libra
Oct 5	12:12 am	Scorpio
Oct 30	3:08 pm	Sagittarius
Nov 9	3:13 pm	Scorpio
Dec 10	9:09 pm	Sagittarius
Dec 31	1:48 am	Capricorn

2000

Jan 18	5:20 pm	Aquarius
Feb 5	3:09 pm	Pisces
Apr 12	7:17 pm	Aries
Apr 29	10:53 pm	Taurus
May 14	2:10 am	Gemini
May 29	11:27 pm	Cancer
Aug 7	12:42 am	Leo
Aug 22	5:11 am	Virgo
Sep 7	5:22 pm	Libra
Sep 28	8:28 am	Scorpio
Nov 7	2:28 am	Libra
Nov 8	2:54 pm	Scorpio
Dec 3	3:26 pm	Sagittarius
Dec 22	9:03 pm	Capricorn

2001

Jan 10	8:27 am	Aquarius
Feb 1	2:10 am	Pisces
Feb 6	3:03 pm	Aquarius
Mar 17	1:06 am	Pisces
Apr 6	2:15 am	Aries
Apr 21	3:09 pm	Taurus
May 5	11:54 pm	Gemini
Jul 12	5:48 pm	Cancer
Jul 30	5:19 am	Leo
Aug 14	12:05 am	Virgo
Aug 31	7:38 pm	Libra
Nov 7	2:54 pm	Scorpio
Nov 26	1:25 pm	Sagittarius
Dec 15	2:56 pm	Capricorn

2002

Jan 3	4:39 pm	Aquarius
Feb 3	11:18 pm	Capricorn
Feb 13	12:22 pm	Aquarius
Mar 11	6:35 pm	Pisces
Mar 29	9:45 am	Aries
Apr 13	5:12 am	Taurus
Apr 30	2:16 am	Gemini

Jul 7	5:37 am	Cancer
Jul 21	5:42 pm	Leo
Aug 6	4:52 am	Virgo
Aug 26	4:11 pm	Libra
Oct 2	4:26 am	Virgo
Oct 11	12:56 am	Libra
Oct 31	5:44 pm	Scorpio
Nov 19	6:30 am	Sagittarius
Dec 8	3:22 pm	Capricorn

2003

Feb 12	8:01 pm	Aquarius
Mar 4	9:05 pm	Pisces
Mar 21	7:17 am	Aries
Apr 5	9:38 am	Taurus
Jun 12	8:35 pm	Gemini
Jun 29	5:18 am	Cancer
Jul 13	7:11 am	Leo
Jul 30	9:06 am	Virgo
Oct 6	8:29 pm	Libra
Oct 24	6:21 am	Scorpio
Nov 12	2:20 am	Sagittarius
Dec 2	4:35 pm	Capricorn
Dec 30	2:54 pm	Sagittarius

2004

Jan 14	6:03 am	Capricorn
Feb 6	11:21 pm	Aquarius
Feb 25	7:59 am	Pisces
Mar 12	4:45 am	Aries
Mar 31	9:28 am	Taurus
Apr 12	8:24 am	Aries
May 16	1:55 am	Taurus
Jun 5	7:49 am	Gemini
Jun 19	2:51 pm	Cancer
Jul 4	9:53 am	Leo
Jul 25	8:59 am	Virgo
Aug 24	8:34 am	Leo
Sep 10	2:39 am	Virgo
Sep 28	9:14 am	Libra
Oct 15	5:58 pm	Scorpio
Nov 4	9:41 am	Sagittarius

2005

Jan 9	11:10 pm	Capricorn
Jan 30	12:38 am	Aquarius
Feb 16	12:47 pm	Pisces
Mar 4	8:35 pm	Aries
May 12	4:15 am	Taurus
May 28	5:45 am	Gemini
Jun 11	2:04 am	Cancer
Jun 27	11:02 pm	Leo
Sep 4	12:54 pm	Virgo
Sep 20	11:41 am	Libra
Oct 8	12:16 pm	Scorpio
Oct 30	4:03 am	Sagittarius
Nov 26	6:55 pm	Scorpio
Dec 12	4:20 pm	Sagittarius

VENUS POSITIONS 1985 – 2005

1985

Jan 4	1:23 am	Pisces
Feb 2	3:29 am	Aries
Jun 6	3:53 am	Taurus
Jul 6	3:01 am	Gemini
Aug 2	4:10 am	Cancer
Aug 27	10:39 pm	Leo
Sep 21	9:53 pm	Virgo
Oct 16	8:04 am	Libra
Nov 9	10:08 am	Scorpio
Dec 3	8:00 am	Sagittarius
Dec 27	4:17 am	Capricorn

1986

Jan 20	12:36 am	Aquarius
Feb 12	10:11 pm	Pisces
Mar 8	10:32 pm	Aries
Apr 2	3:19 am	Taurus
Apr 26	2:10 pm	Gemini
May 21	8:46 am	Cancer
Jun 15	1:52 pm	Leo
Jul 11	11:23 am	Virgo
Aug 7	3:46 pm	Libra
Sep 7	5:15 am	Scorpio

1987

Jan 7	5:20 am	Sagittarius
Feb 4	10:03 pm	Capricorn
Mar 3	2:55 am	Aquarius
Mar 28	11:20 am	Pisces
Apr 22	11:07 am	Aries
May 17	6:56 am	Taurus
Jun 11	12:15 am	Gemini
Jul 5	2:50 pm	Cancer
Jul 30	1:49 am	Leo
Aug 23	9:00 am	Virgo
Sep 16	1:12 pm	Libra
Oct 10	3:49 pm	Scorpio
Nov 3	6:04 pm	Sagittarius
Nov 27	8:51 pm	Capricorn
Dec 22	1:29 am	Aquarius

1988

Jan 15	11:04 am	Pisces
Feb 9	8:04 am	Aries
Mar 6	5:21 am	Taurus
Apr 3	12:07 pm	Gemini
May 17	11:26 am	Cancer
May 27	2:36 am	Gemini
Aug 6	6:24 pm	Cancer
Sep 7	6:37 am	Leo
Oct 4	8:15 am	Virgo
Oct 29	6:20 pm	Libra
Nov 23	8:34 am	Scorpio
Dec 17	12:56 pm	Sagittarius

1989

Jan 10	1:08 pm	Capricorn
Feb 3	12:15 pm	Aquarius

Feb 27	11:59 am	Pisces
Mar 23	1:32 pm	Aries
Apr 16	5:52 pm	Taurus
May 11	1:28 am	Gemini
Jun 4	12:17 pm	Cancer
Jun 29	2:21 am	Leo
Jul 23	8:31 pm	Virgo
Aug 17	8:58 am	Libra
Sep 12	7:22 am	Scorpio
Oct 8	11:00 am	Sagittarius
Nov 5	5:13 am	Capricorn
Dec 9	11:54 pm	Aquarius

1990

Jan 16	10:23 am	Capricorn
Mar 3	12:52 pm	Aquarius
Apr 6	4:13 am	Pisces
May 3	10:52 pm	Aries
May 30	5:13 am	Taurus
Jun 24	7:14 pm	Gemini
Jul 19	10:41 pm	Cancer
Aug 13	5:05 pm	Leo
Sep 7	3:21 pm	Virgo
Oct 1	7:13 am	Libra
Oct 25	7:03 am	Scorpio
Nov 18	4:58 am	Sagittarius
Dec 12	2:18 am	Capricorn

1991

Jan 5	12:03 am	Aquarius
Jan 28	11:44 pm	Pisces
Feb 22	4:02 am	Aries
Mar 18	4:45 pm	Taurus
Apr 12	7:10 pm	Gemini
May 8	8:28 pm	Cancer
Jun 5	8:16 pm	Leo
Jul 11	12:06 am	Virgo
Aug 21	10:06 am	Leo
Oct 6	4:15 pm	Virgo
Nov 9	1:37 am	Libra
Dec 6	2:21 am	Scorpio
Dec 31	10:19 am	Sagittarius

1992

Jan 25	2:14 am	Capricorn
Feb 18	11:40 am	Aquarius
Mar 13	6:57 pm	Pisces
Apr 7	2:16 am	Aries
May 1	10:41 am	Taurus
May 25	8:18 pm	Gemini
Jun 19	6:22 am	Cancer
Jul 13	4:07 pm	Leo
Aug 7	1:26 am	Virgo
Aug 31	11:09 am	Libra
Sep 24	10:31 pm	Scorpio
Oct 19	12:47 pm	Sagittarius
Nov 13	7:48 am	Capricorn
Dec 8	12:49 pm	Aquarius

1993

Jan 3	6:54 pm	Pisces
Feb 2	7:37 am	Aries
Jun 6	5:03 am	Taurus
Jul 5	7:21 pm	Gemini
Aug 1	5:38 pm	Cancer
Aug 27	10:48 am	Leo
Sep 21	9:22 am	Virgo
Oct 15	7:13 pm	Libra
Nov 8	9:07 pm	Scorpio
Dec 2	6:54 pm	Sagittarius
Dec 26	3:09 pm	Capricorn

1994

Jan 19	11:28 am	Aquarius
Feb 12	9:04 am	Pisces
Mar 8	9:28 am	Aries
Apr 1	2:20 pm	Taurus
Apr 26	1:24 am	Gemini
May 20	8:26 pm	Cancer
Jun 15	2:23 am	Leo
Jul 11	1:33 am	Virgo
Aug 7	9:36 am	Libra
Sep 7	12:12 pm	Scorpio

1995

Jan 7	7:07 am	Sagittarius
Feb 4	3:12 pm	Capricorn
Mar 2	5:11 pm	Aquarius
Mar 28	12:10 am	Pisces
Apr 21	11:07 pm	Aries
May 16	6:22 pm	Taurus
Jun 10	11:19 am	Gemini
Jul 5	1:39 am	Cancer
Jul 29	12:32 pm	Leo
Aug 22	7:43 pm	Virgo
Sep 16	12:01 am	Libra
Oct 10	2:48 am	Scorpio
Nov 3	5:18 am	Sagittarius
Nov 27	8:23 am	Capricorn
Dec 21	1:23 pm	Aquarius

1996

Jan 14	11:30 pm	Pisces
Feb 8	9:30 pm	Aries
Mar 5	9:01 pm	Taurus
Apr 3	10:26 am	Gemini
Aug 7	1:15 am	Cancer
Sep 7	12:07 am	Leo
Oct 3	10:22 pm	Virgo
Oct 29	7:02 am	Libra
Nov 22	8:34 pm	Scorpio
Dec 17	12:34 am	Sagittarius

1997

Jan 10	12:32 am	Capricorn
Feb 2	11:28 pm	Aquarius
Feb 26	11:01 pm	Pisces
Mar 23	12:26 am	Aries
Apr 16	4:43 am	Taurus

VENUS POSITIONS 1985 – 2005

May 10	12:20 pm	Gemini
Jun 3	11:18 pm	Cancer
Jun 28	1:38 pm	Leo
Jul 23	8:16 am	Virgo
Aug 17	9:31 am	Libra
Sep 11	9:17 pm	Scorpio
Oct 8	3:25 am	Sagittarius
Nov 5	3:50 am	Capricorn
Dec 11	11:39 pm	Aquarius

1998

Jan 9	4:03 pm	Capricorn
Mar 4	11:14 am	Aquarius
Apr 6	12:38 am	Pisces
May 3	2:16 pm	Aries
May 29	6:32 pm	Taurus
Jun 24	7:27 am	Gemini
Jul 19	10:17 am	Cancer
Aug 13	4:20 am	Leo
Sep 6	2:24 pm	Virgo
Sep 30	6:13 pm	Libra
Oct 24	6:06 pm	Scorpio
Nov 17	4:06 pm	Sagittarius
Dec 11	1:33 pm	Capricorn

1999

Jan 4	11:25 am	Aquarius
Jan 28	11:17 am	Pisces
Feb 21	3:49 pm	Aries
Mar 18	4:59 am	Taurus
Apr 12	8:17 am	Gemini
May 8	11:29 am	Cancer
Jun 5	4:25 pm	Leo
Jul 12	10:18 am	Virgo
Aug 15	9:12 am	Leo
Oct 7	11:51 am	Virgo
Nov 8	9:19 pm	Libra
Dec 5	5:41 pm	Scorpio
Dec 30	11:54 pm	Sagittarius

2000

Jan 24	2:52 pm	Capricorn

Feb 17	11:43 pm	Aquarius
Mar 13	6:36 am	Pisces
Apr 6	1:37 pm	Aries
Apr 30	9:49 pm	Taurus
May 25	7:15 am	Gemini
Jun 18	5:15 pm	Cancer
Jul 13	3:02 am	Leo
Aug 6	12:32 pm	Virgo
Aug 30	10:35 pm	Libra
Sep 24	10:26 am	Scorpio
Oct 19	1:18 am	Sagittarius
Nov 12	9:14 pm	Capricorn
Dec 8	3:48 am	Aquarius

2001

Jan 3	1:15 pm	Pisces
Feb 2	2:15 pm	Aries
Jun 6	5:26 am	Taurus
Jul 5	11:45 am	Gemini
Aug 1	7:19 am	Cancer
Aug 26	11:13 pm	Leo
Sep 20	9:10 pm	Virgo
Oct 15	6:43 am	Libra
Nov 8	8:29 am	Scorpio
Dec 2	6:13 am	Sagittarius
Dec 26	2:26 am	Capricorn

2002

Jan 18	10:43 pm	Aquarius
Feb 11	8:19 pm	Pisces
Mar 7	8:43 pm	Aries
Apr 1	1:41 am	Taurus
Apr 25	12:58 pm	Gemini
May 20	8:28 am	Cancer
Jun 14	3:17 pm	Leo
Jul 10	4:10 pm	Virgo
Aug 7	4:10 am	Libra
Sep 7	10:06 pm	Scorpio

2003

Jan 7	8:08 am	Sagittarius
Feb 4	8:28 am	Capricorn

Mar 2	7:41 am	Aquarius
Mar 27	1:15 pm	Pisces
Apr 21	11:19 am	Aries
May 16	5:59 am	Taurus
Jun 9	10:33 pm	Gemini
Jul 4	12:40 pm	Cancer
Jul 28	11:26 pm	Leo
Aug 22	6:37 am	Virgo
Sep 15	10:59 am	Libra
Oct 9	1:57 pm	Scorpio
Nov 2	4:43 pm	Sagittarius
Nov 26	8:08 pm	Capricorn
Dec 21	1:33 am	Aquarius

2004

Jan 14	12:17 pm	Pisces
Feb 8	11:22 am	Aries
Mar 5	1:13 pm	Taurus
Apr 3	9:58 am	Gemini
Aug 7	6:03 am	Cancer
Sep 6	5:17 pm	Leo
Oct 3	12:21 pm	Virgo
Oct 28	7:40 pm	Libra
Nov 22	8:32 am	Scorpio
Dec 16	12:11 pm	Sagittarius

2005

Jan 9	11:57 am	Capricorn
Feb 2	10:43 am	Aquarius
Feb 26	10:08 am	Pisces
Mar 22	11:26 am	Aries
Apr 15	3:38 pm	Taurus
May 9	11:15 pm	Gemini
Jun 3	10:19 am	Cancer
Jun 28	12:54 am	Leo
Jul 22	8:02 pm	Virgo
Aug 16	10:06 pm	Libra
Sep 11	11:15 am	Scorpio
Oct 7	8:01 pm	Sagittarius
Nov 5	3:12 am	Capricorn
Dec 15	10:59 am	Aquarius

MARS POSITIONS 1985 – 2005

1985

Feb 2	12:19 pm	Aries
Mar 15	12:06 am	Taurus
Apr 26	4:13 am	Gemini
Jun 9	5:40 am	Cancer
Jul 24	11:04 pm	Leo
Sep 9	8:31 pm	Virgo
Oct 27	10:16 am	Libra
Dec 14	1:59 pm	Scorpio

1986

Feb 2	1:27 am	Sagittarius
Mar 27	10:47 pm	Capricorn
Oct 8	8:01 pm	Aquarius
Nov 25	9:35 pm	Pisces

1987

Jan 8	7:20 am	Aries
Feb 20	9:44 am	Taurus
Apr 5	11:37 am	Gemini
May 20	10:01 pm	Cancer
Jul 6	11:46 am	Leo
Aug 22	2:51 pm	Virgo
Oct 8	2:27 pm	Libra
Nov 23	10:19 pm	Scorpio

1988

Jan 8	10:24 am	Sagittarius
Feb 22	5:15 am	Capricorn
Apr 6	4:44 pm	Aquarius
May 22	2:42 am	Pisces
Jul 13	3:00 pm	Aries
Oct 23	5:02 pm	Pisces
Nov 1	7:57 am	Aries

1989

Jan 19	3:11 am	Taurus
Mar 11	3:51 am	Gemini
Apr 28	11:37 pm	Cancer
Jun 16	9:10 am	Leo
Aug 3	8:35 am	Virgo
Sep 19	9:38 am	Libra
Nov 4	12:29 am	Scorpio
Dec 17	11:57 pm	Sagittarius

1990

Jan 29	9:10 am	Capricorn
Mar 11	10:54 am	Aquarius
Apr 20	5:09 pm	Pisces
May 31	2:11 am	Aries
Jul 12	9:44 am	Taurus
Aug 31	6:40 am	Gemini
Dec 14	2:46 am	Taurus

1991

Jan 20	8:15 pm	Gemini
Apr 2	7:49 pm	Cancer
May 26	7:19 am	Leo
Jul 15	7:36 am	Virgo
Sep 1	1:38 am	Libra

Oct 16	2:05 pm	Scorpio
Nov 28	9:19 pm	Sagittarius

1992

Jan 9	4:47 am	Capricorn
Feb 17	11:38 pm	Aquarius
Mar 27	9:04 pm	Pisces
May 5	4:36 pm	Aries
Jun 14	10:56 am	Taurus
Jul 26	1:59 pm	Gemini
Sep 12	1:05 am	Cancer

1993

Apr 27	6:40 pm	Leo
Jun 23	2:42 am	Virgo
Aug 11	8:10 pm	Libra
Sep 26	9:15 pm	Scorpio
Nov 9	12:29 am	Sagittarius
Dec 19	7:34 pm	Capricorn

1994

Jan 27	11:05 pm	Aquarius
Mar 7	6:01 am	Pisces
Apr 14	1:02 pm	Aries
May 23	5:37 pm	Taurus
Jul 3	5:30 pm	Gemini
Aug 16	2:15 pm	Cancer
Oct 4	10:48 am	Leo
Dec 12	6:32 am	Virgo

1995

Jan 22	6:48 pm	Leo
May 25	11:09 am	Virgo
Jul 21	4:21 am	Libra
Sep 7	2:00 am	Scorpio
Oct 20	4:02 pm	Sagittarius
Nov 30	8:58 am	Capricorn

1996

Jan 8	6:02 am	Aquarius
Feb 15	6:50 am	Pisces
Mar 24	10:12 am	Aries
May 2	1:16 pm	Taurus
Jun 12	9:42 am	Gemini
Jul 25	1:32 pm	Cancer
Sep 9	3:02 pm	Leo
Oct 30	2:13 am	Virgo

1997

Jan 3	3:10 am	Libra
Mar 8	2:50 pm	Virgo
Jun 19	3:30 am	Libra
Aug 14	3:42 am	Scorpio
Sep 28	5:22 pm	Sagittarius
Nov 9	12:33 am	Capricorn
Dec 18	1:37 am	Aquarius

1998

Jan 25	4:26 am	Pisces
Mar 4	11:18 am	Aries
Apr 12	8:05 pm	Taurus

May 23	10:42 pm	Gemini
Jul 6	4:00 am	Cancer
Aug 20	2:16 pm	Leo
Oct 7	7:28 am	Virgo
Nov 27	5:10 am	Libra

1999

Jan 26	6:59 pm	Scorpio
May 5	4:32 pm	Libra
Jul 4	10:59 pm	Scorpio
Sep 2	2:29 pm	Sagittarius
Oct 16	8:35 pm	Capricorn
Nov 26	1:56 am	Aquarius

2000

Jan 3	10:01 pm	Pisces
Feb 11	8:04 pm	Aries
Mar 22	8:25 pm	Taurus
May 3	2:18 pm	Gemini
Jun 16	7:30 am	Cancer
Jul 31	8:21 pm	Leo
Sep 16	7:19 pm	Virgo
Nov 3	9:00 pm	Libra
Dec 23	9:37 am	Scorpio

2001

Feb 14	3:07 pm	Sagittarius
Sep 8	12:52 pm	Capricorn
Oct 27	12:20 pm	Aquarius
Dec 8	4:53 pm	Pisces

2002

Jan 18	5:54 pm	Aries
Mar 1	10:06 am	Taurus
Apr 13	12:37 pm	Gemini
May 28	6:44 am	Cancer
Jul 13	10:24 am	Leo
Aug 29	9:39 am	Virgo
Oct 15	12:39 pm	Libra
Dec 1	9:27 am	Scorpio

2003

Jan 16	11:23 pm	Sagittarius
Mar 4	4:18 pm	Capricorn
Apr 21	6:49 pm	Aquarius
Jun 16	9:27 pm	Pisces
Dec 16	8:25 am	Aries

2004

Feb 3	5:05 am	Taurus
Mar 21	2:40 am	Gemini
May 7	3:47 am	Cancer
Jun 23	3:52 pm	Leo
Aug 10	5:15 am	Virgo
Sep 26	4:17 am	Libra
Nov 11	12:12 am	Scorpio
Dec 25	11:05 am	Sagittarius

2005

Feb 6	1:33 am	Capricorn
Mar 20	1:03 pm	Aquarius

MARS POSITIONS 1985 – 2005

Apr 30	9:59 pm	Pisces
Jun 11	9:31 pm	Aries
Jul 28	12:13 am	Taurus

JUPITER POSITIONS 1985 – 2005

Year	Date	Time	Sign	Year	Date	Time		Sign
1985	Feb 6	3:36 pm	Aquarius	1996	Jan 3	7:23 am		Capricorn
1986	Feb 20	4:06 pm	Pisces	1997	Jan 21	3:14 pm		Aquarius
1987	Mar 2	6:42 pm	Aries	1998	Feb 4	10:53 am		Pisces
1988	Mar 8	3:45 pm	Taurus	1999	Feb 13	1:23 am		Aries
1988	Jul 22	0:00 am	Gemini	1999	Jun 28	9:30 am		Taurus
1988	Nov 30	8:55 pm R	Taurus	1999	Oct 23	5:50 am	R	Aries
1989	Mar 11	3:27 am	Gemini	2000	Feb 14	9:40 pm		Taurus
1989	Jul 30	11:51 pm	Cancer	2000	Jun 30	7:36 am		Gemini
1990	Aug 18	7:31 am	Leo	2001	Jul 13	0:04 am		Cancer
1991	Sep 12	6:01 am	Virgo	2002	Aug 1	17:21 pm		Leo
1992	Oct 10	1:27 pm	Libra	2003	Aug 27	9:27 am		Virgo
1993	Nov 10	8:16 am	Scorpio	2004	Sep 25	3:24 am		Libra
1994	Dec 9	10:55 am	Sagittarius	2005	Oct 26	2:52 am		Scorpio

SATURN POSITIONS 1985 – 2005

Year	Date	Time	Sign	Year	Date	Time		Sign
1985	Nov 17	2:10 am	Sagittarius	1998	Jun 9	6:08 am		Taurus
1988	Feb 13	11:51 pm	Capricorn	1998	Oct 25	6:42 pm	R	Aries
1988	Jun 10	5:24 am R	Sagittarius	1999	Mar 1	1:26 am		Taurus
1988	Nov 12	9:26 am	Capricorn	2000	Aug 10	2:26 am		Gemini
1991	Feb 6	6:52 pm	Aquarius	2000	Oct 16	12:47 am	R	Taurus
1993	May 21	4:58 am	Pisces	2001	Apr 20	9:60 pm		Gemini
1993	Jun 30	8:31 am R	Aquarius	2003	Jun 4	1:28 am		Cancer
1994	Jan 28	11:44 pm	Pisces	2005	Jul 16	12:31 pm		Leo
1996	Apr 7	8:50 am	Aries					

URANUS POSITIONS 1985 – 2010

Year	Date	Time	Sign	Year	Date	Time		Sign
1981	Feb 17	8:53	Sagittarius	1995	Jun 9	1:47	R	Capricorn
1981	Mar 20	23:27 R	Scorpio	1996	Jan 12	7:13		Aquarius
1981	Nov 16	12:04	Sagittarius	2003	Mar 10	20:54		Pisces
1988	Feb 15	0:08	Capricorn	2003	Sep 15	3:48	R	Aquarius
1988	May 27	1:22 R	Sagittarius	2003	Dec 30	9:15		Pisces
1988	Dec 2	15:34	Capricorn	2010	May 28	1:50		Aries
1995	Apr 1	12:08	Aquarius	2010	Aug 14	3:31	R	Pisces

NEPTUNE POSITIONS 1984 – 2011

Year	Date	Time	Sign	Year	Date	Time		Sign
1984	Jan 19	2:52	Capricorn	1998	Aug 23	0:27	R	Capricorn
1984	Jun 23	1:16 R	Sagittarius	1998	Nov 28	1:09		Aquarius
1984	Nov 21	13:18	Capricorn	2011	Apr 4	13:37		Pisces
1998	Jan 29	2:46	Aquarius	2011	Aug 5	3:12	R	Aquarius

PLUTO POSITIONS 1984 – 2008

Year	Date	Time	Sign	Year	Date	Time		Sign
1984	May 18	14:19 R	Libra	1995	Nov 10	19:40		Sagittarius
1984	Aug 28	4:59	Scorpio	2008	Jan 26	3:45		Capricorn
1995	Jan 17	9:59	Sagittarius	2008	Jun 14	3:47	R	Sagittarius
1995	Apr 21	2:08 R	Scorpio	2008	Nov 27	2:06		Capricorn

Rising Sign Tables

I have provided **approximate*** rising sign tables for three "zones" in the continental United States as well as Alska and Hawaii. If you were born outside the U.S. you will need to have a chart calculated (see page 286).

1. By looking at the diagram on the facing page, determine which zone you were born in.

2. Turn to the tables for that zone and find the listing for your birth date. If your date is not listed, choose the date just **before** your birth date.

3. Find the time you were born by looking at the time entries to the right of the date. Again, if your birth time is not listed, select the time just before your birth time.

4. Subtract 4 minutes from the time shown for each (if any) day you were born after the listed date to get the sign change time for your birth date. If the adjusted time is **after** your birth time, go one column to the left.

   The sign noted at the top of the column will **probably** be your rising sign.

---

* **PLEASE NOTE, THESE TIMES ARE APPROXIMATIONS**. I cannot stress this enough. If you were born close to the time change or near the edges of the "zone," the table may not give an accurate rising sign. The only way to be sure of your rising sign is to have an astrological chart calculated. Complete date, place **and time** information about your birth are essential to producing an accurate horoscope.

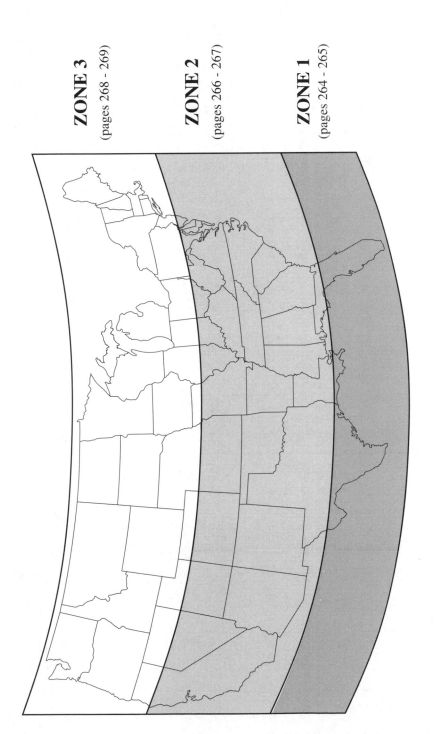

ZONE 3 (pages 268 - 269)

ZONE 2 (pages 266 - 267)

ZONE 1 (pages 264 - 265)

HAWAII TABLES pages 272 - 273

ALASKA TABLES pages 270 - 271

Ascendant Times for Zone 1

	Aries	Taurus	Gemini	Cancer	Leo	Virgo	Libra	Scorpio	Sagittarius	Capricorn	Aquarius	Pisces
Jan 1	11:17 am	12:47 pm	2:28 pm	4:29 pm	6:45 pm	9:06 pm	11:19 pm	1:32 am	3:49 am	6:04 am	8:06 am	9:47 am
Jan 8	10:49 am	12:19 pm	2:01 pm	4:02 pm	6:17 pm	8:38 pm	10:51 pm	1:04 am	3:21 am	5:37 am	7:38 am	9:20 am
Jan 15	10:22 am	11:51 am	1:33 pm	3:34 pm	5:50 pm	8:11 pm	10:24 pm	12:37 am	2:54 am	5:09 am	7:10 am	8:52 am
Jan 22	9:54 am	11:24 am	1:06 pm	3:07 pm	5:22 pm	7:43 pm	9:56 pm	12:09 am	2:26 am	4:42 am	6:43 am	8:25 am
Jan 29	9:27 am	10:56 am	12:38 pm	2:39 pm	4:55 pm	7:16 pm	9:29 pm	11:42 pm	1:59 am	4:14 am	6:15 am	7:57 am
Feb 5	8:59 am	10:29 am	12:11 pm	2:12 pm	4:27 pm	6:44 pm	9:01 pm	11:14 pm	1:31 am	3:47 am	5:48 am	7:30 am
Feb 12	8:32 am	10:01 am	11:43 am	1:44 pm	4:00 pm	6:17 pm	8:34 pm	10:47 pm	1:04 am	3:19 am	5:20 am	7:02 am
Feb 19	8:04 am	9:34 am	11:16 am	1:17 pm	3:32 pm	5:49 pm	8:06 pm	10:19 pm	12:36 am	2:52 am	4:53 am	6:35 am
Feb 26	7:37 am	9:06 am	10:48 am	12:49 pm	3:05 pm	5:22 pm	7:39 pm	9:52 pm	12:09 am	2:24 am	4:25 am	6:07 am
Mar 5	7:09 am	8:39 am	10:20 am	12:22 pm	2:37 pm	4:54 pm	7:11 pm	9:24 pm	11:41 pm	1:57 am	3:58 am	5:39 am
Mar 12	6:42 am	8:11 am	9:53 am	11:54 am	2:10 pm	4:27 pm	6:40 pm	8:57 pm	11:14 pm	1:29 am	3:30 am	5:12 am
Mar 19	6:14 am	7:44 am	9:25 am	11:27 am	1:42 pm	3:59 pm	6:12 pm	8:29 pm	10:46 pm	1:02 am	3:03 am	4:44 am
Mar 26	5:47 am	7:16 am	8:58 am	10:59 am	1:15 pm	3:32 pm	5:45 pm	8:02 pm	10:18 pm	12:34 am	2:35 am	4:17 am
Apr 2	5:19 am	6:49 am	8:30 am	10:32 am	12:47 pm	3:04 pm	5:17 pm	7:34 pm	9:51 pm	12:07 am	2:08 am	3:49 am
Apr 9	4:52 am	6:21 am	8:03 am	10:04 am	12:20 pm	2:37 pm	4:50 pm	7:06 pm	9:23 pm	11:39 pm	1:40 am	3:22 am
Apr 16	4:24 am	5:54 am	7:35 am	9:36 am	11:52 am	2:09 pm	4:22 pm	6:35 pm	8:56 pm	11:12 pm	1:13 am	2:54 am
Apr 23	3:56 am	5:26 am	7:08 am	9:09 am	11:25 am	1:42 pm	3:55 pm	6:08 pm	8:28 pm	10:44 pm	12:45 am	2:27 am
Apr 30	3:29 am	4:59 am	6:40 am	8:41 am	10:57 am	1:14 pm	3:27 pm	5:40 pm	8:01 pm	10:16 pm	12:18 am	1:59 am
May 7	3:01 am	4:31 am	6:13 am	8:14 am	10:30 am	12:46 pm	2:59 pm	5:12 pm	7:33 pm	9:49 pm	11:50 pm	1:32 am
May 14	2:34 am	4:04 am	5:45 am	7:46 am	10:02 am	12:19 pm	2:32 pm	4:45 pm	7:06 pm	9:21 pm	11:23 pm	1:04 am
May 21	2:06 am	3:36 am	5:18 am	7:19 am	9:34 am	11:51 am	2:04 pm	4:17 pm	6:34 pm	8:54 pm	10:55 pm	12:37 am
May 28	1:39 am	3:09 am	4:50 am	6:51 am	9:07 am	11:24 am	1:37 pm	3:50 pm	6:07 pm	8:26 pm	10:28 pm	12:09 am
Jun 4	1:11 am	2:41 am	4:23 am	6:24 am	8:39 am	10:56 am	1:09 pm	3:22 pm	5:39 pm	7:59 pm	10:00 pm	11:42 pm
Jun 11	12:44 am	2:13 am	3:55 am	5:56 am	8:12 am	10:29 am	12:42 pm	2:55 pm	5:12 pm	7:31 pm	9:32 pm	11:14 pm
Jun 18	12:16 am	1:46 am	3:28 am	5:29 am	7:44 am	10:01 am	12:14 pm	2:27 pm	4:44 pm	7:04 pm	9:05 pm	10:47 pm
Jun 25	11:49 pm	1:18 am	3:00 am	5:01 am	7:17 am	9:34 am	11:47 am	2:00 pm	4:17 pm	6:32 pm	8:37 pm	10:19 pm

Ascendant Times for Zone 1

	Aries	Taurus	Gemini	Cancer	Leo	Virgo	Libra	Scorpio	Sagittarius	Capricorn	Aquarius	Pisces
Jul 2	11:21 pm	12:51 am	2:33 am	4:34 am	6:49 am	9:06 am	11:19 am	1:32 pm	3:49 pm	6:05 pm	8:10 pm	9:52 pm
Jul 9	10:54 pm	12:23 am	2:05 am	4:06 am	6:22 am	8:39 am	10:52 am	1:05 pm	3:22 pm	5:37 pm	7:42 pm	9:24 pm
Jul 16	10:26 pm	11:56 pm	1:38 am	3:39 am	5:54 am	8:11 am	10:24 am	12:37 pm	2:54 pm	5:10 pm	7:15 pm	8:57 pm
Jul 23	9:59 pm	11:28 pm	1:10 am	3:11 am	5:27 am	7:44 am	9:57 am	12:10 pm	2:27 pm	4:42 pm	6:43 pm	8:29 pm
Jul 30	9:31 pm	11:01 pm	12:42 am	2:44 am	4:59 am	7:16 am	9:29 am	11:42 am	1:59 pm	4:15 pm	6:16 pm	8:01 pm
Aug 6	9:04 pm	10:33 pm	12:15 am	2:16 am	4:32 am	6:49 am	9:02 am	11:15 am	1:32 pm	3:47 pm	5:48 pm	7:34 pm
Aug 13	8:36 pm	10:06 pm	11:47 pm	1:49 am	4:04 am	6:21 am	8:34 am	10:47 am	1:04 pm	3:20 pm	5:21 pm	7:06 pm
Aug 20	8:09 pm	9:38 pm	11:20 pm	1:21 am	3:37 am	5:54 am	8:07 am	10:20 am	12:37 pm	2:52 pm	4:53 pm	6:35 pm
Aug 27	7:41 pm	9:11 pm	10:52 pm	12:54 am	3:09 am	5:26 am	7:39 am	9:52 am	12:09 pm	2:25 pm	4:26 pm	6:07 pm
Sep 3	7:14 pm	8:43 pm	10:25 pm	12:26 am	2:42 am	4:59 am	7:12 am	9:25 am	11:42 am	1:57 pm	3:58 pm	5:40 pm
Sep 10	6:42 pm	8:16 pm	9:57 pm	11:59 pm	2:14 am	4:31 am	6:44 am	8:57 am	11:14 am	1:30 pm	3:31 pm	5:12 pm
Sep 17	6:15 pm	7:48 pm	9:30 pm	11:31 pm	1:47 am	4:04 am	6:17 am	8:30 am	10:46 am	1:02 pm	3:03 pm	4:45 pm
Sep 24	5:47 pm	7:21 pm	9:02 pm	11:03 pm	1:19 am	3:36 am	5:49 am	8:02 am	10:19 am	12:35 pm	2:36 pm	4:17 pm
Oct 1	5:20 pm	6:49 pm	8:35 pm	10:36 pm	12:52 am	3:08 am	5:21 am	7:34 am	9:51 am	12:07 pm	2:08 pm	3:50 pm
Oct 8	4:52 pm	6:22 pm	8:07 pm	10:08 pm	12:24 am	2:41 am	4:54 am	7:07 am	9:24 am	11:40 am	1:41 pm	3:22 pm
Oct 15	4:24 pm	5:54 pm	7:40 pm	9:41 pm	11:56 pm	2:13 am	4:26 am	6:39 am	8:56 am	11:12 am	1:13 pm	2:55 pm
Oct 22	3:57 pm	5:27 pm	7:12 pm	9:13 pm	11:29 pm	1:46 am	3:59 am	6:12 am	8:29 am	10:44 am	12:46 pm	2:27 pm
Oct 29	3:29 pm	4:59 pm	6:41 pm	8:46 pm	11:01 pm	1:18 am	3:31 am	5:44 am	8:01 am	10:17 am	12:18 pm	2:00 pm
Nov 5	3:02 pm	4:32 pm	6:13 pm	8:18 pm	10:34 pm	12:51 am	3:04 am	5:17 am	7:34 am	9:49 am	11:51 am	1:32 pm
Nov 12	2:34 pm	4:04 pm	5:46 pm	7:51 pm	10:06 pm	12:23 am	2:36 am	4:49 am	7:06 am	9:22 am	11:23 am	1:05 pm
Nov 19	2:07 pm	3:37 pm	5:18 pm	7:23 pm	9:39 pm	11:56 pm	2:09 am	4:22 am	6:39 am	8:54 am	10:56 am	12:37 pm
Nov 26	1:39 pm	3:09 pm	4:51 pm	6:52 pm	9:11 pm	11:28 pm	1:41 am	3:54 am	6:11 am	8:27 am	10:28 am	12:10 pm
Dec 3	1:12 pm	2:41 pm	4:23 pm	6:24 pm	8:44 pm	11:01 pm	1:14 am	3:27 am	5:44 am	7:59 am	10:00 am	11:42 am
Dec 10	12:44 pm	2:14 pm	3:56 pm	5:57 pm	8:16 pm	10:33 pm	12:46 am	2:59 am	5:16 am	7:32 am	9:33 am	11:15 am
Dec 17	12:17 pm	1:46 pm	3:28 pm	5:29 pm	7:49 pm	10:06 pm	12:19 am	2:32 am	4:49 am	7:04 am	9:05 am	10:47 am
Dec 24	11:49 am	1:19 pm	3:01 pm	5:02 pm	7:21 pm	9:38 pm	11:51 pm	2:04 am	4:21 am	6:37 am	8:38 am	10:20 am
Dec 31	11:22 am	12:51 pm	2:33 pm	4:34 pm	6:50 pm	9:11 pm	11:24 pm	1:37 am	3:54 am	6:09 am	8:10 am	9:52 am

Ascendant Times for Zone 2

	Aries	Taurus	Gemini	Cancer	Leo	Virgo	Libra	Scorpio	Sagittarius	Capricorn	Aquarius	Pisces
Jan 1	11:17 am	12:36 pm	2:08 pm	4:05 pm	6:25 pm	8:55 pm	11:19 pm	1:43 am	4:09 am	6:28 am	8:26 am	9:58 am
Jan 8	10:49 am	12:08 pm	1:41 pm	3:38 pm	5:57 pm	8:27 pm	10:51 pm	1:15 am	3:41 am	6:01 am	7:58 am	9:31 am
Jan 15	10:22 am	11:41 am	1:13 pm	3:10 pm	5:30 pm	8:00 pm	10:24 pm	12:48 am	3:14 am	5:33 am	7:31 am	9:03 am
Jan 22	9:54 am	11:13 am	12:46 pm	2:43 pm	5:02 pm	7:32 pm	9:56 pm	12:20 am	2:46 am	5:06 am	7:03 am	8:36 am
Jan 29	9:27 am	10:45 am	12:18 pm	2:15 pm	4:35 pm	7:05 pm	9:29 pm	11:53 pm	2:19 am	4:38 am	6:36 am	8:08 am
Feb 5	8:59 am	10:18 am	11:50 am	1:48 pm	4:07 pm	6:33 pm	9:01 pm	11:25 pm	1:51 am	4:11 am	6:08 am	7:40 am
Feb 12	8:32 am	9:50 am	11:23 am	1:20 pm	3:40 pm	6:06 pm	8:34 pm	10:58 pm	1:24 am	3:43 am	5:40 am	7:13 am
Feb 19	8:04 am	9:23 am	10:55 am	12:53 pm	3:12 pm	5:38 pm	8:06 pm	10:30 pm	12:56 am	3:16 am	5:13 am	6:45 am
Feb 26	7:37 am	8:55 am	10:28 am	12:25 pm	2:45 pm	5:11 pm	7:39 pm	10:03 pm	12:29 am	2:48 am	4:45 am	6:18 am
Mar 5	7:09 am	8:28 am	10:00 am	11:58 am	2:17 pm	4:43 pm	7:11 pm	9:35 pm	12:01 am	2:21 am	4:18 am	5:50 am
Mar 12	6:42 am	8:00 am	9:33 am	11:30 am	1:50 pm	4:16 pm	6:40 pm	9:08 pm	11:34 pm	1:53 am	3:50 am	5:23 am
Mar 19	6:14 am	7:33 am	9:05 am	11:03 am	1:22 pm	3:48 pm	6:12 pm	8:40 pm	11:06 pm	1:26 am	3:23 am	4:55 am
Mar 26	5:47 am	7:05 am	8:38 am	10:35 am	12:55 pm	3:21 pm	5:45 pm	8:12 pm	10:39 pm	12:58 am	2:55 am	4:28 am
Apr 2	5:19 am	6:38 am	8:10 am	10:08 am	12:27 pm	2:53 pm	5:17 pm	7:45 pm	10:11 pm	12:31 am	2:28 am	4:00 am
Apr 9	4:52 am	6:10 am	7:43 am	9:40 am	12:00 pm	2:26 pm	4:50 pm	7:17 pm	9:44 pm	12:03 am	2:00 am	3:33 am
Apr 16	4:24 am	5:43 am	7:15 am	9:13 am	11:32 am	1:58 pm	4:22 pm	6:46 pm	9:16 pm	11:36 pm	1:33 am	3:05 am
Apr 23	3:56 am	5:15 am	6:48 am	8:45 am	11:04 am	1:31 pm	3:55 pm	6:18 pm	8:48 pm	11:08 pm	1:05 am	2:38 am
Apr 30	3:29 am	4:48 am	6:20 am	8:17 am	10:37 am	1:03 pm	3:27 pm	5:51 pm	8:21 pm	10:40 pm	12:38 am	2:10 am
May 7	3:01 am	4:20 am	5:53 am	7:50 am	10:09 am	12:36 pm	2:59 pm	5:23 pm	7:53 pm	10:13 pm	12:10 am	1:43 am
May 14	2:34 am	3:53 am	5:25 am	7:22 am	9:42 am	12:08 pm	2:32 pm	4:56 pm	7:26 pm	9:45 pm	11:43 pm	1:15 am
May 21	2:06 am	3:25 am	4:58 am	6:55 am	9:14 am	11:40 am	2:04 pm	4:28 pm	6:54 pm	9:18 pm	11:15 pm	12:48 am
May 28	1:39 am	2:58 am	4:30 am	6:27 am	8:47 am	11:13 am	1:37 pm	4:01 pm	6:27 pm	8:50 pm	10:48 pm	12:20 am
Jun 4	1:11 am	2:30 am	4:03 am	6:00 am	8:19 am	10:45 am	1:09 pm	3:33 pm	5:59 pm	8:23 pm	10:20 pm	11:53 pm
Jun 11	12:44 am	2:03 am	3:35 am	5:32 am	7:52 am	10:18 am	12:42 pm	3:06 pm	5:32 pm	7:55 pm	9:53 pm	11:25 pm
Jun 18	12:16 am	1:35 am	3:08 am	5:05 am	7:24 am	9:50 am	12:14 pm	2:38 pm	5:04 pm	7:28 pm	9:25 pm	10:58 pm
Jun 25	11:49 pm	1:08 am	2:40 am	4:37 am	6:57 am	9:23 am	11:47 am	2:11 pm	4:37 pm	7:00 pm	8:58 pm	10:30 pm

Ascendant Times for Zone 2

	Aries	Taurus	Gemini	Cancer	Leo	Virgo	Libra	Scorpio	Sagittarius	Capricorn	Aquarius	Pisces
Jul 2	11:21 pm	12:40 am	2:12 am	4:10 am	6:29 am	8:55 am	11:19 am	1:43 pm	4:09 pm	6:29 pm	8:30 pm	10:03 pm
Jul 9	10:54 pm	12:12 am	1:45 am	3:42 am	6:02 am	8:28 am	10:52 am	1:16 pm	3:42 pm	6:01 pm	8:03 pm	9:35 pm
Jul 16	10:26 pm	11:45 pm	1:17 am	3:15 am	5:34 am	8:00 am	10:24 am	12:48 pm	3:14 pm	5:34 pm	7:35 pm	9:07 pm
Jul 23	9:59 pm	11:17 pm	12:50 am	2:47 am	5:07 am	7:33 am	9:57 am	12:21 pm	2:47 pm	5:06 pm	7:07 pm	8:40 pm
Jul 30	9:31 pm	10:50 pm	12:22 am	2:20 am	4:39 am	7:05 am	9:29 am	11:53 am	2:19 pm	4:39 pm	6:36 pm	8:12 pm
Aug 6	9:04 pm	10:22 pm	11:55 pm	1:52 am	4:12 am	6:38 am	9:02 am	11:26 am	1:52 pm	4:11 pm	6:08 pm	7:45 pm
Aug 13	8:36 pm	9:55 pm	11:27 pm	1:25 am	3:44 am	6:10 am	8:34 am	10:58 am	1:24 pm	3:44 pm	5:41 pm	7:17 pm
Aug 20	8:09 pm	9:27 pm	11:00 pm	12:57 am	3:17 am	5:43 am	8:07 am	10:31 am	12:57 pm	3:16 pm	5:13 pm	6:46 pm
Aug 27	7:41 pm	9:00 pm	10:32 pm	12:30 am	2:49 am	5:15 am	7:39 am	10:03 am	12:29 pm	2:49 pm	4:46 pm	6:18 pm
Sep 3	7:14 pm	8:32 pm	10:05 pm	12:02 am	2:22 am	4:48 am	7:12 am	9:36 am	12:02 pm	2:21 pm	4:18 pm	5:51 pm
Sep 10	6:42 pm	8:05 pm	9:37 pm	11:35 pm	1:54 am	4:20 am	6:44 am	9:08 am	11:34 am	1:54 pm	3:51 pm	5:23 pm
Sep 17	6:15 pm	7:37 pm	9:10 pm	11:07 pm	1:26 am	3:53 am	6:17 am	8:40 am	11:07 am	1:26 pm	3:23 pm	4:56 pm
Sep 24	5:47 pm	7:10 pm	8:42 pm	10:39 pm	12:59 am	3:25 am	5:49 am	8:13 am	10:39 am	12:59 pm	2:56 pm	4:28 pm
Oct 1	5:20 pm	6:38 pm	8:15 pm	10:12 pm	12:31 am	2:58 am	5:21 am	7:45 am	10:12 am	12:31 pm	2:28 pm	4:01 pm
Oct 8	4:52 pm	6:11 pm	7:47 pm	9:44 pm	12:04 am	2:30 am	4:54 am	7:18 am	9:44 am	12:04 pm	2:01 pm	3:33 pm
Oct 15	4:24 pm	5:43 pm	7:20 pm	9:17 pm	11:36 pm	2:03 am	4:26 am	6:50 am	9:16 am	11:36 am	1:33 pm	3:06 pm
Oct 22	3:57 pm	5:16 pm	6:48 pm	8:49 pm	11:09 pm	1:35 am	3:59 am	6:23 am	8:49 am	11:08 am	1:06 pm	2:38 pm
Oct 29	3:29 pm	4:48 pm	6:21 pm	8:22 pm	10:41 pm	1:07 am	3:31 am	5:55 am	8:21 am	10:41 am	12:38 pm	2:11 pm
Nov 5	3:02 pm	4:21 pm	5:53 pm	7:54 pm	10:14 pm	12:40 am	3:04 am	5:28 am	7:54 am	10:13 am	12:11 pm	1:43 pm
Nov 12	2:34 pm	3:53 pm	5:26 pm	7:27 pm	9:46 pm	12:12 am	2:36 am	5:00 am	7:26 am	9:46 am	11:43 am	1:16 pm
Nov 19	2:07 pm	3:26 pm	4:58 pm	6:55 pm	9:19 pm	11:45 pm	2:09 am	4:33 am	6:59 am	9:18 am	11:16 am	12:48 pm
Nov 26	1:39 pm	2:58 pm	4:31 pm	6:28 pm	8:51 pm	11:17 pm	1:41 am	4:05 am	6:31 am	8:51 am	10:48 am	12:21 pm
Dec 3	1:12 pm	2:31 pm	4:03 pm	6:00 pm	8:24 pm	10:50 pm	1:14 am	3:38 am	6:04 am	8:23 am	10:21 am	11:53 am
Dec 10	12:44 pm	2:03 pm	3:36 pm	5:33 pm	7:56 pm	10:22 pm	12:46 am	3:10 am	5:36 am	7:56 am	9:53 am	11:26 am
Dec 17	12:17 pm	1:36 pm	3:08 pm	5:05 pm	7:29 pm	9:55 pm	12:19 am	2:43 am	5:09 am	7:28 am	9:26 am	10:58 am
Dec 24	11:49 am	1:08 pm	2:40 pm	4:38 pm	7:01 pm	9:27 pm	11:51 pm	2:15 am	4:41 am	7:01 am	8:58 am	10:31 am
Dec 31	11:22 am	12:40 pm	2:13 pm	4:10 pm	6:30 pm	9:00 pm	11:24 pm	1:48 am	4:14 am	6:33 am	8:30 am	10:03 am

Ascendant Times for Zone 3

		Aries	Taurus	Gemini	Cancer	Leo	Virgo	Libra	Scorpio	Sagittarius	Capricorn	Aquarius	Pisces
Jan	1	11:17 am	12:21 pm	1:42 pm	3:33 pm	5:58 pm	8:41 pm	11:19 pm	1:57 am	4:35 am	7:00 am	8:52 am	10:12 am
Jan	8	10:49 am	11:54 am	1:14 pm	3:06 pm	5:31 pm	8:13 pm	10:51 pm	1:29 am	4:08 am	6:33 am	8:25 am	9:45 am
Jan	15	10:22 am	11:26 am	12:47 pm	2:38 pm	5:03 pm	7:46 pm	10:24 pm	1:02 am	3:40 am	6:05 am	7:57 am	9:17 am
Jan	22	9:54 am	10:59 am	12:19 pm	2:11 pm	4:36 pm	7:18 pm	9:56 pm	12:34 am	3:13 am	5:38 am	7:30 am	8:50 am
Jan	29	9:27 am	10:31 am	11:51 am	1:43 pm	4:08 pm	6:47 pm	9:29 pm	12:07 am	2:45 am	5:10 am	7:02 am	8:22 am
Feb	5	8:59 am	10:04 am	11:24 am	1:16 pm	3:41 pm	6:19 pm	9:01 pm	11:39 pm	2:18 am	4:43 am	6:34 am	7:55 am
Feb	12	8:32 am	9:36 am	10:56 am	12:48 pm	3:13 pm	5:52 pm	8:34 pm	11:12 pm	1:50 am	4:15 am	6:07 am	7:27 am
Feb	19	8:04 am	9:09 am	10:29 am	12:21 pm	2:46 pm	5:24 pm	8:06 pm	10:44 pm	1:23 am	3:48 am	5:39 am	7:00 am
Feb	26	7:37 am	8:41 am	10:01 am	11:53 am	2:18 pm	4:57 pm	7:39 pm	10:17 pm	12:55 am	3:20 am	5:12 am	6:32 am
Mar	5	7:09 am	8:14 am	9:34 am	11:26 am	1:51 pm	4:29 pm	7:11 pm	9:49 pm	12:28 am	2:53 am	4:44 am	6:05 am
Mar	12	6:42 am	7:46 am	9:06 am	10:58 am	1:23 pm	4:02 pm	6:40 pm	9:22 pm	12:00 am	2:25 am	4:17 am	5:37 am
Mar	19	6:14 am	7:19 am	8:39 am	10:31 am	12:56 pm	3:34 pm	6:12 pm	8:54 pm	11:33 pm	1:58 am	3:49 am	5:09 am
Mar	26	5:47 am	6:51 am	8:11 am	10:03 am	12:28 pm	3:07 pm	5:45 pm	8:27 pm	11:05 pm	1:30 am	3:22 am	4:42 am
Apr	2	5:19 am	6:24 am	7:44 am	9:36 am	12:01 pm	2:39 pm	5:17 pm	7:59 pm	10:38 pm	1:03 am	2:54 am	4:14 am
Apr	9	4:52 am	5:56 am	7:16 am	9:08 am	11:33 am	2:12 pm	4:50 pm	7:32 pm	10:10 pm	12:35 am	2:27 am	3:47 am
Apr	16	4:24 am	5:29 am	6:49 am	8:41 am	11:06 am	1:44 pm	4:22 pm	7:04 pm	9:43 pm	12:08 am	1:59 am	3:19 am
Apr	23	3:56 am	5:01 am	6:21 am	8:13 am	10:38 am	1:16 pm	3:55 pm	6:33 pm	9:15 pm	11:40 pm	1:32 am	2:52 am
Apr	30	3:29 am	4:34 am	5:54 am	7:45 am	10:10 am	12:49 pm	3:27 pm	6:05 pm	8:47 pm	11:12 pm	1:04 am	2:24 am
May	7	3:01 am	4:06 am	5:26 am	7:18 am	9:43 am	12:21 pm	2:59 pm	5:38 pm	8:20 pm	10:45 pm	12:37 am	1:57 am
May	14	2:34 am	3:39 am	4:59 am	6:50 am	9:15 am	11:54 am	2:32 pm	5:10 pm	7:52 pm	10:17 pm	12:09 am	1:29 am
May	21	2:06 am	3:11 am	4:31 am	6:23 am	8:48 am	11:26 am	2:04 pm	4:42 pm	7:25 pm	9:50 pm	11:42 pm	1:02 am
May	28	1:39 am	2:43 am	4:04 am	5:55 am	8:20 am	10:59 am	1:37 pm	4:15 pm	6:53 pm	9:22 pm	11:14 pm	12:34 am
Jun	4	1:11 am	2:16 am	3:36 am	5:28 am	7:53 am	10:31 am	1:09 pm	3:47 pm	6:26 pm	8:55 pm	10:47 pm	12:07 am
Jun	11	12:44 am	1:48 am	3:09 am	5:00 am	7:25 am	10:04 am	12:42 pm	3:20 pm	5:58 pm	8:27 pm	10:19 pm	11:39 pm
Jun	18	12:16 am	1:21 am	2:41 am	4:33 am	6:58 am	9:36 am	12:14 pm	2:52 pm	5:31 pm	8:00 pm	9:52 pm	11:12 pm
Jun	25	11:49 pm	12:53 am	2:14 am	4:05 am	6:30 am	9:09 am	11:47 am	2:25 pm	5:03 pm	7:32 pm	9:24 pm	10:44 pm

Ascendant Times for Zone 3

		Aries	Taurus	Gemini	Cancer	Leo	Virgo	Libra	Scorpio	Sagittarius	Capricorn	Aquarius	Pisces
Jul	2	11:21 pm	12:26 am	1:46 am	3:38 am	6:03 am	8:41 am	11:19 am	1:57 pm	4:36 pm	7:05 pm	8:57 pm	10:17 pm
Jul	9	10:54 pm	11:58 pm	1:18 am	3:10 am	5:35 am	8:14 am	10:52 am	1:30 pm	4:08 pm	6:33 pm	8:29 pm	9:49 pm
Jul	16	10:26 pm	11:31 pm	12:51 am	2:43 am	5:08 am	7:46 am	10:24 am	1:02 pm	3:41 pm	6:06 pm	8:01 pm	9:22 pm
Jul	23	9:59 pm	11:03 pm	12:23 am	2:15 am	4:40 am	7:19 am	9:57 am	12:35 pm	3:13 pm	5:38 pm	7:34 pm	8:54 pm
Jul	30	9:31 pm	10:36 pm	11:56 pm	1:48 am	4:13 am	6:51 am	9:29 am	12:07 pm	2:46 pm	5:11 pm	7:06 pm	8:27 pm
Aug	6	9:04 pm	10:08 pm	11:28 pm	1:20 am	3:45 am	6:24 am	9:02 am	11:40 am	2:18 pm	4:43 pm	6:35 pm	7:59 pm
Aug	13	8:36 pm	9:41 pm	11:01 pm	12:53 am	3:18 am	5:56 am	8:34 am	11:12 am	1:51 pm	4:16 pm	6:07 pm	7:32 pm
Aug	20	8:09 pm	9:13 pm	10:33 pm	12:25 am	2:50 am	5:29 am	8:07 am	10:45 am	1:23 pm	3:48 pm	5:40 pm	7:04 pm
Aug	27	7:41 pm	8:46 pm	10:06 pm	11:58 pm	2:23 am	5:01 am	7:39 am	10:17 am	12:56 pm	3:21 pm	5:12 pm	6:33 pm
Sep	3	7:14 pm	8:18 pm	9:38 pm	11:30 pm	1:55 am	4:34 am	7:12 am	9:50 am	12:28 pm	2:53 pm	4:45 pm	6:05 pm
Sep	10	6:42 pm	7:51 pm	9:11 pm	11:03 pm	1:28 am	4:06 am	6:44 am	9:22 am	12:01 pm	2:26 pm	4:17 pm	5:37 pm
Sep	17	6:15 pm	7:23 pm	8:43 pm	10:35 pm	1:00 am	3:38 am	6:17 am	8:55 am	11:33 am	1:58 pm	3:50 pm	5:10 pm
Sep	24	5:47 pm	6:52 pm	8:16 pm	10:07 pm	12:32 am	3:11 am	5:49 am	8:27 am	11:06 am	1:31 pm	3:22 pm	4:42 pm
Oct	1	5:20 pm	6:24 pm	7:48 pm	9:40 pm	12:05 am	2:43 am	5:21 am	8:00 am	10:38 am	1:03 pm	2:55 pm	4:15 pm
Oct	8	4:52 pm	5:57 pm	7:21 pm	9:12 pm	11:37 pm	2:16 am	4:54 am	7:32 am	10:11 am	12:36 pm	2:27 pm	3:47 pm
Oct	15	4:24 pm	5:29 pm	6:49 pm	8:45 pm	11:10 pm	1:48 am	4:26 am	7:05 am	9:43 am	12:08 pm	2:00 pm	3:20 pm
Oct	22	3:57 pm	5:02 pm	6:22 pm	8:17 pm	10:42 pm	1:21 am	3:59 am	6:37 am	9:15 am	11:40 am	1:32 pm	2:52 pm
Oct	29	3:29 pm	4:34 pm	5:54 pm	7:50 pm	10:15 pm	12:53 am	3:31 am	6:09 am	8:48 am	11:13 am	1:05 pm	2:25 pm
Nov	5	3:02 pm	4:07 pm	5:27 pm	7:22 pm	9:47 pm	12:26 am	3:04 am	5:42 am	8:20 am	10:45 am	12:37 pm	1:57 pm
Nov	12	2:34 pm	3:39 pm	4:59 pm	6:51 pm	9:20 pm	11:58 pm	2:36 am	5:14 am	7:53 am	10:18 am	12:10 pm	1:30 pm
Nov	19	2:07 pm	3:11 pm	4:32 pm	6:23 pm	8:52 pm	11:31 pm	2:09 am	4:47 am	7:25 am	9:50 am	11:42 am	1:02 pm
Nov	26	1:39 pm	2:44 pm	4:04 pm	5:56 pm	8:25 pm	11:03 pm	1:41 am	4:19 am	6:58 am	9:23 am	11:15 am	12:35 pm
Dec	3	1:12 pm	2:16 pm	3:37 pm	5:28 pm	7:57 pm	10:36 pm	1:14 am	3:52 am	6:30 am	8:55 am	10:47 am	12:07 pm
Dec	10	12:44 pm	1:49 pm	3:09 pm	5:01 pm	7:30 pm	10:08 pm	12:46 am	3:24 am	6:03 am	8:28 am	10:20 am	11:40 am
Dec	17	12:17 pm	1:21 pm	2:42 pm	4:33 pm	7:02 pm	9:41 pm	12:19 am	2:57 am	5:35 am	8:00 am	9:52 am	11:12 am
Dec	24	11:49 am	12:54 pm	2:14 pm	4:06 pm	6:31 pm	9:13 pm	11:51 pm	2:29 am	5:08 am	7:33 am	9:25 am	10:45 am
Dec	31	11:22 am	12:26 pm	1:46 pm	3:38 pm	6:03 pm	8:46 pm	11:24 pm	2:02 am	4:40 am	7:05 am	8:57 am	10:17 am

Ascendant Times for Alaska

	Aries	Taurus	Gemini	Cancer	Leo	Virgo	Libra	Scorpio	Sagittarius	Capricorn	Aquarius	Pisces
Jan 1	11:16 am	11:45 am	12:29 pm	2:05 pm	4:50 pm	8:05 pm	11:18 pm	2:31 am	5:46 am	8:31 am	10:03 am	10:47 am
Jan 8	10:49 am	11:18 am	12:02 pm	1:33 pm	4:22 pm	7:37 pm	10:50 pm	2:04 am	5:19 am	8:04 am	9:35 am	10:19 am
Jan 15	10:21 am	10:50 am	11:34 am	1:06 pm	3:55 pm	7:10 pm	10:23 pm	1:36 am	4:51 am	7:36 am	9:08 am	9:52 am
Jan 22	9:53 am	10:23 am	11:07 am	12:38 pm	3:27 pm	6:42 pm	9:55 pm	1:09 am	4:24 am	7:09 am	8:40 am	9:24 am
Jan 29	9:26 am	9:55 am	10:39 am	12:11 pm	3:00 pm	6:14 pm	9:28 pm	12:41 am	3:56 am	6:41 am	8:13 am	8:57 am
Feb 5	8:58 am	9:28 am	10:12 am	11:43 am	2:32 pm	5:47 pm	9:00 pm	12:14 am	3:28 am	6:14 am	7:45 am	8:29 am
Feb 12	8:31 am	9:00 am	9:44 am	11:16 am	2:05 pm	5:19 pm	8:33 pm	11:46 pm	3:01 am	5:46 am	7:18 am	8:02 am
Feb 19	8:03 am	8:33 am	9:17 am	10:48 am	1:33 pm	4:52 pm	8:05 pm	11:19 pm	2:33 am	5:19 am	6:50 am	7:34 am
Feb 26	7:36 am	8:05 am	8:49 am	10:21 am	1:06 pm	4:24 pm	7:38 pm	10:51 pm	2:06 am	4:51 am	6:23 am	7:07 am
Mar 5	7:08 am	7:38 am	8:21 am	9:53 am	12:38 pm	3:57 pm	7:10 pm	10:24 pm	1:38 am	4:24 am	5:55 am	6:39 am
Mar 12	6:41 am	7:10 am	7:54 am	9:26 am	12:11 pm	3:29 pm	6:43 pm	9:56 pm	1:11 am	3:56 am	5:28 am	6:12 am
Mar 19	6:13 am	6:42 am	7:26 am	8:58 am	11:43 am	3:02 pm	6:15 pm	9:29 pm	12:43 am	3:28 am	5:00 am	5:44 am
Mar 26	5:46 am	6:15 am	6:59 am	8:31 am	11:16 am	2:34 pm	5:48 pm	9:01 pm	12:16 am	3:01 am	4:33 am	5:17 am
Apr 2	5:18 am	5:47 am	6:31 am	8:03 am	10:48 am	2:07 pm	5:20 pm	8:34 pm	11:48 pm	2:33 am	4:05 am	4:49 am
Apr 9	4:51 am	5:20 am	6:04 am	7:36 am	10:21 am	1:35 pm	4:53 pm	8:06 pm	11:21 pm	2:06 am	3:38 am	4:21 am
Apr 16	4:23 am	4:52 am	5:36 am	7:08 am	9:53 am	1:08 pm	4:25 pm	7:39 pm	10:53 pm	1:38 am	3:10 am	3:54 am
Apr 23	3:56 am	4:25 am	5:09 am	6:40 am	9:26 am	12:40 pm	3:58 pm	7:11 pm	10:26 pm	1:11 am	2:42 am	3:26 am
Apr 30	3:28 am	3:57 am	4:41 am	6:13 am	8:58 am	12:13 pm	3:30 pm	6:44 pm	9:58 pm	12:43 am	2:15 am	2:59 am
May 7	3:01 am	3:30 am	4:14 am	5:45 am	8:31 am	11:45 am	3:03 pm	6:16 pm	9:31 pm	12:16 am	1:47 am	2:31 am
May 14	2:33 am	3:02 am	3:46 am	5:18 am	8:03 am	11:18 am	2:35 pm	5:49 pm	9:03 pm	11:48 pm	1:20 am	2:04 am
May 21	2:06 am	2:35 am	3:19 am	4:50 am	7:36 am	10:50 am	2:08 pm	5:21 pm	8:36 pm	11:21 pm	12:52 am	1:36 am
May 28	1:38 am	2:07 am	2:51 am	4:23 am	7:08 am	10:23 am	1:36 pm	4:53 pm	8:08 pm	10:53 pm	12:25 am	1:09 am
Jun 4	1:11 am	1:40 am	2:24 am	3:55 am	6:40 am	9:55 am	1:09 pm	4:26 pm	7:41 pm	10:26 pm	11:57 pm	12:41 am
Jun 11	12:43 am	1:12 am	1:56 am	3:28 am	6:13 am	9:28 am	12:41 pm	3:58 pm	7:13 pm	9:58 pm	11:30 pm	12:14 am
Jun 18	12:15 am	12:45 am	1:29 am	3:00 am	5:45 am	9:00 am	12:14 am	3:31 pm	6:46 pm	9:31 pm	11:02 pm	11:46 pm
Jun 25	11:48 pm	12:17 am	1:01 am	2:33 am	5:18 am	8:33 am	11:46 am	3:03 pm	6:18 pm	9:03 pm	10:35 pm	11:19 pm

Ascendant Times for Alaska

		Aries	Taurus	Gemini	Cancer	Leo	Virgo	Libra	Scorpio	Sagittarius	Capricorn	Aquarius	Pisces
Jul	2	11:20 pm	11:50 pm	12:34 am	2:05 am	4:50 am	8:05 am	11:18 am	2:36 pm	5:51 pm	8:36 pm	10:07 pm	10:51 pm
Jul	9	10:53 pm	11:22 pm	12:06 am	1:38 am	4:23 am	7:38 am	10:51 am	2:08 pm	5:23 pm	8:08 pm	9:40 pm	10:24 pm
Jul	16	10:25 pm	10:55 pm	11:39 pm	1:10 am	3:55 am	7:10 am	10:23 am	1:37 pm	4:55 pm	7:41 pm	9:12 pm	9:56 pm
Jul	23	9:58 pm	10:27 pm	11:11 pm	12:43 am	3:28 am	6:42 am	9:56 am	1:09 pm	4:28 pm	7:13 pm	8:45 pm	9:29 pm
Jul	30	9:30 pm	10:00 pm	10:44 pm	12:15 am	3:00 am	6:15 am	9:28 am	12:42 pm	4:00 pm	6:46 pm	8:17 pm	9:01 pm
Aug	6	9:03 pm	9:32 pm	10:16 pm	11:48 pm	2:33 am	5:47 am	9:01 am	12:14 pm	3:33 pm	6:18 pm	7:50 pm	8:34 pm
Aug	13	8:35 pm	9:05 pm	9:48 pm	11:20 pm	2:05 am	5:20 am	8:33 am	11:47 am	3:05 pm	5:51 pm	7:22 pm	8:06 pm
Aug	20	8:08 pm	8:37 pm	9:21 pm	10:53 pm	1:38 am	4:52 am	8:06 am	11:19 am	2:38 pm	5:23 pm	6:55 pm	7:39 pm
Aug	27	7:40 pm	8:09 pm	8:53 pm	10:25 pm	1:10 am	4:25 am	7:38 am	10:52 am	2:10 pm	4:55 pm	6:27 pm	7:11 pm
Sep	3	7:13 pm	7:42 pm	8:26 pm	9:58 pm	12:43 am	3:57 am	7:11 am	10:24 am	1:39 pm	4:28 pm	6:00 pm	6:44 pm
Sep	10	6:45 pm	7:14 pm	7:58 pm	9:30 pm	12:15 am	3:30 am	6:43 am	9:57 am	1:11 pm	4:00 pm	5:32 pm	6:16 pm
Sep	17	6:18 pm	6:47 pm	7:31 pm	9:02 pm	11:48 pm	3:02 am	6:16 am	9:29 am	12:44 pm	3:33 pm	5:05 pm	5:48 pm
Sep	24	5:50 pm	6:19 pm	7:03 pm	8:35 pm	11:20 pm	2:35 am	5:48 am	9:02 am	12:16 pm	3:05 pm	4:37 pm	5:21 pm
Oct	1	5:23 pm	5:52 pm	6:36 pm	8:07 pm	10:53 pm	2:07 am	5:21 am	8:34 am	11:49 am	2:38 pm	4:09 pm	4:53 pm
Oct	8	4:55 pm	5:24 pm	6:08 pm	7:40 pm	10:25 pm	1:40 am	4:53 am	8:07 am	11:21 am	2:10 pm	3:42 pm	4:26 pm
Oct	15	4:28 pm	4:57 pm	5:41 pm	7:12 pm	9:58 pm	1:12 am	4:26 am	7:39 am	10:54 am	1:39 pm	3:14 pm	3:58 pm
Oct	22	4:00 pm	4:29 pm	5:13 pm	6:45 pm	9:30 pm	12:45 am	3:58 am	7:12 am	10:26 am	1:11 pm	2:47 pm	3:31 pm
Oct	29	3:33 pm	4:02 pm	4:46 pm	6:17 pm	9:02 pm	12:17 am	3:31 am	6:44 am	9:59 am	12:44 pm	2:19 pm	3:03 pm
Nov	5	3:05 pm	3:34 pm	4:18 pm	5:50 pm	8:35 pm	11:50 pm	3:03 am	6:17 am	9:31 am	12:16 pm	1:48 pm	2:36 pm
Nov	12	2:38 pm	3:07 pm	3:51 pm	5:22 pm	8:07 pm	11:22 pm	2:36 am	5:49 am	9:04 am	11:49 am	1:20 pm	2:08 pm
Nov	19	2:10 pm	2:39 pm	3:23 pm	4:55 pm	7:40 pm	10:55 pm	2:08 am	5:21 am	8:36 am	11:21 am	12:53 pm	1:37 pm
Nov	26	1:39 pm	2:12 pm	2:56 pm	4:27 pm	7:12 pm	10:27 pm	1:40 am	4:54 am	8:09 am	10:54 am	12:25 pm	1:09 pm
Dec	3	1:11 pm	1:40 pm	2:28 pm	4:00 pm	6:45 pm	10:00 pm	1:13 am	4:26 am	7:41 am	10:26 am	11:58 am	12:42 pm
Dec	10	12:43 pm	1:13 pm	2:01 pm	3:32 pm	6:17 pm	9:32 pm	12:45 am	3:59 am	7:14 am	9:59 am	11:30 am	12:14 pm
Dec	17	12:16 pm	12:45 pm	1:29 pm	3:05 pm	5:50 pm	9:04 pm	12:18 am	3:31 am	6:46 am	9:31 am	11:03 am	11:47 am
Dec	24	11:48 am	12:18 pm	1:02 pm	2:37 pm	5:22 pm	8:37 pm	11:50 pm	3:04 am	6:19 am	9:04 am	10:35 am	11:19 am
Dec	31	11:21 am	11:50 am	12:34 pm	2:10 pm	4:55 pm	8:09 pm	11:23 pm	2:36 am	5:51 am	8:36 am	10:08 am	10:52 am

Ascendant Times for Hawaii

	Aries	Taurus	Gemini	Cancer	Leo	Virgo	Libra	Scorpio	Sagittarius	Capricorn	Aquarius	Pisces
Jan 1	11:16 am	12:50 pm	2:38 pm	4:41 pm	6:55 pm	9:09 pm	11:18 pm	1:27 am	3:41 am	5:55 am	7:58 am	9:43 am
Jan 8	10:49 am	12:22 pm	2:11 pm	4:13 pm	6:28 pm	8:41 pm	10:50 pm	1:00 am	3:13 am	5:28 am	7:30 am	9:15 am
Jan 15	10:21 am	11:54 am	1:39 pm	3:46 pm	6:00 pm	8:14 pm	10:23 pm	12:32 am	2:46 am	5:00 am	7:03 am	8:47 am
Jan 22	9:53 am	11:27 am	1:12 pm	3:18 pm	5:32 pm	7:46 pm	9:55 pm	12:05 am	2:18 am	4:33 am	6:35 am	8:20 am
Jan 29	9:26 am	10:59 am	12:44 pm	2:51 pm	5:05 pm	7:19 pm	9:28 pm	11:37 pm	1:51 am	4:05 am	6:08 am	7:52 am
Feb 5	8:58 am	10:32 am	12:17 pm	2:23 pm	4:37 pm	6:51 pm	9:00 pm	11:10 pm	1:23 am	3:38 am	5:40 am	7:25 am
Feb 12	8:31 am	10:04 am	11:49 am	1:52 pm	4:10 pm	6:24 pm	8:33 pm	10:42 pm	12:56 am	3:10 am	5:13 am	6:57 am
Feb 19	8:03 am	9:37 am	11:22 am	1:24 pm	3:42 pm	5:56 pm	8:05 pm	10:14 pm	12:28 am	2:43 am	4:45 am	6:30 am
Feb 26	7:36 am	9:09 am	10:54 am	12:57 pm	3:15 pm	5:29 pm	7:38 pm	9:47 pm	12:01 am	2:15 am	4:18 am	6:02 am
Mar 5	7:08 am	8:42 am	10:27 am	12:29 pm	2:47 pm	5:01 pm	7:10 pm	9:19 pm	11:33 pm	1:48 am	3:50 am	5:35 am
Mar 12	6:41 am	8:14 am	9:59 am	12:02 pm	2:20 pm	4:34 pm	6:43 pm	8:52 pm	11:06 pm	1:20 am	3:22 am	5:07 am
Mar 19	6:13 am	7:47 am	9:32 am	11:34 am	1:48 pm	4:06 pm	6:15 pm	8:24 pm	10:38 pm	12:52 am	2:55 am	4:40 am
Mar 26	5:46 am	7:19 am	9:04 am	11:07 am	1:21 pm	3:39 pm	5:48 pm	7:57 pm	10:11 pm	12:25 am	2:27 am	4:12 am
Apr 2	5:18 am	6:52 am	8:37 am	10:39 am	12:53 pm	3:11 pm	5:20 pm	7:29 pm	9:43 pm	11:57 pm	2:00 am	3:45 am
Apr 9	4:51 am	6:24 am	8:09 am	10:12 am	12:26 pm	2:44 pm	4:53 pm	7:02 pm	9:16 pm	11:30 pm	1:32 am	3:17 am
Apr 16	4:23 am	5:57 am	7:42 am	9:44 am	11:58 am	2:16 pm	4:25 pm	6:34 pm	8:48 pm	11:02 pm	1:05 am	2:50 am
Apr 23	3:56 am	5:29 am	7:14 am	9:16 am	11:31 am	1:45 pm	3:58 pm	6:07 pm	8:21 pm	10:35 pm	12:37 am	2:22 am
Apr 30	3:28 am	5:02 am	6:46 am	8:49 am	11:03 am	1:17 pm	3:30 pm	5:39 pm	7:53 pm	10:07 pm	12:10 am	1:55 am
May 7	3:01 am	4:34 am	6:19 am	8:21 am	10:36 am	12:49 pm	3:03 pm	5:12 pm	7:26 pm	9:40 pm	11:42 pm	1:27 am
May 14	2:33 am	4:07 am	5:51 am	7:54 am	10:08 am	12:22 pm	2:35 pm	4:44 pm	6:58 pm	9:12 pm	11:15 pm	1:00 am
May 21	2:06 am	3:39 am	5:24 am	7:26 am	9:41 am	11:54 am	2:08 pm	4:17 pm	6:30 pm	8:45 pm	10:47 pm	12:32 am
May 28	1:38 am	3:12 am	4:56 am	6:59 am	9:13 am	11:27 am	1:36 pm	3:49 pm	6:03 pm	8:17 pm	10:20 pm	12:05 am
Jun 4	1:11 am	2:44 am	4:29 am	6:31 am	8:46 am	10:59 am	1:09 pm	3:22 pm	5:35 pm	7:50 pm	9:52 pm	11:37 pm
Jun 11	12:43 am	2:17 am	4:01 am	6:04 am	8:18 am	10:32 am	12:41 pm	2:54 pm	5:08 pm	7:22 pm	9:25 pm	11:10 pm
Jun 18	12:15 am	1:49 am	3:34 am	5:36 am	7:51 am	10:04 am	12:14 pm	2:27 pm	4:40 pm	6:55 pm	8:57 pm	10:42 pm
Jun 25	11:48 pm	1:21 am	3:06 am	5:09 am	7:23 am	9:37 am	11:46 am	1:55 pm	4:13 pm	6:27 pm	8:30 pm	10:14 pm

Ascendant Times for Hawaii

	Aries	Taurus	Gemini	Cancer	Leo	Virgo	Libra	Scorpio	Sagittarius	Capricorn	Aquarius	Pisces
Jul 2	11:20 pm	12:54 am	2:39 am	4:41 am	6:56 am	9:09 am	11:18 am	1:28 pm	3:45 pm	6:00 pm	8:02 pm	9:47 pm
Jul 9	10:53 pm	12:26 am	2:11 am	4:14 am	6:28 am	8:42 am	10:51 am	1:00 pm	3:18 pm	5:32 pm	7:35 pm	9:19 pm
Jul 16	10:25 pm	11:59 pm	1:44 am	3:46 am	6:00 am	8:14 am	10:23 am	12:33 pm	2:50 pm	5:05 pm	7:07 pm	8:52 pm
Jul 23	9:58 pm	11:31 pm	1:16 am	3:19 am	5:33 am	7:47 am	9:56 am	12:05 pm	2:23 pm	4:37 pm	6:40 pm	8:24 pm
Jul 30	9:30 pm	11:04 pm	12:49 am	2:51 am	5:05 am	7:19 am	9:28 am	11:38 am	1:51 pm	4:10 pm	6:12 pm	7:57 pm
Aug 6	9:03 pm	10:36 pm	12:21 am	2:24 am	4:38 am	6:52 am	9:01 am	11:10 am	1:24 pm	3:42 pm	5:44 pm	7:29 pm
Aug 13	8:35 pm	10:09 pm	11:54 pm	1:56 am	4:10 am	6:24 am	8:33 am	10:42 am	12:56 pm	3:15 pm	5:17 pm	7:02 pm
Aug 20	8:08 pm	9:41 pm	11:26 pm	1:29 am	3:43 am	5:57 am	8:06 am	10:15 am	12:29 pm	2:47 pm	4:49 pm	6:34 pm
Aug 27	7:40 pm	9:14 pm	10:59 pm	1:01 am	3:15 am	5:29 am	7:38 am	9:47 am	12:01 pm	2:19 pm	4:22 pm	6:07 pm
Sep 3	7:13 pm	8:46 pm	10:31 pm	12:34 am	2:48 am	5:02 am	7:11 am	9:20 am	11:34 am	1:48 pm	3:54 pm	5:39 pm
Sep 10	6:45 pm	8:19 pm	10:04 pm	12:06 am	2:20 am	4:34 am	6:43 am	8:52 am	11:06 am	1:20 pm	3:27 pm	5:12 pm
Sep 17	6:18 pm	7:51 pm	9:36 pm	11:38 pm	1:53 am	4:07 am	6:16 am	8:25 am	10:39 am	12:53 pm	2:59 pm	4:44 pm
Sep 24	5:50 pm	7:24 pm	9:08 pm	11:11 pm	1:25 am	3:39 am	5:48 am	7:57 am	10:11 am	12:25 pm	2:32 pm	4:17 pm
Oct 1	5:23 pm	6:56 pm	8:41 pm	10:43 pm	12:58 am	3:12 am	5:21 am	7:30 am	9:44 am	11:58 am	2:04 pm	3:49 pm
Oct 8	4:55 pm	6:29 pm	8:13 pm	10:16 pm	12:30 am	2:44 am	4:53 am	7:02 am	9:16 am	11:30 am	1:33 pm	3:22 pm
Oct 15	4:28 pm	6:01 pm	7:46 pm	9:48 pm	12:03 am	2:16 am	4:26 am	6:35 am	8:49 am	11:03 am	1:05 pm	2:54 pm
Oct 22	4:00 pm	5:34 pm	7:18 pm	9:21 pm	11:35 pm	1:49 am	3:58 am	6:07 am	8:21 am	10:35 am	12:38 pm	2:27 pm
Oct 29	3:33 pm	5:06 pm	6:51 pm	8:53 pm	11:08 pm	1:21 am	3:31 am	5:40 am	7:54 am	10:08 am	12:10 pm	1:55 pm
Nov 5	3:05 pm	4:39 pm	6:23 pm	8:26 pm	10:40 pm	12:54 am	3:03 am	5:12 am	7:26 am	9:40 am	11:43 am	1:28 pm
Nov 12	2:38 pm	4:11 pm	5:56 pm	7:58 pm	10:13 pm	12:26 am	2:36 am	4:45 am	6:58 am	9:13 am	11:15 am	1:00 pm
Nov 19	2:10 pm	3:43 pm	5:28 pm	7:31 pm	9:45 pm	11:59 pm	2:08 am	4:17 am	6:31 am	8:45 am	10:48 am	12:33 pm
Nov 26	1:39 pm	3:16 pm	5:01 pm	7:03 pm	9:18 pm	11:31 pm	1:40 am	3:50 am	6:03 am	8:18 am	10:20 am	12:05 pm
Dec 3	1:11 pm	2:48 pm	4:33 pm	6:36 pm	8:50 pm	11:04 pm	1:13 am	3:22 am	5:36 am	7:50 am	9:53 am	11:37 am
Dec 10	12:43 pm	2:21 pm	4:06 pm	6:08 pm	8:22 pm	10:36 pm	12:45 am	2:55 am	5:08 am	7:23 am	9:25 am	11:10 am
Dec 17	12:16 pm	1:49 pm	3:38 pm	5:41 pm	7:55 pm	10:09 pm	12:18 am	2:27 am	4:41 am	6:55 am	8:58 am	10:42 am
Dec 24	11:48 am	1:22 pm	3:11 pm	5:13 pm	7:27 pm	9:41 pm	11:50 pm	2:00 am	4:13 am	6:28 am	8:30 am	10:15 am
Dec 31	11:21 am	12:54 pm	2:43 pm	4:46 pm	7:00 pm	9:14 pm	11:23 pm	1:32 am	3:46 am	6:00 am	8:03 am	9:47 am

Bibliography and Resources

Brazelton, T. Berry, M.D., *Toddlers and Parents*, New York:
    Delta Seymore Lawrence, Dell Publishing, 1989.
Fraiberg, Selma H., *The Magic Years*, New York:
    Charles Scribner's Sons, 1959.
Guhl, Beverly and Don H. Fontenell, Ph.D., *Purrfect Parenting*,
    Tucson, Arizona: Fisher Books, 1987.
Johnson, Spencer, M.D., *The One Minute Mother*, New York:
    William Morrow and Co., Inc., 1983.
Spock, Benjamin, M.D., *Dr. Spock on Parenting*, New York:
    Pocket Books, 1988.
Spock, Benjamin, M.D., *Dr. Spock's Baby and Child Care*, New
    York: Pocket Books, 1992.

Other Astrology Books of Special Interest to Parents

Davis, Samantha A., *Understanding Children through Astrology*,
    Largo, Florida: Top of the Mountain Publishing, 1992.
    (Interpretations for Sun, Moon, Mercury, Venus and Mars
    through the signs)
Hand, Robert, *Planets in Youth*, West Chester, Penn.:
    ParaResearch, 1977.
    (Aimed at adolescent and teenager readers, for self-
    understanding. Also useful for parents.)
Star, Gloria, *Optimum Child*, St. Paul, Minn.:
    Llewellyn Publications, 1987.

Books for Learning More About Your Birth Chart

Bloch, Douglas and Demetra George, *Astrology for Yourself,*
Berkeley, Calif.: Wingbow Press, 1987.

Forrest, Steven, *The Inner Sky,* San Diego, Calif.: ACS Publications,
1991.

March, Marion D. and Joan McEvers, *The Only Way to Learn
Astrology, Volume I: Basic Principles*, San Diego, Calif.:
ACS Publications, 1981.

March, Marion D. and Joan McEvers, *The Only Way to Learn
Astrology, Volume II: Math & Interpretation
Techniques*, San Diego, Calif.: ACS Publications, 1981.

March, Marion D. and Joan McEvers, *The Only Way to Learn
Astrology, Volume III: Horoscope Analysis*, San Diego,
Calif.: ACS Publications, 1982.

Negus, Joan, *Basic Astrology: A Guide for Teachers & Students*
and *Basic Astrology: A Workbook for Students*, San Diego,
Calif.: ACS Publications, 1978.

Pottenger, Maritha, *Easy AStrology Guide*, San Diego, Calif.:
ACS Publications, 1991.

Pottenger, Maritha, *Astrology: The Next Step*, San Diego, Calif.:
ACS Publictions, 1986.

Rogers-Gallagher, Kim, *Astrology for the Light Side of the Brain*,
San Diego, Calif.: ACS Publictions, 1995.

Other Astrological Resources

Computer Calculations and Interpretations
Astrology Books and Software

Astro Communications Services, Inc.
5521 Ruffin Road
San Diego, CA 92123-1314

Business Line: 619/492-9919
Toll Free Order Line: 800/888-9983
http://www.astrocom.com
Free catalogs available upon request.

Glossary of Astrological Jargon

ascendant
The **degree** in the zodiac of signs that is rising in the east at the moment of birth. See also degree, Rising Sign, zodiac.

aspect
The angular relationship between points on a circle. Planets or other factors such as Ascendant or Midheaven (let's refer to any and all as "factors") occupying certain points (or degrees) are "in aspect" to each other. Some types of aspects are:

> **conjunction**—factors in the same degree or very close together. An exact conjunction means same degree, and is the strongest aspect.

> **generational**—refers to aspects between outer planets that move so slowly that whole age groups will be born with essentially the same aspects in their birth charts.

> **hard**—generally perceived as stronger in action than soft aspects. Includes conjunction, semi-square, square, sesquare, opposition and quincunx.

> **opposition**—factors that are across from each other in the circle—exactly opposite is 180°apart. Second strongest aspect after the conjunction. Represents a need to balance the themes of the two factors in opposition.

> **out-of-sign**— factors that by degree are in aspect to each other, but are not in the signs in which one would normally expect to find that aspect. See page 357.

> **quincunx**—factors (exactly) 150 degrees apart. Represents a theme where some adjustment is required in order to succeed.

> **semi-sextile**—factors (exactly) 30 degrees apart. Mild, may go unnoticed.

> **semi-square**—factors (exactly) 45 degrees apart. Works similarly to a square. Also sometimes called an **octile**.

> **sesquare**—factors (exactly) 135 degrees apart. Works similarly to a square. Also sometimes called **sesquiquadrate**, or **tri-octile**.

> **sextile**—factors (exactly) 60 degrees apart. Usually considered to represent a theme of opportunity.

> **soft**— aspects that are "softer" in action, and probably will be perceived as less strong, or more passive than the hard aspects. Generally considered to represent themes of ease, and perhaps talent.

square—factors (exactly) 90 degrees apart. Usually considered to be the most dynamic type of aspect after the conjunction and opposition, representing a challenge that needs to be overcome.

trine— factors (exactly) 120 degrees apart. Traditionally said to be a "good" aspect, and it usually does represent a blending of planetary themes that symbolize easy flow or talent. Strongest of the soft aspect series.

birth chart
a chart of the Cosmos as seen from a particular location at a specific time. A birth chart may be calculated for the birth of a person, or the first moment that anything is "born" — an animal, a business, a nation, a question. Also called **horoscope**.

birth data
The factors needed in order to calculate a birth chart, or horoscope: date of birth, time of birth, location (latitude and longitide) of birth.

cardinal
One of the three modes into which signs are categorized. Cardinal means "first" and its signs (Aries, Cancer, Libra and Capricorn) are noted for initiative.

constellations
Groups of stars that have been seen as together in people's imaginations to the point that, throughout time, they have been given names, and mythologies have grown up around them. There are generally considered to be 12, even though a few others intrude on the path. Can be seen at night in an arc across the southern sky.

cycle
In this book, cycle refers to a planet's movement (orbit) around the entire circle of signs. The cycles of the outer planets, and the aspects they make to their starting positions in the birth chart, define major life crisis periods. For example, Saturn takes about 29 to 30 years to go once completely around the circle. At about 14 or so, Saturn will have reached opposition aspect to the degree it was in at the time a person is born. This first "Saturn opposition" represents the "adolescent crisis." At the time of the second opposition of Saturn to its birth position, a person is around 42 years of age, and this is one of the cycles that define the well-known "mid-life crisis."

degrees

A circle has 360 degrees. The zodiac of signs is a circle. Each sign has 30 degrees in it, but we customarily call them by 0 through 29, rather than 1 through 30. The 30th degree of a sign is the same as the 0 degree of the next sign. The fiducial (starting point) of the zodiac circle, by both astrologers and astronomers, is customarily called the 0 degree of the sign Aries. A planet is said to occupy a sign, and also a specific degree of that sign. This is a measurement along the circle of the ecliptic known as celestial longitude. See also ecliptic, signs.

earth

Earth is, of course, the planet we live on. Since a birth chart is a map of the sky drawn from the perspective of we on Earth, Planet Earth does not appear in the birth chart.

In this book the word "earth" is primarily used to designate one of the four elements of the ancients into which the zodiac signs may be categorized. Earth signs (Taurus, Virgo, Capricorn) share charactistics such as pragmatism. They are "grounded," and "down-to-earth" types.

ecliptic

The orbit of Earth around the Sun. As a Great Circle projected out into space, it is more properly called the celestial ecliptic. If you look at the sky at night, over a period of time, you will be able to see the Moon and the planets change their positions along the arc of the southern sky. They are moving through the signs along the ecliptic. A more obvious movement that we all notice is the Sun rising in the east, culminating overhead and then setting in the west. It also seems to be moving along the ecliptic. We see all of this from our vantage point on Earth, so even though we and all of the other planets are really orbiting the Sun, we see their **apparent motion** as around Earth.

elements

Refers to the four ancient elements: fire, earth, air and water. The signs are categorized into four groups according to the elements, and the signs in each group share certain characteristic. See also fire, air, earth, water.

equator

The imaginary circle that goes right around Earth's middle. Projected out into space as a great circle, it is called the celestial equator. Because Earth's polar axis is tipped, the great circles of equator and ecliptic are at an angle to each other, and intersect at two points. The points of intersection are called the equinoxes, and the two points of greatest separation are called solstices. The equinoxes and solstices, then, divide the circles into quarters, and the Sun's apparent movement along the ecliptic marks the beginning of a new season each time it "comes" to the first degree of a new quarter.

fire
One of the four elements. Fire signs are Aries, Leo and Sagittarius. They share "fiery" personality traits such as enthusiasm, drama and romaticism.

fixed
One of the three modes or qualities of action. Fixed signs are Taurus, Leo, Scorpio and Aquarius. All "fixed" in basic nature, they share qualities such as determination and stubbornness.

geocentric
Viewed from Earth, as if Earth were the center of the Universe. Since a person on Earth sees the Cosmos from an earthly perspective, the birth chart or horoscope is drawn with that vantage point. We see the sky (and everything else) relative to ourselves—each of us is the center of our own personal Universe.

glyph
Means symbol. Each planet and sign has a glyph by which we recognize it, thus giving us a shorthand method of writing it, rather than spelling out the word. Glyphs, since they are single digit, also make planetary tables line up much better in space-saving, neat columns—which is why I have asked you to look at glyphs in this book, instead of giving you unneat abbreviations or whole words!

horoscope
Birth chart. "Horo" means hour. Actually, a true horoscope is calculated (cast) for precise time (hour **and minute** of a specific day, month and year) plus precise location (longitude and latitude of birth). Newspaper "horoscope" columns are using the word erroneously, if they only discuss Sun signs, because people who share the same Sun sign do **NOT** have the same horoscope, unless they were born at **exactly** the same moment in the very same location.

houses
Twelve sections of the ecliptic as determined by one of several different mathematical systems. Houses and signs are **NOT** the same! See Chapter 4.

Midheaven
The degree of the ecliptic that is the culminating point in a horoscope. In most house systems, the cusp of House 10. Planets conjunct or opposite the Midheaven are emphasized in a horoscope. Interpretively, it gives information about how a person identifies self, *e.g.*, "I am," how one strives for recognition or seeks fulfillment.

modes
Refers to categories of signs by quality of action: cardinal, fixed and mutable. The cardinal signs are Aries, Cancer, Libra, Capricorn; the fixed are Taurus, Leo, Scorpio, Aquarius; the mutable are Gemini, Virgo, Sagittarius, Pisces.

mutable
The four signs that most express the mode or quality of action of mutability: flexibility, adaptability, versatility.

orb
Refers to the range of degrees within which an aspect is considered to be operative. The closer two bodies are in orb, the stronger the aspect.

polarities
Refers to the division of the 12 signs into two groups, in this book designated as + and – types: + group includes Aries, Gemini, Leo, Libra, Sagittarius, Aquarius; – group includes Taurus, Cancer, Virgo, Scorpio, Capricorn, Pisces.

precession of the equinoxes
The very slow counter-clockwise movement of the zodiac of signs against the backdrop of the zodiac of constellations. The zero point of the signs, 0° Aries (the vernal equinox) coincided approximately with the "beginning" of the constellation Aries about 2000 years ago. Now, 0° Aries of the signs coincides approximately with 4° of Pisces in the constellations. It takes about 26,000 years for the signs to precess all the way around the constellations.

retrograde
The apparent backward motion of a planet.

return
This term was used in the book to refer to the time of a planetary cycle when the planet has moved all the way around the zodiac of signs and returns to the same degree it occupied in the birth chart., *e.g.*: Jupiter takes approximately 12 years to travel through all of the signs, so a person experiences a "Jupiter return" at approximately the age of 12, and again each 12 years thereafter. The "Saturn return" occurs at about age 29 or 30, etc.

Rising Sign
The sign of the zodiac that is rising in the east at the time a person is born.

signs
Twelve equal 30° sectors of the ecliptic circle.

star, in reference to planets
For convenience and "for short," astrologers generally categorize Sun, Moon , Mercury, Venus, Mars, Jupiter, Saturn, Uranus, Neptune and Pluto as "planets," even though everyone knows perfectly well that the Sun is a star and the Moon is a satellite of Earth. Don't ask me why, it just happens.

synastry
The art of comparing one horoscope with another in order to analyze relationship potential.

synthesis
The art of pulling all of the separate themes of a horoscope together, "weighing" them for relative importance, and managing to come up with something that makes sense.

transit
This refers either 1. to the passage of a planet through a sign, *e.g.* "The Sun transits Cancer from June 21 until July 22," or 2. to the passage of a planet in aspect to a position in a horoscope, *e.g.*: Pluto is transiting my Sun by conjunction this year. Transits, according to definition #2, are a primary technique used in astrological forecasting.

vernal equinox
The intersection of ecliptic and equator that occurs when the apparent path of the Sun (ecliptic) crosses the equator at a northward inclination. This is the first day of spring in the northern hemisphere, and this point (degree) of the ecliptic is the designated starting point for the signs: 0° Aries.

water
One of the four elements into which signs are categorized. Water signs are Cancer, Scorpio and Pisces, and they can all be described as emotional, deep, intuitive.

zodiac
This word may refer to any of several systems of dividing up the arc across the sky that is the apparent path of the Sun (ecliptic). For at least the past 2000 years it has been generally agreed by most that there are 12 divisions called Aries, Taurus, Gemini, Cancer, Leo, Virgo, Scorpio, Sagittarius, Capricorn, Aquarius and Pisces. Agreement on which of the 12 are where depends upon which zodiac is being used. There are three:

constellational, tropical and sidereal. The **constellational zodiac** maps the actual constellation that lie approximately beyond the path of the ecliptic. They are decidedly unequal in the number of degrees that would be allotted to each sector—some overlap and there are gaps between others into which some non-zodiac constellations intrude.

The **tropical zodiac** is the equal 30° sections of the ecliptic that are measured from the vernal equinox. This zodiac clearly defines the seasons and is the zodiac most widely used in western astrology, and the one that people are generally referring to when they ask "what's your sign" (even if they mistakenly **think** they mean constellation). Confusion exists because the Greek astrologer/astronomers who devised the tropical system named the equal 30° sectors the same as the constellations that were approximately within them at that time (about 2000 years ago). Due to the precession of the equinoxes, the constellations and signs are no longer "in sync."

The **sidereal zodiac** moves the vernal point in an attempt to keep the signs more in sync with the constellations. A star is selected as the point to which the beginning of the zodiac is referenced, and the signs are measured off from that point, still in equal 30° sectors, which means they still don't really match the unequal constellations, nor do they match the beginning of the seasons. Another problem exists in that there are numerous sidereal systems —disagreement over exactly where that beginning point is. Sidereal systems are most widely used in eastern astrology, but have a few strong advocates in the west.

Index

Also by ACS Publications

All About Astrology Series of booklets
The American Atlas, Expanded 5th Edition (Shanks)
The American Ephemeris Series 2001-2010
The American Ephemeris for the 20th Century [Noon or Midnight] 1900 to 2000, Rev. 5th Ed.
The American Ephemeris for the 21st Century [Noon or Midnight] 2000-2050, Rev. 2nd Ed.
The American Heliocentric Ephemeris 1901-2000
The American Heliocentric Ephemeris 2001-2050
The American Sidereal Ephemeris 1976-2000, 2nd Edition
The American Sidereal Ephemeris 2001-2025
Asteroid Goddesses (George & Bloch)
Astro-Alchemy (Negus)
Astrological Insights into Personality (Lundsted)
Astrology for the Light Side of the Brain (Rogers-Gallagher)
Astrology:The Next Step (Pottenger)
Basic Astrology: A Guide for Teachers & Students (Negus)
Basic Astrology: A Workbook for Students (Negus)
The Book of Jupiter (Waram)
The Book of Neptune (Waram)
The Book of Pluto (Forrest)
The Book of Saturn (Dobyns)
The Book of Uranus (Negus)
The Changing Sky (Forrest)
Cosmic Combinations (Negus)
Dial Detective (Simms)
Easy Astrology Guide (Pottenger)
Easy Tarot Guide (Masino)
Expanding Astrology's Universe (Dobyns)
Finding our Way Through the Dark (George)
Future Signs (Simms)
The International Atlas, Revised 4th Edition
Hands That Heal, 2nd Edition (Bodine)
Healing with the Horoscope (Pottenger)
The Inner Sky (Forrest)
The Michelsen Book of Tables (Michelsen)
Millennium: Fears, Fantasies & Facts
New Insights into Astrology (Press)
The Night Speaks (Forrest)
The Only Way to... Learn Astrology, Vols. I-VI (March & McEvers)
    Volume I, 2nd Edition - Basic Principles
    Volume II - Math & Interpretation Techniques
    Volume III - Horoscope Analysis
    Volume IV- Learn About Tomorrow: Current Patterns
    Volume V - Learn About Relationships: Synastry Techniques
    Volume VI - Learn About Horary and Electional Astrology
Planetary Heredity (M. Gauquelin)
Planets on the Move (Dobyns/Pottenger)
Psychology of the Planets (F. Gauquelin)
Tables of Planetary Phenomena (Michelsen)
Twelve Wings of the Eagle (Simms)
Your Starway to Love, 2nd Edition (Pottenger)

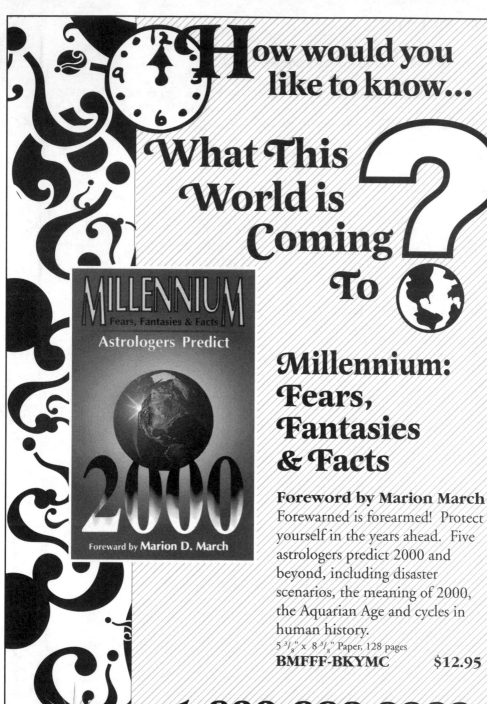